SYMBOLS

COMPLEXES:

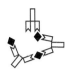 Antigen/antibody complex
(immune complex)

 MHC-peptide complex

 MHC-peptide-TCR/CD3
complex
(Ag recognition complex)

 Fc-antibody
complex

ACTIONS:

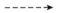 Becomes/yields/
diffuses

 Secretes/stimulates

 Interacts/combines

—×—→ Inhibits/destroys

MISCELLANEOUS:

◆ Antigen (Ag)
(unprocessed,
native)

⬧ Antigenic peptide
(processed antigen)

 Reagent antigen
(antigen-coated particle)

 Carrier particle
(latex or RBC)

 Reagent antibody
(antibody-coated particle)

● Complement (C)

▲ Epitope/soluble antigen
(antigenic determinant)

⬬ Cytokines

 Particulate antigen

 Antibody (Ab)
(immunoglobulin molecule, Ig)

IMMUNOLOGY
Theoretical & Practical Concepts
in Laboratory Medicine

IMMUNOLOGY
Theoretical & Practical Concepts in Laboratory Medicine

Hannah D. Zane

HANNAH D. ZANE, PhD, CLS/SM (NCA), MT (ASCP), SM (AAM)

Professor Emeritus
Board Licensed Bio-Analytical Laboratory Director
Former Department Chairman, Director of Undergraduate
and Graduate Programs, and Clinical Immunology Professor
Department of Clinical Laboratory Sciences
University of Medicine and Dentistry of New Jersey
Newark, New Jersey

with 149 illustrations

W.B. SAUNDERS COMPANY
A Harcourt Health Sciences Company
Philadelphia   London   New York   St. Louis   Sydney   Toronto

W.B. SAUNDERS COMPANY
A Harcourt Health Sciences Company

The Curtis Center
Independence Square West
Philadelphia, Pennsylvania 19106

Editor in Chief: Andrew Allen
Acquisitions Editor: Karen Fabiano
Developmental Editor: Sarahlynn Lester
Project Manager: John Rogers
Senior Production Editor: Helen Hudlin
Designer: Kathi Gosche
Cover Art: Jen Marmarinos

Immunology: Theoretical & Practical Concepts In Laboratory Medicine

ISBN 0-7216-5002-3

NOTICE

Pharmacology is an ever-changing field. Standard safety precautions must be followed, but as new research and clinical experience broaden our knowledge, changes in treatment and drug therapy may become necessary or appropriate. Readers are advised to check the most current product information provided by the manufacturer of each drug to be administered to verify the recommended dose, the method and duration of administration, and contraindications. It is the responsibility of the licensed prescriber, relying on experience and knowledge of the patient, to determine dosages and the best treatment of each individual patient. Neither the publisher nor the editor assumes any liability for any injury and/or damage to persons or property arising from this publication.

W.B. Saunders
A Harcourt Health Sciences Company

Printed in the United States of America

00 01 02 03 04   CL/KPT   9 8 7 6 5 4 3 2 1

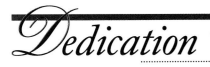

Dedication

To My Grandsons

Todd, Joey, and Chris
Depczynski

Acknowledgments

I am deeply grateful to Dean John Martin who has facilitated my professional growth during my tenure at the University of Medicine and Dentistry of New Jersey (UMDNJ).

In fond memory of my friend and mentor at Rutgers University, Dr. Helen Strausser, I wish to express my deep appreciation for her guidance and encouragement, for providing a nurturing environment for her doctoral students, for understanding each student's needs, and for fully supporting their efforts.

A special acknowledgment is given to Selma Kaszczuk, Senior Editor, Health-Related Professions at W.B. Saunders, for encouraging me to write this book; to Scott W. Weaver, Developmental Editor at W.B. Saunders, for providing editorial assistance, guidance, and encouragement during the initial stages of writing; to Sarahlynn Lester, Associate Developmental Editor, and to Helen Hudlin, Senior Production Editor, Health-Related Professions Editorial, Harcourt Health Sciences (Saunders/Mosby) for their efforts on my behalf; and to Dr. Elaine Keohane, my former student and colleague, for her long-standing friendship and for her invaluable contribution to the development of quality clinical laboratory science programs within the Department of Clinical Laboratory Sciences at UMDNJ.

I wish to convey my special thanks to Karen Novobilski at Monmouth Medical Center, New Jersey, for making available the *actual* test results appearing in this book and for her assistance in selecting procedures comprising current clinical immunology practice.

I would like to particularly acknowledge my son, Andrew Depczynski, and his family for enriching my life and to express my profound appreciation to my husband, Zaki Asaad, for his understanding of my preoccupation with the writing of this book and for his continued encouragement during the process.

I wish to thank all my colleagues for sharing my quest for professional excellence.

Hannah D. Zane

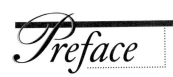

Preface

This book has been written with the primary intent to address the need for *a single immunology textbook for students of clinical laboratory science.* Thus the content has been selected to include current fundamental and advanced immunologic concepts as well as immunologic and molecular laboratory techniques that constitute clinical immunology practice.

Written mainly for undergraduate level students who are preparing for a career in clinical laboratory science at either of two levels of competency (i.e., associate [MLT or CLT] or baccalaureate [MT or CLS] degree levels), this book can be adopted as a clinical immunology textbook in these educational programs. It can also serve as a general immunology textbook for other health science majors, particularly as a prerequisite to a microbiology and blood bank (immunohematology) specialty or as a reference for continuing education of clinical laboratory practitioners.

Therefore, in this context, the selected format includes helpful pedagogical features, such as chapter outlines, numerous original illustrations that clarify the more intricate concepts and mechanisms of immune response to antigens, One Step Further boxes with more advanced information, key words with definitions, student-based learning objectives, and review questions and answers. The text and artwork reflect uniformity in format and organization throughout the book.

The content has been organized into two sections, the first of which contains a comprehensive presentation of fundamental immunologic concepts. The second section includes a concise overview of major immunologic and molecular techniques that have been adopted by the clinical laboratory for the diagnosis and monitoring of infections and various immunologic disease states.

Topics covered in *Section I* include information regarding structure and function of the immune system and fundamental concepts and mechanisms of humoral and cell-mediated immune responses to infectious and other non-self antigens. Included also are cellular and soluble components of the immune system that take part in various responses to antigens, antibody production, and the major mechanisms involved in abnormal or inappropriate responses of the immune system. The concept of tolerance, immunity, response to tissue antigens, MHC-restricted antigen recognition, cytotoxicity, normal cell and tumor markers, and the concept of memory and antibody diversity are examples of the discussions included in this section.

Section II contains discussion of the current scope of clinical immunology laboratory practice in terms of the procedures used for evaluating humoral (e.g., antibody detection and quantification) and cell-mediated immune responses (e.g., microcytotoxicity). Also included are the most frequently used special immunologic methods such as flow cytometry, HLA and tumor cell phenotyping and histocompatibility testing, cell cultures, utilization of DNA probes, and molecular techniques such as PCR, DNA analysis, and identification of microorganisms and various tumor markers.

Specific laboratory protocols, safety measures for laboratory personnel, and discussion of a quality assurance program to ensure reliability of test results introduce the student to important issues in clinical laboratory practice.

Hannah D. Zane

Contents

IMMUNOLOGY
Theoretical & Practical Concepts
in Laboratory Medicine

SECTION I

FUNDAMENTAL CONCEPTS IN IMMUNOLOGY

Section I includes a comprehensive discussion of the structural organization of the immune system and the mechanisms of its responses to a variety of antigenic stimuli.

These mechanisms include:
1. *Natural (non-specific) immune responses*
2. *Acquired (specific) immune responses,* which consist of the humoral and cell-mediated immune responses
3. *Regulation of the immune responses* to maintain homeostasis
4. *Development of tolerance (immunity)* to certain antigens
5. *Tissue injury,* resulting from an exaggerated immune response, such as hypersensitivity or allergy
6. *Immune response to incompatible tissue antigens* in transplantation procedures
7. *Abnormal responses of the immune system,* such as immunodeficiency or autoimmunity

Each immune response is discussed and illustrated in terms of the cells and molecular components (receptors and soluble molecules) and the particular mechanism involved. The major events that occur during a specific immune response (i.e., antigen specific) are discussed, including antigen recognition (cognitive phase), activation of the immune response (cell proliferation and differentiation phase), and resolution of events (effector phase).

Illustrations in this section are designed to elucidate many of these intricate cellular and molecular concepts as well as such concepts as primary and secondary immune responses (memory), structure and acquisition of antibody diversity, cell-to-cell communication, and recognition of self and non-self or foreign an-

tigens (MHC-restricted antigen recognition), among others.

Emphasis is placed on the major cells of the immune system (i.e., lymphocytes, phagocytes, and natural killer [NK] cells) as well as on such soluble molecules as cytokines, immunoglobulins (antibody molecules), and complement.

In addition to normal immune responses (i.e., protective mechanisms against an infection or a disease) also included is discussion of inappropriate or abnormal immune responses. These inappropriate responses of the immune system may lead to the development of secondary infections in situations when the immune system is deficient in its response (e.g., acquired immunodeficiency syndrome [AIDS]) or may cause tissue injury when the immune response is exaggerated (e.g., autoimmunity and allergy).

The theoretic information presented in this section is intended to serve as a foundation for the various immunologic techniques available for evaluating responses of the immune system.

Normal Immune Responses

Learning Objectives

Upon completion of Chapter 1, the student will be prepared to:

INTRODUCTION TO THE IMMUNE SYSTEM
- List recent developments in immunology that reflect its expanding role in research and clinical practice.
- Define general concepts denoted by the following terms: *immunogenicity, specificity, immune response, immunologic memory, effector mechanisms, homeostasis, immunity,* and *tolerance.*
- State the main function of the immune system.
- Differentiate between a natural and specific immune response in terms of the following components or mechanisms: cells and soluble molecules of the immune system, antigen recognition, antigen specificity, memory, and major effector (resolution) mechanisms.
- Describe the events associated with inflammation during a natural immune response.
- State the principal characteristics of a specific immune response.
- Compare and contrast specific humoral immune responses with specific cell-mediated immune responses, using the following major characteristics: site of antigen infectivity, type of antigen presentation, lymphocytes involved in antigen recognition, antigen receptors, major histocompatibility complex (MHC) class, effector cells and molecules, and effector mechanisms.
- Explain the following mechanisms that comprise cell-mediated and humoral immune responses: antigen recognition, activation, cell proliferation and differentiation, and resolution.
- Describe the role of immunologic memory in secondary immune response and immunization.
- List regulators of immune responses.

CONFERRING SPECIFIC IMMUNITY
- Define passive and active immunity.
- Describe the most important points that are considered in vaccine development.
- State situations that require the administration of a vaccine against an infectious agent, such as hepatitis B virus (HBV).

IMMUNOLOGIC TOLERANCE
- List the various mechanisms that may induce a state of tolerance.
- Describe the development of T and B lymphocyte tolerance to self-antigens.
- Name methods used to artificially induce tolerance to foreign antigens.
- Indicate conditions that may induce tolerance to a particular antigen during an immune response to that antigenic stimulus.

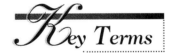

Key Terms

accessory cells - Various cells of the immune system that participate in an immune response to an antigenic stimulus.

activation - Process by which cells on exposure to an antigen are activated (transformed), resulting in increased proliferation known as *blastogenesis, transformation,* or *differentiation.*

anaphylactic - Antigen-specific severe allergic reaction, primarily mediated (moderated) by IgE antibodies, that results in vasodilation (dilation of blood vessels) and contraction of smooth muscle. The reaction may lead to death.

allo - Prefix that can be used to describe genetic dissimilarity in the same species (e.g., allogenic cell is a genetically dissimilar cell of the same species).

auto - Prefix denoting "self," used in identifying such reactions as production of antibodies against self-antigens (autoantibodies) or an autoimmunity, in which the immune system is stimulated and responds to a self-antigen.

anergy - State of unresponsiveness to antigenic stimulation.

antibody - Soluble molecule produced by plasma cell during a humoral immune response, with the capability of specifically binding with a specific epitope on an antigen.

antigen - Any foreign substance or molecule that is capable of inducing an immune response in a host and/or can bind through its epitope(s) to an antibody molecule.

B cell (lymphocyte) - Lymphocyte subset that responds to an antigenic molecule by differentiating into a plasma cell, which can secrete antigen-specific antibodies (effector molecules in a humoral immune response).

cell differentiation - Process by which T and B cells of the immune system are transformed (changed) into effector cells as a result of an antigenic stimulus.

clone - Genetically identical group (family) of cells or organisms.

cluster of differentiation (CD) - Polypeptide molecules, expressed on the surface of cells, that define a particular cell line or a stage of cell maturation.

cytokines - Generic name for a group of soluble molecules involved in the various interactions (signaling) among cells of the immune system during an immune response.

cytolytic (cytotoxicity) - Mechanism by which cells are destroyed or lysed (disruption of cell membrane with release of cell contents).

cytotoxic T cells - Subset of T lymphocytes, bearing a CD8 marker and an antigen receptor on their surface for recognition of antigen, that act as effector cells (have cytotoxic effect on target cells) during a cell-mediated immune response.

effector mechanisms - Effector cells or molecules generated during an immune response that are responsible for resolution (end effect) of the immune response (i.e., elimination or inactivation of an antigenic molecule).

epitope - Part of an antigen, also known as *antigenic determinant,* that combines with a specific antibody or a T cell antigen receptor. More than one epitope may be present on a large antigenic molecule (macromolecule).

helper T cells (lymphocytes) - Subset (subpopulation) of T cells bearing CD4 markers and antigen receptors that recognize antigens and "help" induce a humoral or cell-mediated immune response.

homeostasis - Process of maintaining a stable and uniform normal state within the body.

host - Individual who harbors a microorganism or other foreign material.

humor (extracellular fluid, plasma) - Term not commonly used in immunology except in describing a specific immune response (humoral immune response).

immune response - Response coordinated by cells and soluble components of the immune system to foreign substances, such as infectious agents (microbes) and macromolecules (proteins and polysaccharides).

immune surveillance - Theory that one function of the immune system is to continuously survey the body and destroy any abnormal cells that may develop as a result of an infection or any cellular changes.

immune system - Immune system is composed of a variety of blood and tissue cells, soluble molecules, and lymphoid tissues. Its function is to protect the body against any antigenic molecule by responding through the various mechanisms that comprise the natural and specific immune responses.

immunization - Method of inducing immunity against an infectious agent through administration of specific cells or antibodies from an immunized individual (passive immunity) or through an exposure and immune response to a specific antigen (active immunity).

immunogen - Term used interchangeably with antigen. However, an immunogen is a molecule that is capable of inducing an immune response, whereas the term *antigen* refers to ability to bind with an antibody but not necessarily to evoke an immune response.

immunogenicity - Property of a substance that allows it to initiate a detectable humoral or cell-mediated immune response. Immunogenicity increases with the size and complexity of an immunogen.

infectious - Any agent or disease that is acquired through a contagious or communicable means and produces an immune response and/or a disease state in the host.

interferons (IFNs) - Group of molecules that produce an anti-viral state within a cell, which protects the cell from a viral infection.

interleukin (Il) - Group of molecules that mediate an immune response by "signaling" among cells of the immune system.

lymphokines - Soluble mediators of an immune response, produced by lymphocytes, that are now designated as a subgroup of cytokines.

major histocompatibility complex (MHC) - Genetic region that expresses its products (MHC molecules) on the cell surface of an antigen-presenting cell (APC). The MHC molecules play a role in antigen recognition and in discrimination between self and non-self (foreign) antigens. MHC is also involved in rejection of dissimilar or incompatible grafts (i.e., cell-mediated immune response).

MHC-restriction - Specific recognition of a particular antigen by T cells in the context of MHC (class I or class II MHC molecule). This type of recognition is known as *MHC-restricted recognition.*

memory cells - Memory cells are antigen-stimulated B and T lymphocytes that survive for many years after an initial stimulation with an antigen and which are capable of producing a heightened immune response, known as *secondary immune response,* to a subsequent stimulation with the same antigen.

monoclonal - Term usually used to describe antibodies that have been derived from one clone of cells.

non-self antigen - Any foreign molecule (infectious organism or non-infectious substance) that is recognized by the immune system as foreign (non-self) in the context of the genetically determined MHC molecule.

opsonization - Process by which phagocytosis is facilitated. It involves deposition of opsonins (antibodies or C3b) on the surface of the particular antigen, thus facilitating its ingestion by a phagocyte.

pathogen - Any microorganism that is capable of causing a disease.

phagocytosis - Process by which phagocytic cells (mostly macrophages and granulocytes) engulf and process antigens for elimination or for presentation to T cells for recognition.

primary immune response - Specific response of the immune system (humoral or cell mediated) that is induced (triggered) during an initial encounter with a particular antigen.

primary lymphoid tissue - Lymphoid organs (mainly bone marrow and thymus) or sites where cells of the immune system mature.

receptor - Cell surface molecule that is capable of specifically binding to other extracellular molecules.

resolution - Final stage of an immune response during which the stimulating antigen is eliminated or inactivated, thus bringing the response to an end.

secondary immune response (anamnestic response) - Heightened immune response to a subsequent encounter with the same antigen. It occurs in previously immunized individuals who have immunologic memory as a result of an actual infection or a vaccination.

secondary lymphoid tissues - Structures (lymph nodes, spleen, scattered lymphoid tissue) that house the cells of the immune system and where immune responses occur.

specificity - Characteristic of the specific immune response that refers to specific recognition of a particular antigen by certain cells of the immune system.

suppressor cell - Subpopulation of T lymphocytes, identified by its surface CD8 receptor. Suppressor cells participate in the resolution (inhibition) of an immune response.

target cell - Usually an altered cell against which the products of a specific immune response (effector molecules) are directed.

T cell receptor (TCR) - Antigen receptor, associated with a CD3 complex on the surface of a CD8+ or CD4+ T cell, responsible for recognizing a foreign antigen in the context of a MHC molecule.

tolerance - State of immunologic unresponsiveness.

toxoid - Bacterial toxin that has been made harmless but is still capable of evoking an antibody response.

The current understanding of **immunity** has evolved as a result of years of observations that (1) the body has an ability to defend itself against an infection (**immune response**) and that (2) recovery from an infection is accompanied by a resistance to reinfection by the same infectious agent (**immunity**).

These observations have now been validated through scientific research, particularly within the last 25 years, such as (1) development of recombinant DNA technology and (2) availability of more effective analytic procedures for evaluation of various components of the immune system and mechanisms that comprise immune responses at the cellular and molecular level.

Thus the definition of **immunology** has now been expanded to include the study of:

- The fundamental mechanisms in humoral and cell-mediated immune responses
- Types and characteristics of various immune responses
- Structure and function of the immune system
- The genetic basis for expression of membrane receptors
- The basis for abnormal immune responses (e.g., hyperactivity and immunodeficiency)
- Discovery of tumor and transplantation antigens
- Research and diagnostic procedures

Virtually all current scientific research and practice contains some component related to immunology, making understanding the basic immunologic principles an important foundation for all other related scientific disciplines, such as biotechnology, immunohematology, immunopathology, immunogenetics, immunopharmacology, tumor immunology, transplantation immunology as well as microbiology, hematology, clinical chemistry, and virology.

INTRODUCTION TO THE IMMUNE SYSTEM

THE IMMUNE SYSTEM

Our body is equipped with an immune system, which is composed of lymphoid tissue and a variety of cells and soluble molecules (see Chapters 3 and 4). The immune system has the ability to respond to any antigen, such as a microbe or various macromolecules (proteins and polysaccharides), that is recognized as non-self or foreign (Figure 1-1), in order to protect our body from any potentially infectious organisms.

This response of the immune system to a foreign configuration typically consists of two functionally defined and interrelated immune

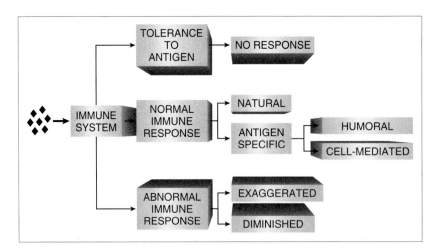

FIGURE **1-1** **Schematic Representation of Host Responses to a Foreign Antigen.** The type of immunologic response that will occur depends on properties of the antigenic stimulus and the constitution (immune status) of the host. Abnormal immune response is observed in such conditions as autoimmune (exaggerated) response and immunodeficient (diminished) response while no response occurs when the host is "tolerant" to a particular antigen.

responses, known as the (1) **natural (non-specific) immune response** and the (2) **specific (acquired) immune response** (described following), which function collaboratively to eliminate or inactivate any antigenic agent. In certain situations, the immune system may also respond abnormally (i.e., an exaggerated or diminished response), thus causing tissue injury or a persistent infection, respectively. Alternatively, the immune system may show no response to a stimulus, a condition that is referred to as **immunologic tolerance.**

Natural or non-specific immune responses are the body's first defense mechanisms against a foreign antigen. However, in situations in which the antigen escapes these natural protective mechanisms and invades the host, another set of antigen-specific and powerful defense mechanisms are triggered. These mechanisms are known as the **specific** or **acquired immune responses** (discussed later in this chapter).

All responses of the immune system are controlled by several **regulatory mechanisms** that maintain homeostasis and return the immune system to a state that existed before the antigenic stimulation. This allows the immune system to respond again to another antigenic stimulus if necessary.

Following a specific immune response to an actual infection or immunization, the host may become **immunized** against the stimulating antigen or develop a state of **tolerance** (non-responsiveness) to that antigenic stimulus. These concepts are described later in the chapter.

The immune system may also be defined in terms of its *functions,* which include:
- **Surveillance:** Recognition of non-self or foreign configuration (antigen)
- **Defense:** Initiation of an immune response (natural or acquired) to eliminate or inactivate a foreign antigen (stimulating agent)
- **Regulation:** Control of immune responses by regulatory mechanisms to maintain homeostasis and to prevent tissue injury that may result from an exaggerated immune response
- **Immunity (immunologic memory):** State of resistance (acquired protection) following exposure to a stimulating agent

- **Tolerance:** Induction of a state of unresponsiveness toward certain antigens (mainly self-antigens), an acquired characteristic of the immune system (specific lymphocytes)

TYPES OF IMMUNE RESPONSES

Although immune responses are categorized mainly into two types, both types of immune responses are a function of one (integrated) immune system (Figure 1-2) that is composed of cells and soluble molecules interacting and functioning cooperatively to eliminate the stimulating antigen (Figure 1-3). The two immune responses are:
- *Natural immune responses*
- *Specific immune responses*

The *natural* and *specific* immune responses represent two ways by which the immune system may respond to a foreign configuration (Table 1-1). However, once the immune response is initiated, both responses function as an integrated defense system, as described following.

Table 1-1 CHARACTERISTICS OF NATURAL AND SPECIFIC IMMUNE RESPONSES

Specific Characteristics	Natural Immune Responses	Specific Immune Responses
Cellular components		
Phagocytic cells	+	+
NK cells	+	+
T lymphocytes	−	+
B lymphocytes	−	+
Soluble components		
Antibodies	−	+
Complement	+	+
Cytokines	+	+
Physical barrier	+	−
Local barrier	−	+
Antigen stimulation	−	+
Specificity	−	+
Immunologic memory	−	+
Amplification	−	+

+, present; −, absent; *NK,* natural killer cells.

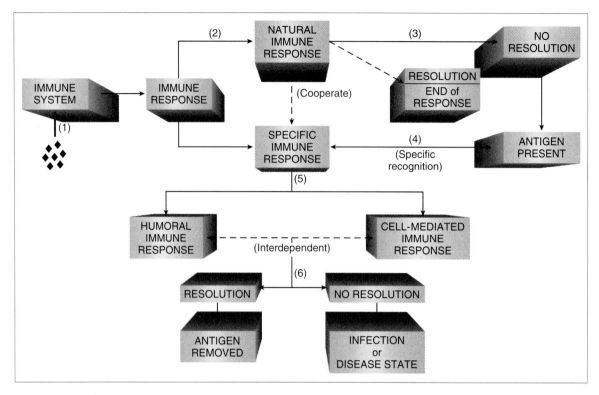

FIGURE **1-2** **Series of Events During Host Encounter with an Antigenic Stimulus.** When the immune system encounters an antigen *(1)* and effectively responds with mechanisms that make up the natural immune response *(2)*, the response is ended. However, if an antigen evades a natural immune response *(3)* but is recognized by the immune system, a specific immune response is triggered *(4)*. Depending on the type of antigen *(5)*, the response may be humoral (response to extracellular antigen, such as various bacteria, with secretion of antibodies), or it may be cell mediated (response to intracellular antigens, such as viruses, or to abnormal cells). Resolution of events occurs when the antigen is removed, while ineffective removal of antigen results in infection or a disease state *(6)*.

The type of immune response that may occur (i.e., **natural** or **specific**) depends on such factors as:

- Recognition of the foreign antigen or antigenic peptides
- Characteristics of the antigenic stimulus
- Site of infection (extracellular or intracellular site)

Natural (Non-Specific) Immune Responses

This type of a response of the immune system to an antigen may be viewed as **natural immunity** because it is the body's first line of natural defense against a foreign antigen. The mechanisms of natural immunity are present in all humans as a product of evolution, are not acquired, and do not require specific recognition of an antigen by the immune system for initiation of the response.

The natural immune responses are also considered to be **non-specific** because they have the following characteristics (see Table 1-1):

- Do not require prior exposure to a foreign antigenic configuration to be effective
- Do not have the ability to recognize a foreign antigenic structure
- Do not have "memory" and are not enhanced by subsequent exposures to an antigenic structure
- May be enhanced by specific immune responses

Components of Natural Immune Responses

The components of natural immune responses are present in all humans. The most impor-

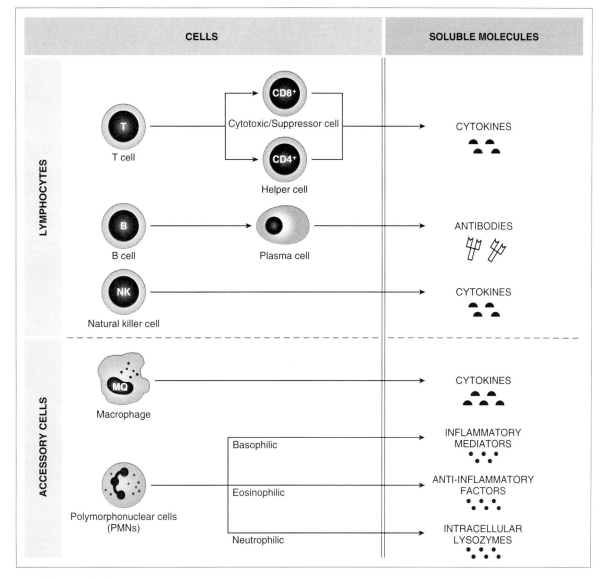

FIGURE **1-3** **Major Cells and Soluble Molecules of the Immune System.**   (See text in Chapter 4.)

tant natural immune responses include the following.

physical barriers. Skin and mucous membranes protect the body from invasion of various microorganisms through such mechanisms as (1) continuous renewal of epithelial cells lining the skin surface, (2) normal bacterial flora on the skin, (3) pH of the skin surface, stomach, intestinal tract, and vagina, (4) trapping of microorganisms in mucus, (5) antibodies on mucosal surface (sIgA, see Chapter 5), (6) bacterial enzymes (lysozyme) in saliva and tears.

cells of the immune system. Examples of such cells include phagocytic cells and natural killer cells (see Figure 1-3).

soluble molecules. Examples include complement, type I interferon (IFN), and tumor necrosis factor (TNF) (Table 1-2).

other factors. Other factors include genetic factors (i.e., the gene complex known as the *major histocompatibility complex [MHC]*) that control immune responsiveness and expression of histocompatibility antigens as well as age that is associated with de-

Table 1-2   SELECTED MEDIATORS OF SPECIFIC AND NON-SPECIFIC IMMUNITY

Cytokine	Origin	Target Cell	Effect on Immune Response
MEDIATORS OF SPECIFIC IMMUNITY			
IL-2	T cell	T cell	Growth/cytokine production
		B cell	Growth/antibody synthesis
		NK cell	Growth/activation
Gamma IFN	T cell/NK cell	MQ/NK cell/endothelial cell	Activation
IL-3 (CSF)	T cell	All progenitor cells	Growth/differentiation
IL-4	Helper cell	B cell	Growth/stimulation
	T cell	T cell	Growth
MEDIATORS OF NON-SPECIFIC IMMUNITY			
Type I IFN	Phagocyte	All cells	Antiviral
	Other cells	NK cells	Activation
TNF	Phagocyte	Neutrophils,	Inflammation
	T cells	Endothelial cells	Activation
IL-6	Phagocytes, endothelial cells	B cells, thymocytes	Growth

IFN, interferon; *TNF*, tumor necrosis factor; *IL*, interleukin; *NK*, natural killer; *CSF*, colony-stimulating factor; *MQ*, macrophage.

creased responsiveness in the elderly and the very young.

Mechanisms of Natural Immune Responses

The primary mechanisms that are triggered during a natural immune response to an invading microorganism consist of various components that are naturally present and available in all humans. These mechanisms include phagocytosis, complement activation, and inflammation.

phagocytosis. Neutrophils, monocytes, and macrophages are cells of the immune system that are capable of phagocytic activity (Figure 1-4). This is the primary mechanism by which the body defends itself against extracellular microorganisms and other antigenic molecules (see Chapter 2). Bacterial resistance to phagocytosis and degradation (digestion) within the phagocyte is an important indicator of bacterial virulence (pathogenicity); the more virulent the bacteria the more it can evade this natural defense mechanism of the immune system.

complement activation. In the absence of specific antibodies that can eliminate antigens through promoting phagocytosis in a *natural immune response* by opsonizing bacteria (see

Figure 1-4) or through eliminating antigen by binding with it and forming antigen/antibody complexes (see *humoral immune response* on pp. 15-16), a variety of complement components or fragments (see One Step Further Box 4-2) can also play an important role in eliminating extracellular bacteria. The complement components involved in natural immune responses are:

- *C3b:* Although less widely acknowledged than T cell recognition of non-self antigens, the complement system also plays a role in discriminating non-self antigens by binding to foreign particles (immune complexes and microorganisms) that have sites allowing deposition of C3b molecules. This non-specific binding of C3b to foreign antigens is known as *opsonization,* a process that enhances phagocytosis (see Figure 1-4) and degradation of the foreign antigenic particles to which C3b fragments are bound (see Chapter 4).

- *C3a and C5a (also known as anaphylotoxins):* These complement activation products participate in an inflammatory response by triggering degranulation of basophils and mast cells, with release of histamines and leukotrienes that cause (1) vascular smooth muscle contraction,

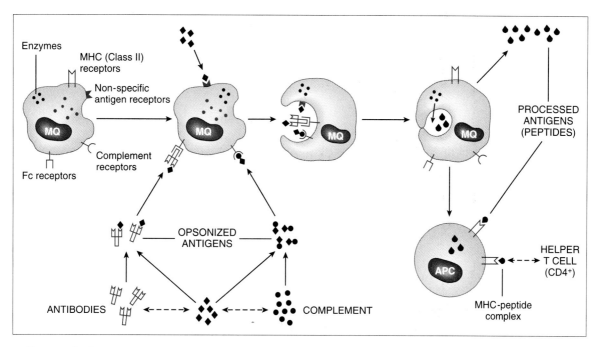

FIGURE **1-4**   **Antigen Processing by Macrophages.**   *Phagocytosis:* Mononuclear phagocytes bind free (extracellular) antigen, such as bacteria, by their non-specific surface antigen receptors. The bound antigen is internalized and degraded by the macrophages *(MQ),* thus removing foreign antigens through phagocytosis (natural immune response). *Antigen-presenting cells (APCs):* The degraded antigen (peptides) are expressed on the MQ surface, bound to class II major histocompatibility complex *(MHC)* molecule, and presented for specific recognition by the immune system (CD4+ cells) in the specific humoral immune response. Opsonization by secreted antibodies and by complement (C3b fraction) facilitates phagocytosis. This is an example of collaboration between the natural and specific immune responses.

(2) increased vascular permeability, and (3) migration of neutrophils and monocytes from blood vessels. Anaphylotoxins are also responsible for the chemotactic attraction (chemotaxis) of neutrophils to the site of inflammation (see Chapter 4).

inflammation. The cellular and systemic events that are associated with tissue injury or infection as the host attempts to restore homeostasis (stability in the area of injury) are discussed in One Step Further Box 1-1.

Specific Immune Responses

The specific immune response, also referred to as a **specific** or **acquired immunity,** is initiated (triggered) by an exposure to a specific antigen that has successfully evaded natural immune responses and is subsequently recognized by the immune system (certain lymphocytes) as foreign or non-self (see Figure 1-2).

"Immunity" in this context refers to specific mechanisms of the immune system that are available for response to a particular antigen. It differs from the concept of an *active or passive "immunity" or resistance* to a particular antigen that resides in antigen-specific "memory" cells of the immune system (see discussion of immunologic memory on p. 25).

Also the term *specific* in this context refers to the recognition of a particular epitope on an antigenic molecule by the CD4+ and CD8+ T lymphocytes of the immune system through their surface antigen receptors. The concepts of specificity and antigen recognition are described further in subsequent sections.

Acquired is another designation for a specific immune response, used to differentiate it from the naturally occurring (non-specific) defense mechanisms (see Table 1-1 and discussion of types of specific immune responses).

Box 1-1

Inflammation

Inflammation occurs in response to any type of tissue injury (physical) or to an invasion with an infectious agent (immunologically induced inflammation). Although the latter is initiated following specific recognition of antigen, the events that follow have no immunologic specificity. Thus **inflammation is a nonspecific immune response.**

Events During Inflammation

There are several main cellular and systemic events that occur during inflammation as the body attempts to reverse the inflammatory condition to a normal state that existed before tissue injury (Figure 1-5).

1. *Systemic inflammatory events include:*
   - Increase in blood supply to area of injury
   - Increased capillary permeability, allowing transport of a variety of larger molecules (e.g., antibodies, complement, and various plasma enzyme systems) across endothelium to the site of inflammation
   - Increase in acute phase reactants, such as serum proteins (e.g., C-reactive protein) associated with acute phase response (discussed following)

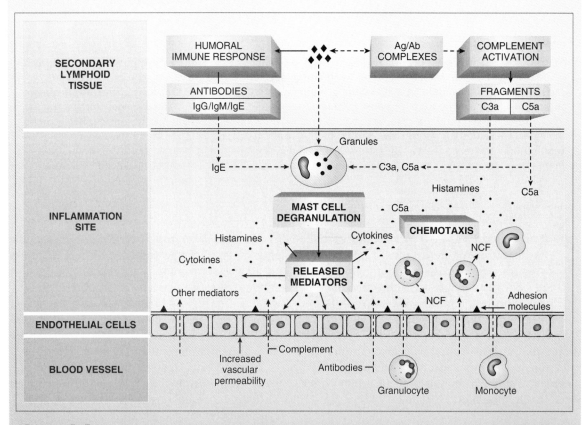

FIGURE **1-5** **Immunologic Events During Inflammation.** Inflammatory response to an antigen results in tissue damage at the site of inflammation. Main soluble molecules involved in the response are mediators (vasoactive amines) released by mast cells (activated by IgE and C3a), such as histamine, cytokines and C5a fragments from complement activation. Other mediators of inflammation (kinins) enter the site from blood vessels. Granulocytes (neutrophils, basophils) and monocytes also enter the inflammation site because of increased vascular permeability and attraction by chemotaxis. These cells contribute to inflammation by elaborating NCF and other cytokines. Adhesion molecules (new receptors on endothelial cells) promote retention of these cells at the site, also contributing to inflammation and tissue damage. *Ig*, immunoglobulin (antibody); *Ag*, antigen; *Ab*, antibody; *C*, complement; *NCF*, neutrophil chemotactic factor.

Box 1-1—cont'd

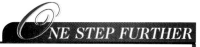
ONE STEP FURTHER

2. *Hematologic changes include:*
   - Increased blood leukocyte count with a "shift to the left" (increase in immature neutrophils)
   - Increase in blood fibrinogen levels
   - Activation of Hegemon factor (XII) of the blood coagulation system
   - Increase in erythrocyte sedimentation rate
3. *Cellular (immunologic) events include:*
   - Migration of leukocytes (macrophages, neutrophils, lymphocytes) out of capillaries into the site of inflammation (known as *cellular infiltration*) under the attraction of chemotactic molecules (see Figure 4-3)
   - Accumulation of leukocytes at the site of inflammation, promoted by the presence of adhesion molecules (new surface receptors) expressed by endothelial cells in response to the action of tumor necrosis factor (TNF); these adhesion molecules make the cells adhesive to leukocytes

Even though inflammation is one of the natural protective mechanisms against invading organisms and is important in recovery from an infection, the cells and mediators that participate in the inflammatory reaction may actually be the cause of tissue injury. The immunologic disorders that follow inflammation are known as **hypersensitivity** (see Chapter 7) and are classified according to the same events that initiate immune responses.

Types of Inflammatory Reactions

The first inflammatory response studied almost 100 years ago was a localized cutaneous reaction to an intradermal injection of an antigen. This experimental model, known as the **skin test,** even now provides valuable information regarding various types of immunologically induced inflammation. Inflammation can be classified as follows:

- **Antibody (IgE)-mediated inflammation** (type I hypersensitivity, immediate hypersensitivity)
- **Immune complex–mediated inflammation** (type III hypersensitivity)
- **T cell–mediated inflammation** (type IV hypersensitivity, delayed type hypersensitivity [DTH])

ANTIBODY-MEDIATED INFLAMMATION

This is a common inflammatory response that can be observed as an immediate skin test reaction and is caused by mediators (histamine, prostaglandins, cytokines) released by mast cells or basophils in response to a reaction of antigen with IgE antibodies bound to IgE receptors on the surface of mast and basophilic cells.

Mechanism of IgE-mediated response. Surface-bound antibodies are first secreted into plasma in response to stimulation with an inherently harmless antigen or allergen (e.g., inhaled pollen or dust particles, ingested food, chemicals in contact with skin, or drugs), from where they pass into the inflammation site and bind to the cell surface IgE receptors on mast cells and basophils. As an antigen and the specific antibody (IgE) bind to the IgE receptors, the cells release inflammatory mediators that increase vascular permeability. These changes promote cellular infiltration (neutrophils, degranulated mast cells/basophils, and eosinophils), erythema (redness of skin), heat, and itching in the area of inflammation. A clinical expression of antibody-mediated inflammation includes such reactions as immediate hypersensitivity, asthmatic reactions, allergy, and hay fever.

IMMUNE COMPLEX–MEDIATED INFLAMMATION

Antigen/antibody-mediated inflammation occurs when immune complexes are formed in circulation by antigen reacting with specific antibodies, being deposited in various tissues, and triggering an inflammatory event.

Mechanism of antigen/antibody-mediated response. IgM or IgG class antibodies, capable of activating complement, react with an antigen to form antigen/antibody immune complexes within the circulation. These immune complexes are deposited in various tissues, such as the basement membrane of the glomerulus (Goodpasture's syndrome) and blood vessels, triggering complement activation. Resulting complement fragments, known as *inflammatory mediators* (e.g., C3a, C4a, and particularly C5a) are chemotactic for neutrophils (see Chapter 4). Changes in vascular permeability and aggregation of platelets and infiltration with mononuclear cells at the site of immune complex deposition result in an inflammatory state. Two clinical expressions of this type of inflammation are:

- **Arthus reaction,** which is a localized edema (presence of increased amount of fluid in the intercellular tissue spaces) and tissue inflammation, seen in intradermal injection of antigen (e.g., immunotherapy for allergy), which serves as a model system for all immune complex–mediated diseases
- **Systemic serum sickness,** caused in some instances by therapeutic injection of foreign material (e.g., immunization with horse serum)

Continued

Box 1-1—cont'd

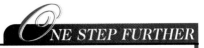

T Cell–Mediated Inflammation

This inflammation is produced by an interaction of antigen with a specific T lymphocyte in the context of a class II MHC (major histocompatibility complex). Discussion of specific antigen recognition and induction of cell-mediated immune response is presented in this chapter and Chapter 6.

Mechanism of T cell–mediated reaction. Lymphocytes and inflammatory cells (monocytes, granulocytes) infiltrate the site of antigenic stimulation, where the coagulation/kinin system is activated. The resulting fibrin formation and deposition produces a typical cutaneous induration (hardened fibrous tissue), which is associated with a delayed type of hypersensitivity (DTH) (discussed in Chapter 7).

Regulation of Inflammation

Inflammation is controlled by various mediators, released by leukocytes (see cytokines, Chapter 4), plasma enzyme products (complement, fibrinolytic system, kinin system, and coagulation system), and vasoactive mediators (amines, kinins) released from basophils, mast cells, and platelets.

The main regulation of inflammation, however, is by the antigen responsible for the inflammatory reaction. As the stimulating antigen is eliminated, the inflammation also subsides. In cases of persisting stimulus, the inflammation becomes chronic.

Acute Phase Response

This rapid response to inflammation consists of an increase in concentration of certain plasma proteins (e.g., acute phase reactants) such as (1) C-reactive protein (CRP), a non-specific opsonin that facilitates phagocytosis of bacteria, (2) alpha 2 macroglobulins (anti-proteinases), (3) fibrinogen (protein involved in coagulation), and (4) serum amyloid A protein (SAA) (elevated in viral and bacterial infections).

The exact function of the acute phase reactants has not been fully defined, although opsonization by CRP and anti-proteinase activity does encourage natural immunity, thus protecting against tissue injury.

Laboratory Diagnosis of Inflammation

The following biologic markers may be of value in diagnosing inflammation:
- Plasma fibrinogen level
- Erythrocyte sedimentation rate (ESR)
- C-reactive protein (CRP)
- Interleukin 6 (IL-6)
- Serum amyloid A (SAA)

Detection of increased **plasma fibrinogen** level (mediated by cytokine IL-6) is of clinical significance in that the resulting in vitro rouleaux formation of red blood cells causes increased **erythrocyte sedimentation rate (ESR).**

Although ESR may be used as a marker for the presence of an acute phase response (a sign of inflammation), other indicators of inflammation (e.g., **C-reactive protein [CRP]** and **IL-6 [interleukin-6]**) may be of value. Because increase in both CRP and IL-6 is seen in acute and chronic inflammation (e.g., rheumatoid arthritis), disease-specific laboratory evaluation is required.

Table 1-3	FUNDAMENTAL DIFFERENCES BETWEEN HUMORAL AND CELL-MEDIATED IMMUNE RESPONSES	
Differential Characteristics	Humoral Immune Response	Cell-Mediated Immune Response
Stimulating Ag	Extracellular (exogenous)	Intracellular (endogenous)
Ag presentation	Phagocyte, B lymphocyte	Altered cell (infected or tumor)
Ag recognition	Class II MHC restricted	Class I MHC restricted
Cells involved in Ag recognition	CD4+ (helper T cell)	CD8+ (cytotoxic T cell)
Ag receptor	T cell receptor (TCR)	T cell receptor (TCR)
Effector cells	B lymphocyte (plasma cell)	T lymphocyte (cytotoxic T cell)
Effector molecules	Antibodies (immunoglobulins)	Cytotoxins
Resolution of infection	Ag/Ab complex formation; opsonization	Cytotoxicity and cell lysis (cytolysis)

Ag, antigen; *Ab,* antibody; *MHC,* major histocompatibility complex; *CD,* cluster of differentiation.

Types of Specific Immune Responses

Specific immune responses are some of the most powerful defense mechanisms available for inactivation or removal of a potentially immunogenic molecule before it can have a damaging effect on the host. These responses may occur during the first or second (and subsequent) encounters with the particular antigen and are designated as **primary** or **secondary immune responses,** respectively.

Two mechanisms by which the immune system specifically responds to a particular immunogen are (Figure 1-6):

- *Humoral immune response*
- *Cell-mediated immune response*

Although both humoral and cell-mediated immune responses function as one integrated (interdependent) response to an antigenic stimulus (Table 1-3), each response has specific characteristics that differentiate it from the other, as follows:

- Response to a different type of antigen and its site of infectivity (see Chapter 2)
- Mechanisms that are triggered during the response
- Components of the immune system, such as effector cells and molecules involved in eliminating the antigenic stimulus (see Table 1-2)

The induction (initiation) of both humoral and cell-mediated immune responses, however, depends on the ability of the immune system to differentiate between self and non-self antigens. This is an important feature of the immune system because it determines whether a specific immune response will or will not occur.

humoral immune responses. Humoral immune responses are brought about by various

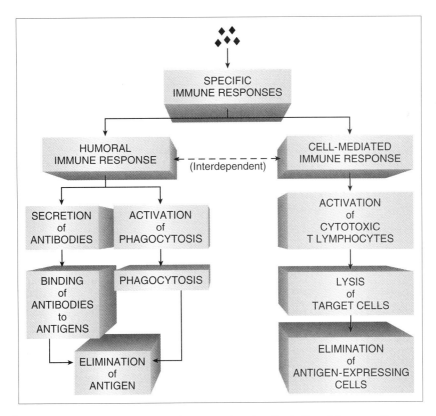

FIGURE **1-6** **Schematic Representation of Humoral and Cell-Mediated Immune Responses.** The immune system responds specifically to a foreign (antigenic) molecule in one of two ways: (1) by secreting specific antibodies (humoral immune response) that bind the antigen or enhance phagocytosis through opsonization to remove the stimulating antigen or, alternatively, (2) by activating cytotoxic T lymphocytes to lyse target cells that bear the specific antigen (cell-mediated immune response).

extracellular (exogenous) foreign organisms (mainly bacteria) and by certain *intracellular antigens* as they migrate between cells. The extracellular location of these antigens makes them directly accessible to the immune system and available for elimination by specific antibodies produced during a humoral immune response (Figure 1-7).

mechanism. The extracellular antigens are processed by a phagocytic cell (see Figure 1-4), known as an antigen-presenting cell (APC) and are expressed on their cell surface bound to the surface-self class II MHC molecules (major histocompatibility complex molecules) (Figure 1-8). The MHC-antigenic peptide complex is presented to the class II–restricted helper T lymphocytes (CD4+) for specific antigen recognition by their surface antigen receptors (T cell receptors). The T cell receptor (TCR) is in association with CD3 receptor (TCR/CD3 complex). The CD4 receptor participates in antigen recognition as an accessory molecule. This type of antigen recognition is referred to as a *MHC-restricted recognition* or *class II MHC-restriction* (Figure 1-9).

Alternatively, B cells may serve as antigen-presenting cells (APCs) in specific recognition of the antigenic molecule by CD4+ cells (see Figure 1-8). This mechanism involves two steps: (1) specific binding of antigen by B cells through

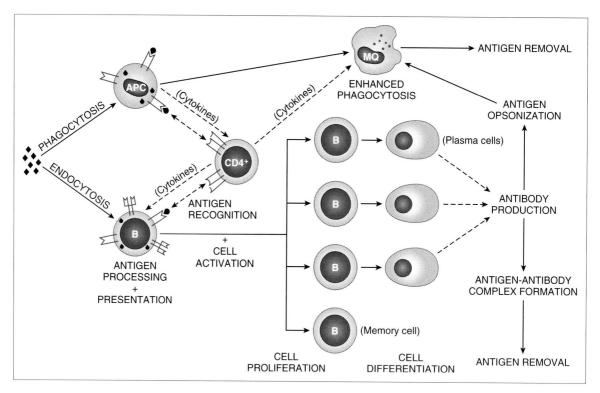

FIGURE **1-7** **Schematic Representation of Immunologic Events During Humoral Immune Response.** Note that extracellular antigens (mainly bacteria) are internalized and processed by antigen-presenting cells (macrophages and resting B lymphocytes). The processed antigens (peptides) are then expressed bound to class II MHC molecules and presented for recognition by the CD4+ (helper) T lymphocytes through their surface antigen receptors (TCRs). Cytokines, elaborated by macrophages and recognition of antigen by the CD4+ cell, activate the CD4+ cell. The activated cell elaborates cytokines that, in turn, activate B lymphocytes and macrophages. Antigen-specific activated B lymphocytes proliferate and differentiate into antibody-secreting plasma cells. Resolution of events and elimination of antigen is accomplished by binding of antigens by antibodies (forming of antigen/antibody complexes) and by phagocytosis (facilitated by opsonization). *TCR,* T cell receptor; *CD,* cluster of differentiation.

their surface immunoglobulin receptors (sIgs) and (2) antigen presentation to CD4+ T cell, which has been processed and bound to the MHC molecule on a B lymphocyte.

The CD4+ cells become activated upon recognizing the antigenic stimulus as non-self and in turn (1) activate macrophages to phagocytose and destroy the antigen and to mediate the humoral immune responses through secreted cytokines (see Table 1-2), (2) stimulate B cells to differentiate into antibody-secreting plasma cells, (3) enhance phagocytosis, and (4) promote inflammation.

The secreted antigen-specific antibodies participate in the elimination of antigenic stimulus by forming antigen/antibody complexes, neutralizing bacterial toxins, and by opsonization of antigen to promote phagocytosis (see Figure 1-4). These specific antibodies may also activate complement, with resulting production of various complement fragments (i.e.,

C3b) that promote bacterial phagocytosis through opsonization (see Chapter 4).

cell-mediated immune response. Immune response to the *intracellular (endogenous)* microorganisms, such as bacteria, parasites, or viruses, is principally cell mediated. Viruses and certain microorganisms are obligatory (compulsory) intracellular microorganisms that replicate within a cell, causing changes in the cell's characteristics. Since these organisms are not readily accessible to the circulating antibodies (in the blood) for binding and elimination, the humoral immune responses are ineffective.

However, the host's immune system has an effective defense mechanism that is capable of eliminating intracellular (endogenous) antigens and cells expressing these antigens as well as eliminating cells expressing mutant or abnormal protein antigens on their surface. The mechanism involves destruction (lysing) of any

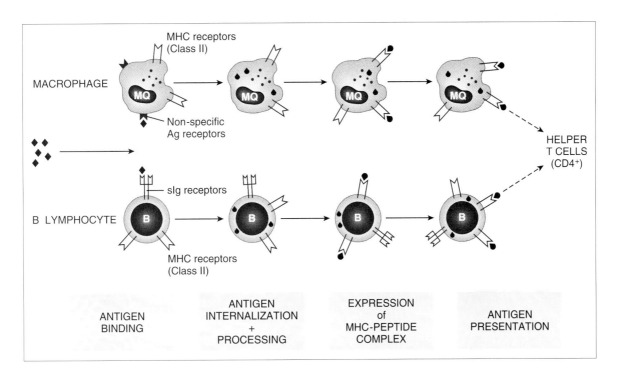

FIGURE **1-8** **Antigen-Presenting Cells (APCs).** Macrophages and B lymphocytes function as APCs in the humoral immune response because both types of cells are able to internalize and process foreign antigen (extracellular) and express self class II MHC molecules that bind processed antigen for presentation to CD4+ T lymphocytes for recognition. CD4+ T cells recognize MHC-bound peptides and trigger a humoral immune response. *MHC,* major histocompatibility complex; *Ag,* antigen; *sIg,* surface immunoglobulin.

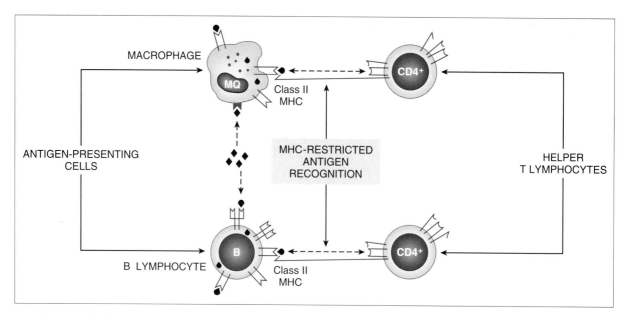

FIGURE **1-9** **Class II MHC–Restricted Antigen Recognition.** Antigen recognition by CD4+ T lymphocytes is limited to processed antigen (peptides), presented by APC in the context of self class II MHC complex (peptide bound to MHC molecule). CD4+ cells recognize antigen through their surface antigen receptors, consisting of the TCR/CD3 complex (recognition complex). CD4 receptor serves as an accessory molecule for the recognition complex. *MHC*, major histocompatibility complex; *APC*, antigen-presenting cell; *TCR*, T cell receptor; *CD*, cluster of differentiation.

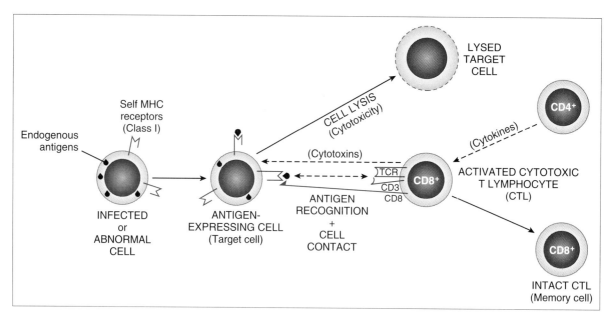

FIGURE **1-10** **Schematic Representation of Immunologic Events During Cell-Mediated Immune Response.** Note that intracellular antigenic molecules (mainly viruses) are expressed on the surface of abnormal or infected cells bound to self MHC molecules as MHC-peptide complexes that are specifically recognized by cytotoxic (CD8+) T lymphocytes through their antigen receptors (TCR/CD3). CD8 receptor is an accessory molecule to the TCR complex. The CD8+ cells become activated by the antigen (and by cytokines secreted by CD4+ cell) and respond by releasing cytotoxins that lyse antigen-expressing cells (target cells), thereby removing the stimulating antigen. Cytotoxic cells, which function as both the antigen-presenting cells (APCs) and target cells, remain unaltered and are available to continue their cytotoxic function. *MHC*, major histocompatibility complex; *CTL*, cytotoxic T lymphocyte; *TCR*, T cell receptor; *CD*, cluster of differentiation.

antigen-bearing cells (also referred to as *target cells*). This defense mechanism against endogenous antigens is known as the *cell-mediated immune response* (Figure 1-10).

mechanism. During the immune response, the CD8+ T lymphocytes specifically recognize antigenic molecules that are expressed on the surface of an antigen bearing abnormal or infected cells (see Figure 1-10) and initiate cell lysis (cytotoxicity) of the antigen-expressing cell.

The expressed antigenic molecules consist of endogenously processed microbial (mainly viral) or abnormal (mutant) protein located within an infected or abnormal (tumor) cell and displayed as a peptide (degraded protein) in association with the class I MHC (major histocompatibility complex) on the surface of the antigen-containing cell (Figure 1-11). Antigen-specific CD8+ lymphocytes, when specifically recognizing the displayed antigen (Figure 1-12) through their antigen receptors (T cell receptors present in association with CD3 receptor and the accessory CD8 molecule), become activated and differentiate into cytotoxic T lymphocytes (CTLs) with "help" (cytokine secretions) from the CD4+ helper T lymphocytes (see Figure 1-10).

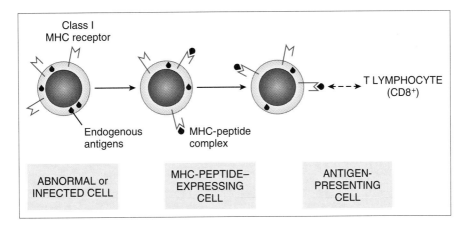

FIGURE **1-11** **Antigen-Presenting Cell in Cell-Mediated Immune Response.** An infected or an abnormal cell may serve as an antigen-presenting cell (APC) by expressing endogenous antigens bound to self class I MHC molecules for recognition by CD8+ cells. Any cell expressing such an MHC-peptide complex on its surface serves as both an APC and a target cell in a cell-mediated immune response. Target cell lysis occurs as the means of eliminating any abnormal cell containing the stimulating antigen. Cell lysis occurs by the action of cytotoxins (effector mechanism) elaborated by the antigen-activated CD8+ cell, with "help" from CD4+ cells. *MHC,* major histocompatibility complex; *CD,* cluster of differentiation.

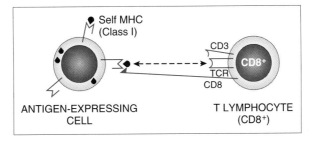

FIGURE **1-12** **Class I MHC–Restricted Antigen Recognition.** Antigen recognition by CD8+ T lymphocytes is limited to intracellular antigens (peptides), expressed by an abnormal or infected cell (APC) bound to self class I MHC molecule. CD8+ cells recognize antigen through their surface antigen receptors, consisting of the TCR/CD3 complex (recognition complex). CD4 receptor serves as an accessory molecule for the recognition complex. *MHC,* major histocompatibility complex; *APC,* antigen-presenting cell; *TCR,* T cell receptor; *CD,* cluster of differentiation.

Elaboration of cytotoxins by the antigen-activated cytotoxic T cell (CD8+) and destruction of any antigen-expressing cell (target cell) by an effector mechanism, known as *cytotoxicity* (Figure 1-13), resolves (ends) the immune response by eliminating the particular antigen. This is the major route for eliminating virally infected or abnormal (tumor) cells.

Other possible protection against certain intracellular infections includes (1) phagocytosis by macrophages that have been activated by T helper cell–derived cytokine (IFN-gamma), (2) action of natural killer cells (NK cells), and (3) opsonization of antigens by specific antibodies during an early stage of an infection (see Figure 1-7).

primary vs. secondary specific immune responses. It has been shown that the immune system has the ability to mount a specific immune response to an antigen that enters into the host's internal environment and is recog-

nized as non-self or foreign. The response to the foreign configuration may be either in the form of *a primary immune response* (first encounter with an antigen), or *a secondary immune response* (second or subsequent encounter with the same antigen) as discussed following and in Figure 1-14.

primary immune response. This type of a specific response of the immune system occurs on exposure to an antigen, either through an *actual infection* or a *vaccination* that the T cells of the immune system specifically recognize as foreign. The immune response that follows antigen recognition consists of a variety of events (described following) that leads to the elimination of the stimulating antigen.

However, not all antigen-stimulated cells (T and B lymphocytes) differentiate into effector cells during the immune response. Instead, some of these cells develop into antigen-specific "memory" cells by poorly understood mecha-

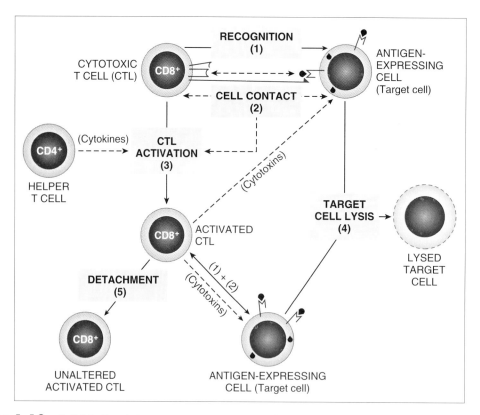

FIGURE **1-13** **Cell-Mediated Cytotoxicity.** This main effector mechanism in cell-mediated immune response involves removal of abnormal (antigen-bearing) cells through *(1)* CD8+ cell recognition of cell-bound antigen in the context of self class I MHC molecule, *(2)* activation of CTL through cell contact and by cytokines from helper T cells, *(3)* secretion of cytotoxins by CTL, *(4)* lysis of target cell by cytotoxins, and *(5)* disengagement of CTL from contact and its availability for other cell-to-cell interactions.

nisms. The "memory" cells, having the ability to specifically recognize a previously encountered antigen, are responsible for conferring a long-lasting immunity (protection) against the stimulating antigen (see Figure 1-14). The conferred immunity may last for as long as 20 years.

secondary immune response. "Memory" T and B lymphocytes that are produced during a primary immune response remain inactive until a repeated encounter with the same antigen occurs. Upon a second or subsequent antigenic stimulation, the "memory" cells proliferate and differentiate into effector cells (e.g., cytotoxic T cells), which are capable of eliminating the stimulating antigen through various effector mechanisms, described following.

This *secondary (anamnestic) immune response* (see Figure 1-14) is a heightened response, occurring more rapidly than the pri-

mary immune response and offers a more effective protection against a variety of infectious agents. Thus the secondary immune response occurs in situations in which (1) the antigen has been previously encountered and (2) the host has been immunized against that particular antigenic structure during the primary immune response.

Major Immunologic Events During Specific Immune Response

As the immune system encounters an antigen and specifically recognizes it as a foreign configuration, certain specific immune responses (humoral or cell mediated) are triggered (see Figures 1-7 and 1-10). These specific immune responses consist of various mechanisms and follow a definite sequence of events (Figure 1-15). Thus, the immunologic events that occur

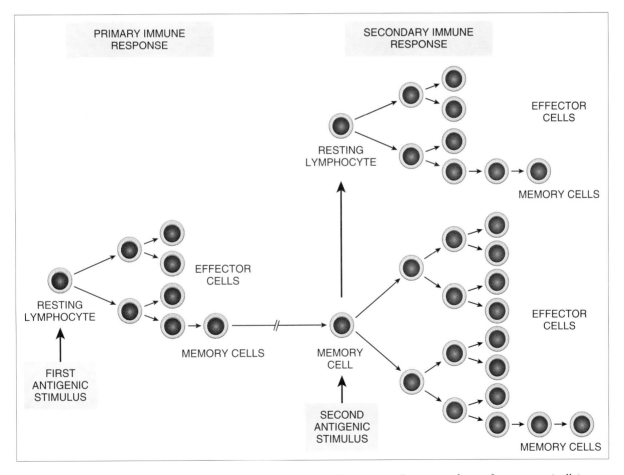

FIGURE **1-14** **Cellular Events in Secondary Immune Response.** Presence of specific memory (cells) is responsible for a more rapid and greater immune response to a second and subsequent exposure to the same antigen than is observed in the primary immune response.

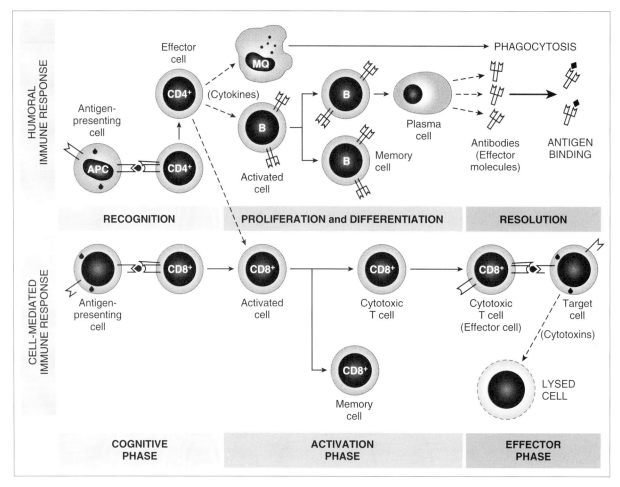

FIGURE **1-15**   **Phases of the Immune Response.**   Three phases or events that occur during a humoral and cell-mediated immune response are (1) antigen recognition *(cognitive phase)*, which initiates all immune responses and involves antigen processing, presentation, and recognition by T lymphocytes (CD4+ and CD8+); (2) proliferation and differentiation of antigen-activated T and B lymphocytes into cytotoxic and plasma cells, respectively *(activation phase);* and (3) elimination or inactivation of antigens through various effected mechanisms, mainly cytolysis, phagocytosis, and binding by antibodies *(effector phase).*

during an immune response (humoral and cell mediated) can be categorized into three main stages or phases (Table 1-4) and include:

- *Cognitive phase (antigen recognition)*
- *Activation phase (cell proliferation/cell differentiation)*
- *Effector phase (resolution of immune response)*

cognitive phase. Specific recognition of a foreign antigen by T lymphocytes (CD4+ and CD8+ cells) occurs as a foreign antigen binds to the antigen-specific T lymphocyte and triggers the events that constitute an immune response (humoral or cell mediated).

The recognition of an antigen depends on presence of a self major histocompatibility (MHC) molecule on the surface of an antigen-presenting cell (APC) and is referred to as *MHC-restricted antigen recognition* (see Figures 1-9 and 1-12). Recognition also depends on the form in which the antigen is presented, that is, only peptides processed and expressed as a MHC-peptide complex on the surface of an antigen-presenting cell are recognized by antigen receptors (TCR/CD3 and CD4 or CD8 accessory molecules) located on the surface of CD4+ and CD8+ lymphocytes (see Chapter 3). Either a humoral or cell-mediated

Table 1-4 CATEGORIZATION OF EVENTS OCCURRING DURING AN IMMUNE RESPONSE

Phase	Mechanism (Process)	Humoral Response	Cell-Mediated Response
COGNITIVE PHASE	Ag processing Ag presentation Ag recognition	Extracellular antigens MQ, B cells Class II MHC restriction	Intracellular antigens Abnormal, infected cells Class I MHC restriction
ACTIVATION PHASE	Cell activation Cell proliferation Cell differentiation	B lymphocyte Activated B lymphocyte Plasma cell (effector cells)	T lymphocyte Activated T lymphocyte Cytotoxic T lymphocyte
EFFECTOR PHASE	Secretion of effector molecules Resolution of events	Antibodies, cytokines, other Formation of Ag/Ab complex, phagocytosis	Cytotoxins, cytokines, other Cytotoxicity (cell lysis)

Ag, antigen; MQ, macrophage (phagocytic cell); MHC, major histocompatibility complex: Ag/Ab, antigen/antibody.

Table 1-5 KEY FEATURES IN ANTIGEN RECOGNITION BY THE IMMUNE SYSTEM

Feature	T Cells CD4+	CD8+	B Cells
Type of recognition	Specific	Specific	Non-specific
Antigen receptor	TCR	TCR	sIg
Antigen presentation	Macrophage, B cell	Altered cell	Free peptides, native proteins, and other molecules
Pattern of Ag presentation	MHC-bound peptides	MHC-bound peptides	Free native molecules
Type of MHC restriction	Class II MHC	Class I MHC	None
Type of immune response	Humoral, cell mediated	Cell mediated	*

*B cells are a component of humoral immune responses and differentiate into antibody-secreting cells (plasma cells) on stimulation with mediators secreted by CD4+ T cells. B cells may also function as APCs (see text).
CD4+, helper T lymphocyte; CD8+, cytotoxic T lymphocyte (CTL); Ag, antigen; TCR, T cell receptor for antigen recognition; sIg, surface immunoglobulin (antibody) molecule on B cells; APC, antigen-presenting cell; MHC, major histocompatibility complex; CD, cluster of differentiation.

immune response follows specific antigen recognition.

The type of immune response that is initiated (i.e., humoral or cell mediated), therefore, depends on the antigenic molecule that is encountered by the immune system and on the type of MHC-restricted antigen recognition by antigen-specific T cell that occurs (Table 1-5).

activation phase (proliferation and differentiation). Activation of the immune system is initiated during the specific recogni-tion of a foreign antigen by resting T lymphocytes (see Figures 1-9 and 1-12) and is promoted by the various mediator molecules that are elaborated by lymphocytes and accessory cells of the immune system (see Figure 1-3 and Table 1-2). The T lymphocytes become activated by binding to the specific antigen bound to their self MHC molecule while B lymphocytes bind with free antigen and become activated with help from the CD4+ T cells (see Figure 1-15).

Activation of T and B cells may also occur through an in vitro (tissue culture) exposure to different mitogens, most common of which are T cell–activating lectins, lipopolysaccharide (PHA) and Concanavalin-A (Con-A) and B cell–activating pokeweed mitogen (PWM).

Two events occur following antigen recognition and lymphocyte activation: cell proliferation and differentiation.

cell proliferation. This occurs as an increase in antigen-specific lymphocytes through expansion (induction of mitosis) of specific clones and an increased expression of existing surface molecules as well as an appearance of new activation markers.

The new markers are *adhesion molecules* that promote a better interaction between cells and *receptors for growth and differentiation factors,* such as IL-2 receptor and MHC molecules on T cells, and IL-2 receptor, CD23 molecules, and other receptors on B cells. Interaction of cells through these receptors and corresponding cytokines leads to proliferation and maturation of lymphocytes.

cell differentiation. Specific clones differentiate into effector cells whose primary function is to eliminate the stimulating antigen through elaboration of effector molecules.

In a humoral immune response, the helper T lymphocytes (CD4+) that participate in antigen recognition also stimulate B lymphocytes to proliferate and differentiate into antibody-secreting cells (plasma cells) that elaborate antigen-specific antibodies (effector molecules), which can then bind with the extracellular antigens, thus inactivating or eliminating them through formation of antigen/antibody complexes, or through opsonization, which promotes phagocytosis of the particular antigen (see Figures 1-7 and 1-15).

During a cell-mediated immune response, the cytotoxic T lymphocytes that recognize an antigenic molecule also induce the T lymphocytes to proliferate and differentiate into cytotoxic T cells (CTLs). The CTLs function as effector cells by destroying altered (abnormal) cells through a mechanism known as *cytotoxicity* or *cytolysis* (see Figures 1-13 and 1-15).

effector phase. During this stage, the immune response is resolved (completed) as the stimulating antigen is eliminated or inacti-vated, and the immune system returns to a state that existed before the encounter with a particular antigen.

The resolution of events in an immune response is the result of various effectors in immune responses (i.e., cells and mediator [soluble] molecules). For example, the effector cell in a cell-mediated immune response is the cytotoxic/suppressor T cell (CD8+), whereas in the humoral immune response, the specific antibody (secreted by B cell–derived plasma cells) is an effector molecule. Helper T cells (CD4+), in addition to their ability to recognize antigens, also function as effector cells by elaborating various cytokines (signals) that activate B lymphocytes and "assist" in the activation of CD8+ cells (see Figure 1-15).

Other effector cells (e.g., mononuclear phagocytes, dendritic cells) and certain defense mechanisms in natural immunity (e.g., phagocytosis and complement activation) also participate in eliminating microbes although they do not specifically recognize any antigen.

Characteristics of Specific Immune Response

Characteristics that differentiate natural from specific immune responses are presented in Table 1-1. Among those that are most characteristic of a specific immune response are:

- *Specific recognition of self and foreign antigens*
- *Lymphocyte diversity*
- *Immunologic memory*
- *Regulation of immune response*

specific antigen recognition. One of the most important characteristics of the immune system is its ability to specifically recognize an antigen, thus determining whether an immune response will or will not occur.

Normally, the immune system discriminates between self and non-self antigens in the context of self major histocompatibility complex (MHC) molecules that are encoded by the MHC gene, responding only to non-self or foreign antigens. It does so by the following mechanisms.

antigen recognition by T lymphocytes. Helper (CD4+) and cytotoxic (CD8+) T lymphocytes are the only cells of the immune system that have the ability to specifically recognize antigens. This is because T lymphocytes are the only cells that have surface antigen-specific receptors (TCR/CD3, CD4 or CD8 serving as accessory molecules) capable of antigen recognition (see Figures 1-9 and 1-12).

Antigen recognition is limited to recognition of small peptide fragments (degraded protein) that have been processed by other cells (antigen-presenting cells [APCs]) and bound on their surface through a cleft on a specialized group of molecules. These surface molecules are a product of an inherited set of MHC genes and are known as the class I and class II MHC molecules (see Figures 1-9 and 12).

Thus recognition of foreign antigens by CD4+ cells is associated with the *class II MHC molecule* (MHC-antigenic peptide complex) on an antigen-presenting cell (APC), whereas CD8+ cells recognize antigens that are associated with the *class I MHC-antigenic peptide complex* on an abnormal or altered cell. This type of specific antigen recognition by the helper (CD4+) and cytotoxic (CD8+) T lymphocytes activates events that constitute the humoral and cell-mediated immune response, respectively, and is referred to as a *MHC-restricted antigen recognition* (see Table 1-5 and Figure 1-12).

T lymphocytes do not recognize "free" antigenic peptides or membrane proteins that may become associated with the self MHC molecule.

antigen recognition by B lymphocytes. B lymphocytes do not have the ability to specifically recognize foreign molecules, although they may specifically bind with an antigenic molecule (see following).

This inability of B cells to specifically recognize antigens, discriminate between self and non-self antigens, and trigger an immune reaction is because they lack specialized surface antigen receptors (TCR/CD3 complex on T cells) that are responsible for specific antigen recognition and for discriminating between self and non-self antigens (see Table 1-5 and Figure 1-12).

Specificity of antigen recognition by the B cells, therefore, is limited to their "recognition" of the complementary configuration of an antigenic molecule. This allows for a specific binding of that antigen by the antigen-binding site of the surface membrane–bound immunoglobulins (Igs), known as *B cell receptors*

(BCRs) (see discussion of surface Igs in Chapter 5).

Unlike the specific antigen recognition by T cells, B cell antigen recognition is not MHC-restricted (see Figure 1-9). Thus B cells cannot initiate an immune response but are involved in the humoral immune responses and may serve as antigen-presenting cells in certain situations (see Chapter 3). Their participation in a humoral immune response depends on their activation by helper T cells, which are able to recognize a foreign configuration in the MHC context (see previous discussion). Once activated, B cells proliferate and differentiate into antibody-producing cells (plasma cells) that secrete antibodies with a specificity for the stimulating antigen that has been recognized by the helper T cells.

lymphocyte diversity. The immune system has the ability to recognize almost a limitless number of antigens; however, each lymphocyte can recognize only one particular antigen (epitope) through the mechanisms described previously and in Chapter 5.

As the antigen binds through its epitope to the antigen receptor (TCR) on a lymphocyte, the lymphocyte is stimulated by the antigen, proliferates (multiplies), and produces a sufficient number of antigen-specific lymphocyte clones that are necessary to mount a successful immune response.

This process of activating T cell clones (a line of cells with the same genetic make-up [i.e., originating from one cell]) that express the specific receptors for a particular antigen is known as **clonal selection.** Clonal selection is unlike **clonal deletion** of self-reactive T cell clones, which occurs in the thymus in the context of their MHC molecules (Figure 1-16).

immunologic memory. Immunologic memory is a function of T and B lymphocytes. During a primary immune response, antigen-stimulated T and B cells develop (differentiate) into effector cells, which participate in the removal of the stimulating antigen. Some of these antigen-stimulated T and B lymphocytes, however, do not differentiate into effector cells during the primary immune response but instead (by some yet unclear mechanism) become T and B "memory" cells.

Subsequent stimulation with the same antigen leads to a heightened and more rapid

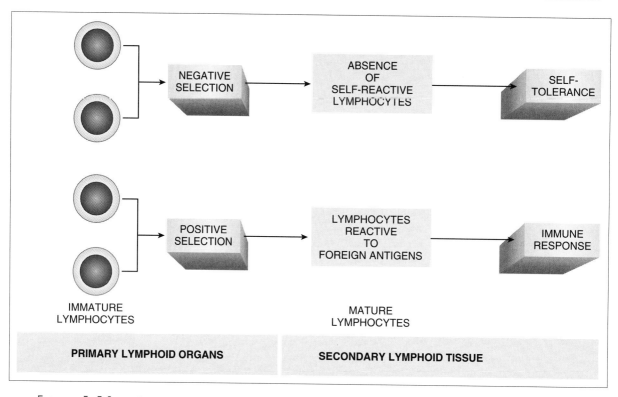

FIGURE 1-16 **Selection of Lymphocyte Clones.**   Cells with specificity for self-antigens are inactivated or deleted by "negative selection" in the primary lymphoid organs (bone marrow, thymus). Absence of self-reactive clones prevents the immune system from responding to self-antigens. Lymphocytes, expressing antigen receptors capable of reacting with non-self (foreign antigens) but lacking specificity for self-antigens, are selected by "positive selection" and mature in the secondary lymphoid tissues and are able to produce an immune response to foreign antigens. Immune responses to foreign or non-self antigens occur in secondary lymphoid tissue (peripheral tissue, spleen, lymph nodes).

response, known as *secondary immune response* (see Figure 1-14), and to the differentiation of the "memory" cells and other resting lymphocytes into effector cells with same effector functions as those generated during a primary immune response.

regulation of immune responses. Positive selection of cells that can recognize antigens in the context of the self major histocompatibility (MHC) molecule through *clonal selection* and elimination of self-reacting T lymphocytes through *clonal deletion* constitute a powerful mechanism that regulates the immune response by recognizing self from non-self antigens, thus determining if an immune response will or will not occur (see Figure 1-16).

As the immune system recognizes and responds to foreign (non-self) antigens, various immune mechanisms are triggered that activate antigen-specific lymphocyte clones and initiate an immune response. This immune response is normally self-limiting.

The following mechanisms are involved in the regulation of immune responses and maintenance of homeostasis.

self-regulation. As the antigen is removed from a host by effectors of the immune response (effector cells, cytokines, and antibodies), the intensity of the response decreases with time. This self-limiting process is a normal phenomenon that maintains homeostasis and ensures that the immune response lasts for only as long as it is needed.

Participating in the self-limiting mechanisms are (1) *cytokines* and *antibodies* (immunoglobulins), which are secreted for only a short period of time and are shut off after the antigen is eliminated and (2) *effector cells of the immune responses* (i.e., cytotoxic/suppressor T lymphocytes and plasma cells) that are also short-lived and are not self-renewing. Therefore another exposure to the *same* antigen is necessary to initiate another immune response, known as a *secondary immune response* or *anamnestic response* (see Figure 1-14). During this secondary immune response, the resting and memory cells are stimulated to generate new effector cells and soluble molecules.

genetic control. This refers to the MHC-linked immune response genes, which play a particularly important role by providing a mechanism for recognition of self and non-self (foreign) antigens in the context of their gene product, known as the *major histocompatibility complex (MHC) molecules.* This ensures that the immune response occurs only in response to a foreign molecule, thereby avoiding such an abnormal immune reaction as autoimmunity (reactivity to self-antigens).

other regulators. Although not fully understood, regulation of an immune response also takes place through other regulators of the immune response such as (1) stimulating antigen, (2) lymphocytes, (3) soluble molecules, (4) accessory cells, (5) idiotypic interactions, and (6) neuroendocrine modulation.

CONFERRING SPECIFIC IMMUNITY

Immunity or a state of resistance to a particular antigen may be conferred on an individual in either of two ways (i.e., passively or actively), and the resulting immune state is known as either:

- *Passive immunity* or
- *Active immunity*

Passive immunity is conferred "passively" by administration of preformed cells or antibodies from another previously actively immunized individual. In active immunity, the individual becomes immunized by actually mounting an immune response to the stimulating antigen.

PASSIVE (NATURAL) IMMUNITY

Passively acquired immunity is a type of specific immunity that may be conferred upon an individual by transferring cells or antibodies from another individual who has been previously successfully and specifically immunized.

This type of immunity offers a rapid way of conferring resistance to a particular antigen without an actual exposure or an immune response of the recipient. However, because there is no induction of "memory cells" (see previous discussion), this type of immunity is short-lived, lasting only as long as the transferred cells or antibodies are present. Passive immunity is a most useful tool for quickly providing neutralizing antibodies (antitoxins) against such toxins as tetanus and snake venoms and as a preventive (antiviral) measure against hepatitis B infection (One Step Further Box 1-2).

ACTIVE (SPECIFIC) IMMUNITY

Exposure of an individual to either an infectious or non-infectious foreign configuration triggers a humoral or cell-mediated immune response that results in an actively acquired specific immunity.

Immunity Induced by Infection
An individual becomes immunized by "actively" responding to an antigenic stimulation through the mechanisms of a specific immune response.

The molecular and cellular mechanisms comprising specific immune responses involved in conferring specific (active) immunity and the evaluation of these responses with the use of medical laboratory technology (immunologic procedures) form the basis for the content of this textbook.

Immunity Induced by Vaccination
The purpose of a vaccination (immunization) is to induce the recipient's immune system to respond specifically to an (altered) infectious organism or to a non-infectious antigenic configuration that is administered to the individual in the form of a vaccine. During the immune response that follows this deliberate stimulation of the immune system, the host develops a protective state (active immunity) against re-infection with the same antigen.

Vaccine Development
Acceptance of vaccination as a prophylactic (preventive) measure against many infectious diseases has generated interest in the mechanisms by which immunity can be conferred as well as interest in the development of vaccines

Box 1-2

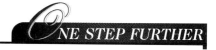

Hepatitis B Vaccine

The first vaccine against hepatitis B virus (HBV) was approved in the USA and made available as a world-wide prophylactic application in 1982. The vaccine consisted of a purified suspension of inactivated surface hepatitis B antigen (HBsAg) particles obtained from plasma of chronic carriers of HBsAg.

A more recent development in the formulation of the HBV vaccine is the use of recombinant HBV antigen, produced by recombinant DNA technology. Use of this type of vaccine is now a standard practice for pre- and post-exposure prophylaxis of medical workers, hemodialysis patients, patients requiring on-going transfusion therapy (hemophilia, sickle cell anemia, and aplastic anemia patients), homosexually active men, intravenous drug users, individuals in contact with HBV carriers (household and sexual), and international travelers.

Indications for Vaccination

PRE-EXPOSURE VACCINATION

Various health care professionals, such as medical, dental, and laboratory personnel, are at risk of contracting hepatitis B virus (HBV). Individuals who are exposed or have a potential for exposure to blood-borne pathogens by the nature of their occupation are referred to as "high-risk" personnel. Under the Occupational Safety and Health Administration (OSHA) regulations (see Chapter 9), these individuals are encouraged to accept vaccination against HBV infection as a pre-exposure prophylactic (preventive) measure.

Administration of a recombinant vaccine, consisting of the hepatitis B surface antigen (HBsAg) protein, has been proven to be non-infective and yet an effective means of inducing active specific immunity. Protective antibodies in response to HBsAg appear in more than 90% of healthy individuals when the vaccine is administered in three intramuscular doses: two doses 1 month apart and one dose 6 months later (boosters).

AFTER ACCIDENTAL EXPOSURE

Recombinant HBV vaccine is administered within a 24-hour period of exposure and 1 month later to induce an immune response.

In order to provide a quick prophylactic measure against HBV, a hepatitis B immunoglobulin (HBIg) containing preformed antibodies against HBsAg and a standard immunoglobulin (Ig) from immunized individuals may also be administered at the time of vaccination. The standard Ig preparation, however, is a less effective measure than HBIg because of the lower concentration of available specific antibodies against HBV.

FOR PERINATAL EXPOSURE

An infant born to a mother who tests positive for HBsAg at delivery is treated in the same way as someone after an accidental exposure.

Laboratory Testing

PRE- AND POST-VACCINATION SCREENING

Immune status (i.e., existence of previous exposure to HBV) must be established before administration of a vaccine. This may be accomplished by testing for presence of specific antibodies to HBV antigen by currently available techniques (see Chapter 13). Presence of antibodies to HBc (core) and to HBs (surface) antigens confirms the existence of a prior exposure to HBV that has occurred through an actual infection. Vaccine is not administered in such situations.

However, if no specific antibodies to HBV are detected, the individual is encouraged to receive a vaccination. Testing for the presence of HBV antibodies should be performed again after vaccination. If immunity has been conferred, HBs antibodies will be present, but HBc antibodies will be absent. A state of active immunity may be induced by (1) an actual infection with a microbe or (2) administration of a vaccine.

---

against a variety of bacterial and viral infective agents, such as hepatitis B virus (see One Step Further Box 1-2) and the human immunodeficiency virus (HIV).

Because each infectious agent is capable of producing a different specific immune response according to its infectivity, a vaccine must be designed in such a way as to elicit the desired immune response necessary to confer long-

lasting immunity against the infectious agent. The elements that are essential in vaccine development are:

- *Design of the vaccine*
- *Ability of vaccine to stimulate "memory" cells*
- *Infectivity of the microbe or virus*

vaccine design. Several types of vaccine formulations or designs as well as a variety of stimulating agents have been used in ongoing research in the area of vaccine development to confer specific immunity against an infectious agent or its specific epitopes (antigenic determinants). A summary of these research efforts is presented in One Step Further Box 1-3.

immunologic memory. Immunologic "memory" is responsible for the long-lasting immunity that is conferred by vaccination and is attributed to T and B "memory cells."

mechanism. During a primary immune response to a stimulating antigen, certain T and B lymphocytes do not develop into effector cells that participate in the resolution of an infection but instead become "memory" cells.

Upon subsequent stimulation with the same antigenic molecule, a secondary immune response is triggered (see Figure 1-14), resulting in differentiation of the existing "memory" cells into effector cells, capable of secreting soluble effector molecules (e.g., antibodies and cytokines), which are responsible for a more rapid resolution of an infection (removal of antigenic stimulus).

infectivity of microorganisms. There are two basic patterns of microbial infectivity that must be considered before formulating an effective vaccine. These are the **intracellular** and **extracellular infectivity** by intracellular and extracellular microorganisms, respectively (see Chapter 2). Each type of infectivity is a function of the organism's characteristics that determines its accessibility to the immune system and the type of an immune response that will be effective in eliminating the infectious antigen.

In *extracellular infections* (e.g., bacterial), a *humoral immune response* is triggered, which results in the production of antigen-specific antibodies that will eliminate the infectious bacterial antigen (see Figure 1-7).

Intracellular infections (e.g., viral) trigger a *cell-mediated immune response,* which mainly consists of production of cytotoxic T cells (see Figure 1-10) that eliminate (lyse) antigen-containing cells.

IMMUNOLOGIC TOLERANCE

The immune system has the potential for specifically recognizing and responding to an almost limitless number of antigens, including self-antigens. The antigen recognition is in the con-

text of the self major histocompatibility complex (MHC), which indicates that the immune system (T lymphocytes) has the ability to discriminate between self and non-self (foreign) antigens. It does so by reacting to foreign antigens in the form of an immune response and tolerating self-antigens (self-tolerance), thus preventing autoimmune reactions (see autoimmunity discussion in Chapter 7).

As the immune system encounters an antigen, one of two events may occur in response to self or to a particular non-self (foreign) antigen (see Figure 1-1):

- *Immune response*
- *Immunologic tolerance*

Tolerance to self-antigens is *naturally acquired.* However, it is also possible to *artificially induce* tolerance against a particular foreign antigen by a variety of mechanisms. As research in this area continues, artificially induced tolerance may become an important tool in reducing rejection of foreign tissue (grafts) by the host (see Chapter 6) and preventing hyperactivity of the immune system (e.g., autoimmunity and allergic reactions discussed in Chapter 7).

Several mechanisms responsible for producing natural and artificial tolerance to self or foreign antigens have been proposed and are presented in Table 1-6.

Typically, tolerance to a specific antigen is maintained for as long as that stimulating antigen persists. As the antigen concentration diminishes below a certain level, the responsiveness returns. In tolerance to self-antigens, resulting from a clonal deletion or anergy (see discussion following), the induced tolerance lasts only until the new lymphocytes are generated.

TOLERANCE TO SELF-ANTIGENS

Tolerance to self-antigens (recognition of self vs. non-self) is one of the most important features of the immune system because it prevents an immune response against the body's self-antigens and the development of autoimmunity.

Self-tolerance is an acquired characteristic of the immune system by which self-reactive lymphocytes (immature lymphocyte clones specific for self-antigens) are destroyed (deleted) or blocked from maturing or becoming activated as they encounter a self-antigen in the primary

Box 1-3

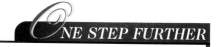

Vaccine Design

Several types of vaccine designs (formulations) and various stimulating agents are a focus of an ongoing research in the area of vaccine development for the purpose of conferring specific immunity (resistance) against an infectious agent or, more specifically, against its antigenic determinants (epitopes). Currently available vaccine formulations (designs) used as prophylactic measures and those still in a research phase of development are:

- *Attenuated vaccines*
- *Synthetic antigen vaccines*
- *Live viral vectors*
- *Subunit vaccines*
- *"Naked" DNA*

Attenuated Vaccines

Attenuated (weakened) vaccines were the first vaccines to be developed (Louis Lister). This type of vaccine is used even now to confer specific immunity and includes *Mycobacterium tuberculosis bacilli*, Calmette-Guerin (BCG), mutants of *Salmonella typhi*, and an inactivated *Bordetella pertussis* against whooping cough.

Many of these vaccines, however, confer only a short-lived and limited protection. More recently, the use of live attenuated viral vaccines (from long-term cell cultures) has proven to be a more effective and longer-lasting means of conferring protection against such infectious diseases as polio and measles.

Synthetic Antigen Vaccines

Synthetic antigen vaccines, which consist of synthetic peptides corresponding to an antigenic determinant on a particular infectious organism, have been made available as an outcome of such recent advances in biotechnology as (1) identification of sequences of bacterial antigenic proteins, (2) availability of recombinant DNA technology for production of large quantities of proteins (peptides) that are necessary for formulating a vaccine, and (3) identification of various antigenic determinants (epitopes).

This type of vaccine is used to confer protection against such infectious diseases as the hepatitis B virus and herpes simplex.

Live Viral Vectors

This vaccine design uses a live recombinant viral vector (carrier). The procedure is a relatively novel and technically difficult approach to vaccine design and involves insertion of a selected gene (DNA), which codes for the desired microbial or viral antigen, into a non-pathogenic virus (viral genetic material) by a process of recombination. The resulting altered virus is then used as an antigen to induce in the host (1) neutralizing antibodies (humoral immune response) and (2) specific cytotoxic T lymphocytes (cell-mediated immune response).

These live viral vaccines represent the newest approach to production of vaccines, particularly against the human immunodeficiency virus (HIV).

Recombinant vaccinia viruses, such as hepatitis B surface antigen and herpes simplex virus proteins, are also currently being investigated in this category of vaccines.

Subunit Vaccines

These are a new generation of vaccines that consist of specific, defined regions of a pathogen, which are capable of inducing a protective immune response. The subunit vaccines, also known as *purified antigen vaccines,* use highly purified proteins or synthetic peptides representing an immunologically important region of these proteins.

Recent research in subunit vaccine development has focused on the method of vaccine delivery for viral diseases, using liposome technology. Artificial phospholipid vesicles (membranes), known as *liposomes,* are prepared and used for encapsulating various proteins and peptides for presentation to evoke an immune response in the host.

Among the available subunit vaccine preparations are (1) diphtheria or tetanus toxin (toxoid), which has effectively controlled both of these diseases, (2) bacterial polysaccharide antigens against *Hemophilus influenzae* and pneumococcal infections, which, although of short duration, have proven to be effective in high-risk situations, and (3) purified hepatitis B surface antigen (HBsAg) against the hepatitis B virus.

"Naked" DNA

As a vaccine vector, "naked" DNA is the most novel approach to research in vaccine design. It is hoped that this vaccine formulation will overcome the barrier of HIV-1 diversity (i.e., persistent viral replication and high mutation rate) that has until now prevented the development of a successful prophylactic vaccine against HIV-1 infection. The proposed use of "naked" DNA is to inoculate it directly into muscle tissue, where the DNA can be delivered to the nucleus of the cells and where it will direct the expression of the vaccine antigens. The intracellular expression would produce both the antibody and cytotoxic T lymphocyte (CTL) responses, similar to responses observed in live recombinant viral vectors.

Table 1-6	INDUCTION OF NATURAL AND ARTIFICIAL TOLERANCE
Mechanism	Description
Clonal deletion (self-reactive cells)	Prevents an immune response to self-antigens (self-tolerance)
Lack of MHC molecule	Precludes binding and presentation of certain antigens (MHC-restricted antigen recognition)
Clonal abortion	Prevents cell maturation
Block in cytokine signals	Interrupts immune response
High dose of administered antigen	Favors tolerance (artificially induced tolerance)
Oral or intravenous administered antigen	Lowers immune response
Antigen without adjuvant	May be non-immunogenic
Clonal exhaustion	Result of repeated antigenic stimuli

lymphoid organs. Only immature lymphocyte clones lacking specificity for self-antigens are selected to mature and have the ability to respond to any foreign antigen which they encounter. These T and B lymphocytes will not respond to self-antigens, thus exhibiting tolerance to self (see Figure 1-16), which is discussed following.

T Lymphocyte Tolerance to Self-Antigens

During maturation in the thymus, T cells acquire antigen receptors (T cell receptors [TCR]) for recognition of a variety of antigenic molecules. T cells are also "educated" in the thymus to respond to antigens only in the context of self MHC molecules that are encoded by the MHC genes (MHC-restricted antigen recognition, see Chapter 3).

As the T cells mature and proliferate in the thymus, many of the self-reactive T cells, instead of developing to maturity, are destroyed by a process known as **clonal deletion** or **negative selection.** Only those T cells expressing antigen receptors (TCRs) that are capable of recognizing antigenic peptides bound to self MHC molecule will be selected to mature **(positive selection)** (see Figure 1-16).

B Lymphocyte Tolerance to Self-Antigens

The most obvious explanation for non-reactivity of B cells against self-antigens is the *lack of T cell help* (CD4+ lymphocytes), which is necessary for the production of antibodies during a humoral immune response.

B cells may also be made tolerant to self-antigens during their maturation in the bone marrow, where the immature B cells (bearing only IgM antigen receptors) interact with a self-

antigen and are eliminated by **clonal abortion.** Alternatively, B cells may be inactivated or made unresponsive to an antigenic stimulation, creating a **state of anergy** (unresponsiveness).

Any B cells that do not encounter a self-antigen will develop to maturity, acquire IgM and IgD antigen receptors, and enter secondary lymphoid tissue where they may encounter a foreign antigen and respond (see Figure 1-16).

TOLERANCE GENERATED DURING AN IMMUNE RESPONSE

There are several mechanisms that induce a state of immune unresponsiveness (tolerance) following an encounter with an antigenic stimulus.

clonal exhaustion. Lymphocyte depletion occurs mainly during a vigorous immune response and repeated antigenic stimulation, so that a subsequent antigenic stimulus may be met with unresponsiveness.

development of anti-idiotypic antibodies. Antibodies formed against an antibody-combining site (serving as an antigen) may physically block the site, thereby causing unresponsiveness (see Chapter 5).

feedback inhibition of immune response. Certain molecules generated during an immune response may also contribute to tolerance by inhibiting lymphocyte activation and effector functions through a mechanism not yet fully understood. These molecules include antibodies, suppressor T lymphocytes (see following), cytokines, and anti-idiotypic antibodies.

suppressor T cells. Characterization of "suppressor" T cells is a focus of current research. Although "suppressor" cells were originally considered to be CD8+ cells, some researchers now believe that they may not represent a unique cell population (CD8+) but be lymphocytes that inhibit immune response by different mechanisms, such as inhibitory cytokine activity.

ARTIFICIALLY INDUCED TOLERANCE

It has been shown that certain forms of protein antigens are capable of inhibiting specific immune response (humoral and cell mediated) by inducing tolerance in peripheral helper T cells (CD4+ cells), which are required for both responses.

Following are several examples of artificial induction of tolerance to foreign antigens, such as transplanted tissue and allogeneic (genetically different) cells, in both neonatal (newborn) and adult hosts:

- Administration of anti-lymphocyte monoclonal antibodies (e.g., anti-lymphocyte globulin, antibodies against CD4+ and CD8+ markers)
- Immunosuppressive regimens (e.g., total body irradiation drugs, cyclosporin A)
- Inoculation of allogeneic cells
- Administration of soluble protein antigens

Suggested Readings

Abbas AK, Lichtman AH, Pober JS: General properties of immune response (pp 3-16); Activation of T lymphocytes (pp 161-180). In *Cellular and molecular immunology,* Philadelphia, 2000, WB Saunders.

Ada G: Twenty years into the saga of MHC-restriction, *Immunol Cell Biol* 72:447, 1994.

Emini EO: Hurdles in the path to an HIV-1 vaccine, *Scient Am Sci Med* 2:38-47, 1995.

Roitt I, Male D, Brostoff J: *Immunology,* St Louis, 1998, Mosby.

Review Questions

INTRODUCTION TO THE IMMUNE SYSTEM

1. Specific immune response *differs* from non-specific (natural) immune response in that the specific immune response:
   a. involves phagocytic cells
   b. has "memory" and specificity
   c. is naturally occurring
   d. is less effective

2. Immunologic memory is a function of:
   a. T and B lymphocytes
   b. T lymphocytes only
   c. macrophages
   d. T lymphocytes and natural killer cells

3. The host's first defenses directed against any foreign antigen are a product of evolution (inborn) and do not require specific antigen recognition by the immune system. These are the:
   a. natural immune responses
   b. cell-mediated immune responses
   c. humoral immune responses
   d. acquired immune responses

4. The following are all components of the natural immune response (naturally present in all humans) *except* for:
   a. skin and mucous membranes
   b. phagocytes and natural killer cells
   c. tumor necrosis factor and complement
   d. helper and cytotoxic T lymphocytes

5. A mechanism that is a component of both the natural and acquired immune response:
   a. phagocytosis
   b. inflammation
   c. endocytosis
   d. cell differentiation

6. Which of the complement activation products, known as *anaphylotoxins*, participate in inflammatory response by triggering mast cell degranulation?
   a. C3b and C5b
   b. C3a and C5a
   c. membrane attack complex
   d. C3a and C5b

7. Cells *not* involved in specific immune responses are:
   a. helper T cells
   b. cytotoxic T cells
   c. natural killer (NK) cells
   d. plasma cells

8-10. Match the major events that occur during a specific immune response with the appropriate descriptive statement:

   ____ activation phase
   ____ cognitive phase
   ____ effector phase

   a. cell-mediated cytotoxicity
   b. production of antibodies
   c. antigen recognition by T cells in context of MHC molecule
   d. T and B cell proliferation
   e. T and B cell differentiation
   f. resolution of infection
   g. activation of immune response

11-14. Match the following main characteristics of specific immune response with their descriptions:

   ____ specificity
   ____ self-regulation
   ____ diversity
   ____ memory

   a. responsible for secondary immune response
   b. ability to selectively respond to a particular antigen
   c. ability to respond to a variety of antigenic molecules
   d. abnormality leads to autoimmunity

15-21. Match the appropriate immune response to each listed characteristic:

   a. humoral immune response
   b. cell-mediated immune response

   ____ antibodies are effector molecules
   ____ cytotoxic T cells cause lysis of antigen-bearing cells
   ____ response is to extracellular antigens
   ____ phagocytes present antigens for recognition
   ____ antigen recognition is class I MHC–restricted
   ____ helper T cell (CD4+) recognizes antigens
   ____ requires assistance from helper T lymphocyte

22. Which of the following phrases describes primary function of the humoral immune response?
    a. graft rejection
    b. resistance to bacterial infections
    c. resistance to viral and fungal infections
    d. tumor immunity

23. Immunoglobulins are secreted by:
    a. neutrophils
    b. macrophages
    c. T lymphocytes
    d. plasma cells

24. Which cells function as effector cells in a cell-mediated immune response?
    a. macrophages
    b. natural killer (NK) cells
    c. T cells
    d. B cells

25. An altered or virally infected cell, against which a cytotoxic (cytolytic) cell-mediated immune response is directed, is known as:
    a. cytotoxic T cell
    b. opsonized cell
    c. target cell
    d. memory cell

26. All the following statements define the role of helper T cells in an immune response *except:*
    a. are antigen-presenting cells
    b. activate B cells and cytotoxic T cells
    c. recognize antigens in context of class II MHC molecule
    d. need cytokines from macrophages for activation

27. The complex involved in recognition of self vs. non-self is:
    a. antigen bound to an antigen-presenting cell (APC)
    b. antigen receptor (TCR) on a macrophage
    c. major histocompatibility complex (MHC)
    d. surface immunoglobulin (sIg)–antigen complex

28. Class II MHC molecule is present on the surface of which of the following cells of the immune system?
    a. B lymphocytes
    b. mononuclear phagocytes
    c. cytotoxic T lymphocytes (CD8+)
    d. helper T lymphocytes (CD4+)

29. Class I MHC molecules are found on which cell type(s)?
    a. tumor cells
    b. cytotoxic T lymphocytes (CTLs)
    c. neutrophils
    d. all of the above

30. Class I MHC molecule is required for antigen recognition by which of the following cells?
    a. cytotoxic T cells (CD8+)
    b. helper T cells (CD4+)
    c. natural killer (NK) cells
    d. B cells

31. Which of the following are soluble mediators of an immune response released during T cell activation?
    a. complement
    b. thymosin
    c. immunoglobulins (Igs)
    d. cytokines

32. Which specific receptors located on the surface of a T cell are responsible for antigen recognition?
    a. surface immunoglobulins (sIg)
    b. major histocompatibility complex (MHC-peptide complex)
    c. antigen receptor (TCR/CD3) in association with CD8 or CD4 molecules
    d. all of the above

33-40. Match the specific cell type with following key features associated with antigen recognition:

    a. CD4+ T lymphocytes
    b. CD8+ T lymphocytes
    c. B lymphocytes

    ____ express surface immunoglobulins (sIgs)
    ____ initiate cell-mediated immune response
    ____ involved in class I–restricted antigen recognition
    ____ show no MHC restriction in antigen recognition
    ____ bind with free antigen molecules
    ____ recognize class II MHC-peptide complex on an antigen-presenting cell
    ____ recognize MHC-bound antigen on surface of an abnormal (tumor) or infected cell
    ____ initiate humoral immune response

41. Cells that assist B cells in responding to antigenic molecules are:
    a. cytotoxic T cells (CD8+)
    b. helper T cells (CD4+)
    c. mononuclear phagocytes
    d. natural killer (NK) cells

42. Production of antigen-specific antibodies during a humoral immune response is triggered by:
    a. extracellular organisms
    b. exogenous antigens
    c. bacterial antigens
    d. all of the above

43. In a secondary immune response, the cells responsible for promoting a stronger and faster reaction to an antigenic stimulus are:
    a. resting T cells
    b. resting B cells
    c. memory T and B cells
    d. all of the above

44. All the following mediators are involved in tissue injury at the site of inflammation *except:*
    a. vasoactive amines
    b. prostaglandins
    c. histamines
    d. cytokines

45. All of the following terms represent a type of inflammation *except:*
    a. antibody mediated
    b. immune complex mediated
    c. T cell mediated
    d. complement mediated

46. Laboratory evaluation of inflammation includes detection of *specific* indicators of inflammation. Select all that apply:
    a. C-reactive protein (CRP) concentration in serum
    b. plasma fibrinogen level
    c. interleukin 6 (Il-6)
    d. erythrocyte sedimentation rate

47-52. Match the following cell markers with the appropriate cell type (each cell type may be used more than once):

    ____ CD4   a. helper T cell
    ____ CD8   b. B cell
    ____ class II MHC   c. cytotoxic T cell
    ____ class I MHC
    ____ TCR/CD3   d. macrophages
    ____ sIg

53. The primary regulation of an immune response is inhibition (shutting-off) of the responses through the following mechanisms. Select all that apply:
    a. removal of the stimulating antigen from the host
    b. recognition of self and non-self antigens (MHC linked)
    c. genetic control (MHC gene products) ensuring that response is only to foreign molecule
    d. removal of self-reactive cells by clonal deletion

CONFERRING SPECIFIC IMMUNITY

54. Specific immunity may be conferred on an individual either passively or actively. Select all statements that are *true*:
    a. active immunity is induced by an actual infection or vaccination with a particular antigen
    b. active immunity is a result of a humoral or cell-mediated immune response to a particular antigen
    c. passive immunity is short lived because there is no induction of "memory" cells
    d. passive immunity confers specific immunity through administration of preformed cells or antibodies (from an immunized individual)

55. Health care personnel, such as clinical laboratory employees, are at risk of contracting hepatitis B virus (HBV). Such individuals should receive the HBV vaccine:
    a. prior to exposure to HBV infection
    b. as a prophylactic measure
    c. within a 24-hour period of an accidental exposure
    d. all of the above

56. The following HBV vaccine formulation is now used as a standard practice:
    a. recombinant HBV (HBsAg protein) vaccine produced by DNA technology (synthetic antigen vaccine)
    b. inactivated surface hepatitis B antigen (HBsAg) particles from chronic carriers of HBsAg (attenuated vaccine)
    c. live genetically altered recombinant virus (live recombinant viral vectors)
    d. "naked" DNA as a vaccine vector

IMMUNOLOGIC TOLERANCE

57. Select the term that best describes tolerance:
    a. regulation
    b. immunocompetence
    c. unresponsiveness
    d. immunodeficiency

58. Tolerance to self-antigens is one of the most important features of the immune system in that it prevents occurrence of all of the following *except*:
    a. immunodeficiency
    b. specific immune response
    c. overactivity of the immune system
    d. autoimmunity

59. Immunosuppressive regimens (e.g., total body irradiation, drugs) are an example of what type of artificially induced tolerance?
    a. self-tolerance in newborns
    b. T cell tolerance during cell maturation
    c. tolerance to foreign antigens
    d. tolerance to self-antigens

60. T cell tolerance to self-antigens is established by elimination of clones of T cells (before maturation in the thymus) that are reactive to self-antigens. This process of eliminating T cell clones is known as:
   a. T cell "education" to respond to antigens only in context of self-MHC
   b. clonal deletion
   c. negative selection
   d. all of the above

61. Positive selection describes a process by which only certain T cells that recognize antigenic peptides bound to self-MHC are selected to mature. This selection is based on acquiring which type of T cell receptors?
   a. CD3
   b. surface immunoglobulin (sIg)
   c. antigen receptors (TCR)
   d. major histocompatibility complex (MHC)

62. State of tolerance, resulting from an immune response, may be established by the following mechanism(s):
   a. clonal exhaustion
   b. feedback inhibition of immune response
   c. "suppressor" T cells activity
   d. all of the above

CHAPTER 2

Stimulators of Immune Response

Learning Objectives

Upon completion of Chapter 2, the student will be prepared to:

TERMINOLOGY

- Define the following terms: *antigen, hapten, immunogenic molecule, adjuvant, epitope, specificity, non-self molecule.*
- State the main characteristic that differentiates an antigen from an immunogen.

TYPES OF ANTIGENS

- State two main functions of histocompatibility antigens (MHC molecules).
- Define class I and class II MHC molecules.
- Name two types of tumor markers (antigens), stating their general classification, site of origination, use in clinical diagnosis.
- Discuss the basic concept (principle) involved in detection of tumor antigens.
- Classify the following tumor markers (antigens) according to their site of origination: (PSA), (hCT), (sIg), CD 10 (CALLA), (CEA).

ANTIGEN CLASSIFICATION ACCORDING TO SITE OF INFECTIVITY

- Differentiate between extracellular and intracellular antigens in terms of the type of: T lymphocytes that recognize the antigen, immune response that is induced by each class of antigen, MHC-restriction for each antigen, effector cells or molecules that are generated during an immune response.
- Describe recognition of antigenic peptides in terms of the type of T cell and its receptors and the MHC molecule involved.

FACTORS DETERMINING IMMUNOGENICITY

- Describe five properties of an antigenic molecule that define it as immunogenic.

SITES OF ANTIGEN ELIMINATION BY HOST

- Name three sites where elimination of foreign antigens occurs during an immune response.

DETECTION OF ANTIGENS IN HOST

- Name two laboratory procedures used to detect antigens in plasma and in cells.

Key Terms

antigen - Molecule that is recognized by the immune system as foreign. Capable of inducing an immune response and/or binding with a specific antibody.

epitope (antigenic determinant) - Smallest antigenic site on an antigen that is capable of combining with a specific complementary antibody (forming antigen/antibody complex) or with a surface immunoglobulin (antibody) on a B cell. When recognized by T cells (CD4+ and CD8+) as foreign, it can trigger an immune response.

cell-mediated immune response - Specific immune response to an antigen-altered cell (mainly viral) that is recognized by the immune system as foreign and is destroyed by a mechanism known as *cell-mediated immunity (cytotoxicity).*

humoral immune response - Response of the immune system, mainly to extracellular microorganisms (e.g., bacteria), that results in production of specific antibodies directed against the stimulating antigen.

immunogen (immunogenicity) - Antigen that is capable of inducing (triggering) an immune response.

major histocompatibility complex (MHC) - MHC molecules are products of the MHC genes. They are expressed on the surface of T cells of the immune system and are categorized as class I and class II MHC molecules. They participate in antigen recognition and distinguish self from non-self (foreign) antigens.

malignant - Refers to "transformed" (e.g., malignant tumors) cells that have lost the ability to regulate their cell cycle.

specificity - Characteristic of the acquired (specific) immune system, which refers to the ability of the T cells (T cell receptors on CD8+ and CD4+ T cells) to recognize only a particular antigenic determinant (epitope). Each T cell shows specificity for one epitope. The term is also used to describe affinity of antibody molecules for the specific antigen (epitope) that

40   PART I   FUNDAMENTAL CONCEPTS IN IMMUNOLOGY

induced their production. An antibody will only bind (specifically) with its complementary antigen. This reaction is referred to as *antigen specific*.

tumor - Structurally or functionally abnormal cell growth.

tumor marker - Also referred to as *tumor antigen*. Is expressed on the surface of a specific tumor cell, thought to be an expression of a mutated or viral gene or an abnormal expression of a normal gene. Tumor markers may be shed into plasma.

Our body is continuously exposed to a variety of infectious agents within our environment, such as bacteria, viruses, fungi, and other parasites, that are capable of accessing our internal environment to cause an infection if not contained.

Fortunately, as we have seen in Chapter 1, the body is equipped with a powerful defense mechanism that is capable (in most instances) of protecting itself from these invaders. This mechanism is known as the **immune response.** The immune response persists for as long as antigenic stimulation exists and stops only when the stimulus is removed.

In this context, antigens function as initiators and powerful regulators of the immune response.

Most antigens enter the body through the skin and mucosal epithelial cells of the gastrointestinal and the respiratory tract. Some antigens are transported from these sites of entry to the regional lymphoid organs mainly by the lymphatic system and may then enter the circulatory system. Antigens remaining at the site of entry become the target for the effectors of an immune response because the body defends itself against these antigens (see discussion of immune response in Chapter 1).

TERMINOLOGY

Infectious agents that invade the host are most commonly referred to as **antigens** but may also be designated as *immunogens, antigenic molecules or stimuli, stimulating agents, foreign configurations or substances, foreign agents, foreign molecules, allergens, pathogens,* or *pathogenic or infectious organisms,* depending on the role that they play in a particular situation.

All the previous designations refer to a foreign antigen that may be defined as *any foreign molecule that is specifically recognized by the host's immune system as foreign (non-self) and is capable of triggering an immune response.* Certain antigens can also specifically bind to an antibody molecule.

The type of immune response that occurs in response to an antigenic stimulus depends on several factors (see discussion following). In general, antibodies are produced in response to extracellular antigens (bacteria) and are the effectors of humoral immune response, whereas cytotoxic T cells and other effectors are a product of cell-mediated immune responses that are induced by intracellular antigens (viruses).

Although the term *antigen* and *immunogen* are often used interchangeably, an antigen that is capable of producing an immune response is most appropriately referred to as an **immunogen** and that term is used, for example, when describing immunization (vaccination) procedure. The term **antigen,** properly used, is applied to a molecule that is only capable of binding to an antibody but that does not induce an immune response. Therefore *not all antigens are immunogens, but all immunogens are considered antigens.*

For example, the term *antigen* is most commonly used in clinical laboratory practice, particularly when referring to an antigen binding with an antibody (antigen/antibody reaction). Other terms (e.g., *allergen*) may be used when describing the immune response (allergic reaction) that will occur in response to this type of antigenic stimulation.

TYPES OF ANTIGENS

Virtually every biologic molecule, such as sugars, lipids, hormones, intermediary metabolites, and macromolecules (e.g., phospholipids, nucleic acids, complex carbohydrates, and proteins), may function as an antigen or possess the potential for being antigenic.

The portion of an antigen that is recognized by the T and B lymphocytes and also binds to

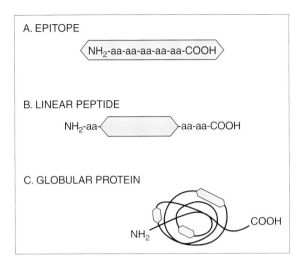

A. EPITOPE

NH₂-aa-aa-aa-aa-aa-COOH

B. LINEAR PEPTIDE

NH₂-aa-‹___›-aa-aa-COOH

C. GLOBULAR PROTEIN

COOH

NH₂

FIGURE **2-1** **Illustration of an Epitope (Antigenic Determinant).** **A,** An epitope consisting of 5 amino acid (aa) residues with a carboxyl (COOH) and amine (NH₂) ends. **B,** A peptide containing one epitope. **C,** Three epitopes on a globular protein molecule. Two (outside) epitopes are accessible.

the specific antibodies is known as an **antigenic determinant** or an **epitope,** the latter being a newer designation. An epitope, which serves as the smallest biochemical unit of an antigen that is capable of eliciting an immune response (Figure 2-1), consists of 4 to 6 amino acids (aa). The size and structure of an epitope varies according to the type of antigen.

It is now possible to determine the presence of multiple epitopes on an antigen by using specific antibodies (as reagents) that are directed against an epitope. However, because of stearic hinderance (position or configuration of a molecule), not all epitopes are readily accessible to the antibodies (see Figure 2-1) and, therefore, will not bind with the antibody. This may limit the detection of all existing epitopes on a molecule. The same principle governs immunogenicity in that not all epitopes are available to the immune system for recognition and a subsequent immune response.

In antigen recognition by the immune system, the antigenic epitopes are recognized by antigen-specific T cell receptors (TCRs), located on the surface of T and B cells, which are genetically determined and develop without any antigenic stimulation. This ensures that lymphocytes are available for recognition and response to foreign antigens even in an unim-

munized individual (see antigen recognition in Chapter 3).

T lymphocytes generally are selected and stimulated by an antigen to respond. The newly generated antigen-specific lymphocyte clones (see *clonal selection* discussed in Chapter 3) play a vital role in the immune response that is directed against the stimulating antigen (see discussion of immune responses, Chapter 1).

Although in the past, antigens were classified as **thymic-dependent antigens** (requiring T cells for induction of an immune response) or **thymic-independent antigens** (stimulating antibody production, mainly IgM, without T cell interaction), it is now believed that even the thymic-independent antigens require participation of helper T cells.

PROTEIN ANTIGENS

The protein component of certain bacteria and most viruses induce strong *humoral* and *cell-mediated responses* and produce a long-lasting immunologic memory. Recognition of protein antigens by T lymphocytes is MHC restricted (see Chapter 3 and the discussion following).

Peptides

Peptides consist of segments of amino acids, which are derived from protein antigens that have been processed (degraded) by antigen-presenting cells. These peptides bind to class I or class II MHC molecules, depending on the type of antigenic stimulation (described following) before recognition by the immune system (i.e., T lymphocytes):

- *Peptides bound to class I MHC molecules* are mainly peptides derived from intracellular proteins and organisms (viruses) and are displayed on the surface of the cell for recognition by antigen-specific T cell receptors (TCR), located on the CD8+ cytotoxic T lymphocytes (CTLs). Following antigen recognition as foreign, a specific immune response *(cell mediated)* is triggered against the displayed intracellular organisms (mostly viruses) and any abnormal cells, resulting in cytolysis (cell lysis) of the abnormal (antigen-altered) cell produced by the activated CTL.
- *Peptides bound to class II MHC molecules* are peptides derived from extracellular

organisms (mainly bacteria) that are processed by an antigen-presenting cell (APC). They are displayed on the surface of antigen-presenting cells (APCs) in association with the class II MHC molecules. These MHC-bound peptides are recognized by specific antigen receptors (TCRs) on CD4+ T lymphocytes (helper T cells). Specific antigen recognition is required for the activation of *humoral* and *cell-mediated immune responses,* which result in the production of antigen-specific antibodies and appropriate cell-mediated effectors necessary to eliminate the stimulating antigen, respectively.

POLYSACCHARIDES AND LIPIDS

These antigenic molecules (e.g., capsular polysaccharide antigens) are not recognized by T cells and, therefore, are not capable of inducing cell-mediated immune response by stimulating MHC-restricted T cells. However, an induction of *T cell–independent humoral immune response* may occur with a production of mainly IgM antibodies, which provide only a short-lived immunity.

HAPTEN-CARRIER COMPLEX

Low molecular weight antigens, known as **haptens,** in order to be immunogenic, must first be attached to a larger molecule (macromolecule, usually a protein), which serves as a **carrier molecule:**

hapen + carrier→hapten/carrier complex
(immunogenic complex)

The resulting hapten-carrier complex serves as an immunogen for initiating *a humoral immune response* (see discussion of macromolecules and synthetic antigens following), which can be directed against the hapten, the carrier, or both components of the complex.

MACROMOLECULES

Large immunogenic molecules have the ability to initiate a *humoral immune response.* These macromolecules are larger than the antigen-binding region on an antibody molecule (discussed in Chapter 5) and possess multiple epi-topes, each of which may be bound to an antibody. Therefore binding of a macromolecule by an antibody occurs through these epitopes (specific sites) located on an antigenic molecule.

SYNTHETIC ANTIGENS

Synthetic antigens consist of chemically synthesized short peptides that correspond to the known amino acid sequence of a protein that is a part of an infectious organism. The synthesized peptides (haptens) can be linked to a "carrier" molecule and used as a synthetic antigen in vaccine formulations (see One Step Further Box 1-3). The expected immune response to the stimulating synthetic antigen is the production of specific antibodies (during humoral immune response), which, on subsequent exposure, specifically react with an equivalent (native) antigenic sequence on an infectious organism.

"Immunologic memory," resulting from an immunization with a synthetic antigen, relates to the carrier molecule of the hapten-carrier conjugate not to the specific antigenic peptide, thus limiting the use of these antigens. However, new approaches to the use of synthetic antigens are currently under investigation (e.g., bifunctional immunogen formulations) that may eliminate this limiting factor.

HISTOCOMPATIBILITY ANTIGENS

Human leukocyte antigens (HLA-A, HLA-B, HLA-C molecules), also referred to as *tissue antigens* (self-antigens) or *alloantigens* (genetically dissimilar antigens in the same species), are now known as *class I MHC antigens* (discussed in One Step Further Box 3-3 and Chapter 6).

Human major histocompatibility complex (MHC) is the current terminology used to identify the HLA gene region on a human chromosome. The HLA-A, -B, and -C gene products (tissue antigens) are now called **class I MHC molecules,** while the **class II MHC molecule** designation is equivalent to the HLA-DR, -DP, and -DQ gene products.

Of the various genes that comprise the human genome (a complete set of genes in an individual), MHC genes are the most polymorphic (many forms) genes. Their protein products (class I and II MHC molecules) can bind fragments of antigenic protein (peptides) to form MHC-peptide complexes that can be recognized by T lymphocytes of the immune system as foreign (non-self) or self.

HLA tissue antigens (class I MHC antigens), representing the MHC gene products, are expressed on the surface of a variety of human cells. These cell surface antigens reflect the specific genetic make-up of an individual, thus serving as *specific tissue markers* that can be identified by tissue typing (microcytotoxicity) tests. Panels of allosera (reagent antibodies against alloantigens) obtained from individuals previously immunized against these gene products, or monoclonal antibodies (see HLA phenotyping in Chapter 14), may be used as reagents in tissue typing.

Histocompatibility antigens (MHC molecules) are important in immunology in that they:

- Participate in recognition of self and non-self antigens
- Trigger rejection of incompatible tissue grafts (see discussion of antigen recognition in Chapter 1)
- Serve as specific tissue markers, thus reflecting a specific genetic make-up of an individual (see Chapter 6 and molecular fingerprinting, One Step Further Box 15-1)

THYMUS-INDEPENDENT ANTIGENS

Thymus-independent antigens (e.g., bacterial polysaccharides and some polymerized protein) seem to have the ability to stimulate B lymphocytes (humoral immune response) to produce antibodies (mainly IgM class with no memory) without any participation of the T lymphocytes.

Recent studies, however, indicate that even in these thymus-independent immune responses, some T cell help is involved.

TUMOR ANTIGENS

Although the immune system is able to limit the occurrence of tumors (to some extent) through such anti-tumor responses as surveillance and other effector mechanisms of the humoral and cell-mediated immune responses, it is clear that certain tumors evade the immune system and develop into malignant tumors.

It is believed that **malignant tumors** (neoplasms, carcinomas, cancers), consisting of a clone (mass) of abnormal cells, are derived from normal self-tissue by such malignant transformation as mutations in tumor suppressor genes, regulatory genes, or oncogenes. These transformations may result in a loss of mechanisms that control normal cells, causing unregulated proliferation of tumor or abnormal cell clones. As the abnormal cells proliferate, they may infiltrate adjacent tissue and spread to other parts of the body (metastasize) to establish secondary tumors.

The abnormal cell clones (tumor cells) show loss of their specific functions and biochemical characteristics as well as normal cellular morphology (appearance) and may express certain gene products (molecules) known as **tumor markers.**

These tumor markers (antigens) can be expressed on the surface of specific tumor cells and may be analyzed by immunophenotyping (see Chapter 14). Tumor markers may also be shed into blood, urine, or other body fluids, which can be analyzed for the presence of tumor marker in the form of biochemical substances.

Although many tumor cell surface markers have been identified, there are only few that have the ability to stimulate the immune system and are truly **tumor-specific antigens** (One Step Further Box 2-1 and Table 2-1).

Most tumor antigens expressed by a tumor cell are also expressed by different tumors arising from the same type of cell or from normal cells. Consequently, these tumor antigens or markers, known as **tumor-associated antigens (TAA)** (see Table 2-1 and One Step Further Box 2-1), are not recognized as foreign by the immune system and, therefore, do not induce an immune response against the antigen-bearing cells to eliminate these abnormal cells or stop their proliferation. However, TAAs are important in clinical or tumor immunology because their detection may support an already established diagnosis, monitor progression or regression, and establish prognosis for malignant tumors.

RED BLOOD CELL SURFACE ANTIGENS

The two most important constituents of a blood cell (erythrocyte) membrane are the glycophorin (integral) and spectrin (peripheral) membrane proteins.

The glycophorin (integral membrane protein) is the main red blood cell (RBC) glycoprotein, consisting of carbohydrate and protein

Box 2-1

Tumor Markers

Tumor markers are thought to be an expression of a mutated or viral gene or an abnormal expression of a normal gene.

The first tumor marker to be associated with a malignancy was an atypical protein detected in urine of some cancer patients by a physician named Sir Henry Bence-Jones (1847). This atypical protein, later named *Bence-Jones protein,* was found to consist of light chains of immunoglobulin G (IgG), which are secreted by transformed B lymphocytes and are detectable in serum and urine. It became a tumor marker for a B lymphocyte malignancy (multiple myeloma).

More recently (1960s), with the development of a variety of immunoassays, certain markers previously used as indicators of certain cancers (e.g., acid phosphatase indicator of prostate cancer, alkaline phosphatase marker for bone cancer, and serum and urine amylase indicator of pancreatic cancer) were replaced with other tumor markers identified by this new technology.

Currently the most widely used tumor markers in diagnosis and monitoring of malignant tumors are:
- **Tumor antigens or antigenic molecules** expressed on the surface of a specific tumor cell and identified by specific antibodies
- **Biochemical substances,** expressed by a tumor cell and shed into various body fluids such as blood and urine

Other tumor markers, showing a tremendous potential for serving as indicators of genetic alterations and as identifiers of tumor-causing genes and which have become the target of intensive research in tumor immunology, are the *molecular* and *gene tumor markers.*

Classification of Tumor Markers
Tumor markers are typically classified according to the site of their origination, although some references list tumor markers on the basis of their biochemical characteristics or their tumor specificity.

The following classification is based on the site of origination of the tumor markers:
- **Tumor-specific markers:** Expressed by tumor cells
- **Tumor-associated markers:** Expressed by certain normal host tissue or by various tumor cells originating from the same cell line
- **Tissue-specific tumor markers:** Expressed by a particular tissue

TUMOR-SPECIFIC MARKERS
Tumor-specific markers may develop through various molecular mechanisms, most direct of which is a transformation (structural change) of a normal cell into an abnormal or tumor cell, resulting in the production of a *new antigenic protein.*

Other mechanisms that have been proposed are genetic mutations that code for *altered protein structure* or cause an *inappropriate assembly of membrane proteins.*

Therefore tumor-specific markers, expressed on a surface of a particular tumor cell, may consist of:
- New antigenic protein
- Altered cellular protein
- Abnormal membrane structure antigens

There are only a few of these tumor-specific antigens (markers) that are unique to a particular tumor and that are detectable by antibodies produced in other species (see Table 2-1).

Example of tumor-specific markers are:
- *Tumor specific transplantation antigens:* Animal experiments show that these antigens are capable of stimulating a specific rejection of transplanted tumor. The rejection is mediated by tumor-specific cytotoxic T lymphocytes (CTLs), which function as effector cells for antitumor immunity (cell-mediated immunity).
- *Terminal deoxynucleotidyl transferase (TdT):* This DNA enzyme marker is used to diagnose a particular type of blood dyscrasia (abnormality), known as *acute lymphocytic leukemia (ALL),* and to differentiate it from acute myeloid leukemia. This clinical application of TdTf marker is possible because TdT-containing cells (lymphoblastic cells) are found in an increased number in the blood of patients with ALL but are not detected in patients with non-lymphocytic leukemias or in healthy individuals. Another application of the TdT marker in clinical diagnosis is in classification of non-Hodgkin's lymphoma.

TUMOR-ASSOCIATED ANTIGENS (TAAs)
Tumor-associated antigens are tumor markers that may be expressed as surface molecules by different tumors that originate from the same cell type. In fact, several different types of TAAs may be expressed by the same tumor. The TAAs may also appear on normal cells and some benign (non-malignant) tumor cells.

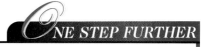

Box 2-1—cont'd

With the availability of monoclonal antibodies, generated in large quantities by hybridoma technology (see One Step Further Box 14-1), it is now possible to isolate and characterize various tumor-associated antigens. Because the expression of TAAs on tumor cells is higher than the expression of these markers on normal tissue, it is also now possible to differentiate between transformed (abnormal) and non-transformed (normal) cells.

In ongoing cancer research, TAAs have also been used as targets for anti-tumor antibodies that have been coupled (bound) to various molecules (e.g., radioisotopes, drugs, toxic substances) as a form of immunotherapy. Although this type of therapy seems promising, there are numerous difficulties that still need to be resolved.

The best characterized of the various tumor-associated antigens are the **oncofetal antigens.** These tumor markers are glycoproteins that are normally produced by developing (fetal) tissue during embryogenesis (development of the embryo) but are not present in an adult. Oncofetal antigens are expressed on tumor cells by some undefined mechanism and are shed into the serum of patients with certain cancers (see discussion following).

- *Alpha-fetoprotein (AFP):* AFP is an oncofetal antigen that is secreted in a high concentration (2 to 3 mg/mL, serum level) in fetal life. In adults, AFP is replaced by albumin and only an insignificant amount is detected in serum. However, elevated serum levels of AFP are detectable in liver cancer (hepatocellular carcinoma), germ cell tumor, and occasionally in gastric and pancreatic cancer. Therefore AFP can be used as an indicator (tumor marker) in such cancers. However, there are limitations in the use of AFP as a tumor marker because it is also associated with liver disease such as cirrhosis.
- *Carcinoembryonic antigen (CEA)* CEA is an oncofetal antigen, consisting of a large membrane glycoprotein that is also expressed (shed) into extracellular fluid (e.g., serum). Normally, during pregnancy (first two trimesters), high levels of CEA are found in the gastrointestinal tract, liver, and pancreas, with reduced levels also observed in the mucosa of the colon and the lactating breast. Increased serum levels of CEA are observed in association with carcinomas of the colon, lung, liver, pancreas, bladder, cervix, and prostate. CEA, therefore, is not specific

enough to be considered a marker for screening or diagnosing any particular tumor type. However, in cancer of the colon and in breast cancer, high CEA levels are present in patients with recurring tumors and metastasis. In this context, therefore, CEA may be used to monitor the recurrence of colon cancer, particularly after initial treatment. Recent research indicates that CEA functions as an adhesion molecule that binds one tumor cell to another and may be involved in tumor cell-to-cell interaction and in interaction between tissues in which the cells are located.

TISSUE-SPECIFIC TUMOR MARKERS

These tumor markers are antigens that are characteristic of a particular tissue type and may also be expressed by tumors that develop from that tissue. These antigens do not induce an immune response because they bear the same antigens (self) as normal tissue.

Tissue-specific antigens are clinically significant in that they may serve as targets in immunotherapy. Their identification may require the use of antibody probes, described following.

Examples of tissue-specific tumor antigens are:
- *CD10 marker:* This marker was previously known as *common acute lymphoblastic leukemia antigen (CALLA)*, which is a characteristic pre–B cell stage (immature B lymphocyte) surface tumor marker (known as *differential antigen*) for B cell lineage tumors. Mature B lymphocytes express surface immunoglobulins (sIgs). These differential antigens indicate a particular stage of normal cell development (differentiation), and, when found on tumors arising from a particular normal tissue, they do not stimulate an immune response against the cells that express them.
- *Prostate specific antigen* (PSA): This is a small glycoprotein molecule that can be detected in the serum of patients with prostatic cancer, inflammation, and prostatic hypertrophy (overgrowth of cells). It is specific for prostate tissue but not for cancer of the prostate, thus its usefulness is mainly limited to prognosis and monitoring of therapy in established cases of prostatic cancer. However, as a result of several studies, which indicate that PSA identifies a certain percentage of men with prostatic cancer, PSA may be useful in such screening programs. Elevated serum levels of PSA have been seen more frequently rather than an in-

Continued

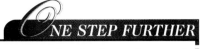

Box 2-1—cont'd

crease in acid phosphatase in prostatic cancer; thus, PSA is now used in a screening program that surpasses the use of the latter as a marker of prostatic cancer.

Detection of Tumor Markers

Tumor markers may be detected in tissues obtained from abnormal or new growth (neoplasia) and in certain body fluids (mainly serum). For example, carcinoembryonic antigen (CEA) may be detected in tumor tissue of the liver and in serum by various immunologic, biochemical, and molecular tech-

niques, (see discussion of testing for malignancy in Chapter 8).

Although tumor markers are an invaluable tool in cancer research, their use in clinical diagnosis is limited to prognosis and monitoring of tumors previously diagnosed by other methods. This is because (1) many markers are not specific for a particular tumor (occurring also in other malignancies or conditions), (2) the quantity present does not directly relate to the mass (size) of the tumor, and (3) many techniques used to detect tumor markers are not approved for clinical use.

---

components, that spans the entire membrane lipid bilayer and protrudes to the outer surface of the RBC membrane.

The majority of the membrane glycoproteins carry the RBC antigens, such as the blood group antigens. These antigens are capable of evoking an immune response during an incompatible blood transfusion.

ADJUVANTS

Adjuvants are substances that non-specifically *enhance* an immune response (humoral or cell mediated) by forming insoluble complexes, thus increasing the surface area of the antigen. They are usually introduced into the host together with an antigen and produce the enhancement by:

- Increasing the size of the antigenic molecule
- Prolonging the antigen retention
- Stimulating macrophages and/or lymphocytes

The most potent of a number of available adjuvants is Freund's complete adjuvant (CFA), which consists of killed mycobacteria in water-oil emulsion. In humans, the most commonly used adjuvant is a suspension of aluminum hydroxide (alum precipitate), on which an immunogen is adsorbed.

ANTIGEN CLASSIFICATION ACCORDING TO SITE OF INFECTIVITY

The immune system specifically responds to a foreign configuration in one of two ways, either

by *cell-mediated* or *humoral immune response,* depending on the site of microbial infectivity (Figure 2-2). These responses can be used to classify the antigenic molecule as an *extracellular* or *intracellular* antigen (Table 2-2).

EXTRACELLULAR ANTIGENS (EXOGENOUS)

In an *extracellular infection* (mainly bacterial), infectious organisms (and certain intracellular organisms as they migrate between cells) are directly accessible to the immune system for recognition and subsequent elimination. As the immune system responds **(humoral immune response)** to the stimulating antigen, specific antibodies (effector molecules) are produced with the capability of binding to and inactivating or eliminating the stimulating antigen.

INTRACELLULAR ANTIGENS (ENDOGENOUS)

In an *intracellular infection* (mainly viruses and certain intracellular bacteria and parasites), the organisms replicate within a cell, causing changes in the cell's characteristics. These altered infected cells (and tumor cells) are recognized by the immune system as abnormal or foreign and are eliminated together with the antigen, mainly by the cytotoxic T lymphocytes (effector cells)) generated during a **cell-mediated immune response.**

Natural killer cells (NK) and type I interferons (see Table 1-2), both a part of natural immunity, also participate in protecting the host against viral infection during its early stages.

Table 2-1 SELECTED TUMOR MARKERS	
Tumor Marker	Type of Tumor Detected
TUMOR-SPECIFIC MARKERS	
Cell Enzyme Markers	
TdT	Acute lymphocytic leuk
Cell Surface Markers	
CA 125	Ovarian cancer
CA 19-9*	Pancreatic cancer
TUMOR-ASSOCIATED MARKERS	
Serum Markers	
CEA	Adult malignant tissue (colorectal cancer)
$B_2 M$*	Multiple myeloma and inflammation (systemic lupus erythematosus, rheumatoid arthritis)
AFP	Liver cell carcinoma and testicular tumors
TAG-72*	Breast, stomach, colon, lung, and ovarian tissue
TISSUE-SPECIFIC MARKERS	
Cell Surface Markers	
CD 10 (CALLA)	B cell leukemia (lymphoblastic)
Surface immunoglobulins (sIgs)	B cell leukemia and lymphoma
IL-2 receptor*	T cell leukemia (virus associated)
Serum Markers	
Prostate specific antigen (PSA)	Prostatic cancer
Calcitonin (hCT)	Thyroid (medullary) cancer
GENE/CHROMOSOME MARKERS	
p53 gene (mutated)*	Colorectal tumors
Ph^1 chromosome	Chronic myelogenous leukemia

*Investigative use.

TdT, deoxynucleotidyl transferase (expressed by immature lymphocytes); *CA*, cancer antigen; *CEA*, carcinoembryonic antigen (expressed by normal fetal cells); B_2M, beta$_2$-microglobulin (expressed by normal nucleated cells); *AFP*, alpha-fetoprotein; *TAG*, tumor-associated antigen; *CD*, cluster of differentiation; *CALLA*, common acute lymphocytic leukemia antigen; *IL*, interleukin; Ph^1, Philadelphia.

FACTORS DETERMINING IMMUNOGENICITY

A key feature in the initiation of a specific immune response is the specific recognition of a foreign antigen (bound to MHC molecule, a product of MHC genes) by the T cells (helper and cytotoxic) through their surface antigen receptors (specific for each antigen), which triggers the events of an immune response.

Although the exact properties required for a molecule to be immunogenic (able to induce an immune response) are not fully understood, certain criteria have been defined and include the following.

HOST'S GENETIC COMPOSITION

The ability of the immune system to specifically recognize and respond to a foreign molecule depends on the host's inheritance of a specific set of major histocompatibility (MHC) genes. The MHC genes, originally described as immune response (Ir) genes and a HLA gene region (see discussion of histocompatibility antigens) code for class I and class II MHC molecules that are expressed on the surface of all nucleated and immunocompetent cells, respectively (see Chapter 3).

Antigens are recognized by the cytotoxic T lymphocytes (CD8+) and helper T lympho-

Table 2-2	DIFFERENTIAL CHARACTERISTICS OF INTRACELLULAR AND EXTRACELLULAR ANTIGENS	
Characteristics	Intracellular Antigens (Endogenous)	Extracellular Antigens (Exogenous)
Type of antigen	Virus or altered cell (processed antigens)	Bacteria (intact antigens)
Antigen-presenting cell (APC)	Altered (target) cell (virally infected or tumor cell)	Phagocytes (macrophages)
MHC restriction complex	Class I MHC–antigenic peptide	Class II MHC–antigen complex
Antigen recognition cell	Cytotoxic T lymphocyte (CD8+ cell)	Helper T Lymphocyte (CD4+ cell)
Antigen receptor	T cell receptor (TCR) on CD8+ cell	T cell receptor (TCR) on CD4+ cell
Effector cell	Cytotoxic T lymphocyte (CTL)	B lymphocyte (plasma cell)
Effector molecules	Cytotoxins	Antibodies (immunoglobulins)
Resolution (antigen removal)	Cell lysis (cytolysis)	Antigen-antibody complexes
Type of immune response	Cell mediated	Humoral

MHC, major histocompatibility complex; *CD,* cluster of differentiation; *Ag,* antigen; *CTL,* cytotoxic T lymphocyte; *TCR,* T cell receptor.

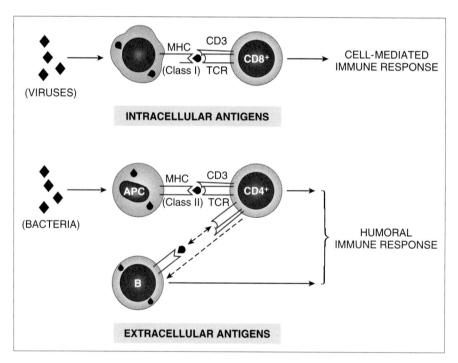

FIGURE **2-2**   **Representation of Intracellular and Extracellular Antigens in the Context of a Site of Infectivity (Intracellular or Extracellular).**   Context determines the type of recognition by the immune system (T lymphocytes) and the immune response that will be evoked (see also Chapter 4). *MHC,* major histocompatibility complex; *CD3,* receptor on T cell involved in recognition; *TCR,* T cell receptor specific for recognition of each antigen; *CD8+,* cytotoxic T cell; *APC,* antigen-presenting cell; *CD4+,* helper T cell.

cytes (*CD4+*) expressing antigen receptors on their surface, known as T cell receptors (TCR), which recognize the MHC-antigenic peptide complex on the antigen-presenting cell (APC). These TCRs are specific for each antigen that is recognized in the context of the MHC class I and II molecules (see One Step Further Box 3-3).

GENETIC DISSIMILARITY

An immunogenic molecule must be recognized as foreign (non-self) by the host's immune system (T lymphocytes, in the context of the MHC molecules).

ACCESSIBILITY

Epitopes (antigenic determinants) must be readily accessible to the immune system for recognition.

SIZE OF THE MOLECULE

Generally accepted minimal size of a molecule that is able to induce an immune response is 10,000 molecular weight. Smaller molecules, such as amino acids and monosaccharides, are not immunogenic. Other small molecules may be only weakly immunogenic. Molecules with larger molecular weight (greater than 100,000 macromolecules) are potent immunogens, most potent of which are the macromolecular proteins.

STRUCTURE OF THE MOLECULE

Although no definite structural characteristics have been established, the general rule is that the more complex the molecule, the greater is its immunogenicity. For example, synthetic polymers with repeating units of single amino acids are poor immunogens, whereas aromatic amino acids enhance immunogenicity of large protein molecules.

Small peptides (degraded proteins) must first be bound to a MHC molecule for recognition and response by the immune system. These small peptides cannot be recognized in a free state. This is not the case with the free unaltered antigens (not bound to MHC), such as bacteria, because these are recognized in a free state and are capable of inducing an immune response. This concept is discussed earlier under intracellular and extracellular antigens.

ANTIGEN DOSE

The optimal dose (amount of antigen) for immunogenicity depends on the type of antigen. Large doses or repeated administration of an antigen may produce a state of specific unresponsiveness, known as *immunologic tolerance* (T cells become tolerant). Large doses may also inhibit antibody production (specific B cells become tolerant).

SITES OF ANTIGEN ELIMINATION BY HOST

The immune system has the capability of recognizing a foreign molecule and directing its response against it, thereby eliminating the stimulating antigen through a variety of available mechanisms (natural and specific immune responses). The removal of antigens occurs during the **effector phase of a humoral or cell-mediated immune response** and is a primary function of the immune system (see Figures 1-2 and 1-6).

As the immune system encounters an antigen for the first time, a *primary immune response* is triggered. Upon subsequent encounter with the same antigen, a *secondary immune response* will occur. The secondary immune response is a more effective mechanism (see Figure 1-14). However, both the primary and secondary immune responses, initiated by the immune system, are effective mechanisms for eliminating the stimulating antigens.

For example, elimination of antigen occurs during a humoral immune response that produces specific antibodies (effector molecules) against the stimulating antigen. These antibodies are capable of binding with that antigen and forming immune complexes (antigen/antibody complex) that are then eliminated by the lymphatic system. This is an example of one of the most direct effector mechanisms studied. Alternatively, antibodies can bind to the stimulating antigen (opsonization), making it more susceptible to phagocytosis. Both mechanisms for removing antigenic material from the host are seen in the effector phase of the humoral immune response (see Figure 1-7).

The fate (elimination) of any immunogenic molecule that evades the natural immune response (first line of defense) is determined by its route of entry. The following are several available ways for elimination of antigens from the main sites of antigen entry.

BLOOD CIRCULATION

A foreign molecule is carried via blood to the **spleen,** *a principal site of immune response to blood-borne antigens,* where it is recognized as foreign by T cells of the immune system, thus stimulating a specific immune response. During the effector phase of the immune response, the stimulating antigenic molecule becomes the target for the effectors of the response (see Chapter 1, Figure 1-15) and is eliminated or inactivated.

SKIN

Local inflammatory response occurs as the antigen is recognized as foreign (see One Step Further Box 1-1 and Figure 1-5). The antigen is typically carried from this site of entry to the regional lymph nodes draining the affected area, where the T cells within the **lymph nodes** recognize it as foreign and where the main event of the immune response and antigen elimination occurs. Therefore, even though the response is initially local, it may eventually spread throughout the body.

GASTROINTESTINAL OR RESPIRATORY TRACT MUCOSA

Lymphoid tissue (e.g., Peyer's patches) located in the mucosa of the gastrointestinal or respiratory tract is capable of mounting an immune response to the invading antigen by producing specific antibodies that are deposited at the site and are capable of binding to and eliminating the stimulating antigen. Also, committed (activated) lymphocytes in the area of antigen entry are transported via the thoracic duct to other regional lymphoid organs where they can respond to antigens arriving from the original

site of entry (gastrointestinal or respiratory tract) via the lymphatic system.

DETECTION OF ANTIGENS IN HOST

In the past, detection of various infectious organisms has been limited to the identification of an organism mainly by its morphologic and biochemical characteristics, using laboratory procedures that represent an area of laboratory medicine known as *microbiology.*

With recent developments in all areas of *clinical laboratory technology,* including *biotechnology* (e.g., DNA probes), and with the availability of such new tools as antigen-specific monoclonal antibodies for use as reagents in immunologic procedures (see One Step Further Box 14-1), detection of infectious organisms has been greatly expanded. We now can detect specific epitopes (antigenic determinants) on a microorganism, against which an immune reaction is mounted to eliminate the infectious organism. These tests represent a powerful and reliable tool for diagnosing the presence of an infection (see testing for immune response to infectious agents in Chapter 8).

For example, by using **monoclonal antibodies,** we can now detect both the specific antigens (cellular or in plasma) and the specific antibodies directed against these antigens.

The basic principle of using monoclonal antibodies is to establish the existence of an antigen/antibody reaction, which can be detected by immunofluorescence or by examining for formation of a specific color (see Chapters 13 and 14). Presence of antigen/antibody complex indicates that the antigen (unknown) or the antibody have combined with the specific reagent antibody or antigen.

ANTIGEN DETECTION IN SERUM OR PLASMA

Antigens may be detected by several laboratory methods that employ antigen-specific monoclonal antibodies as reagents and other immunologic procedures and molecular techniques that use the same principles as methods for antibody detection (described in Chapters 13, 14, and 15).

ANTIGEN DETECTION IN CELLS

Antigens can be detected by labeling specific antibodies with fluorescent molecules and reacting the labeled antibody with antigens present within a cell or tissue (see immunofluorescence method, Chapter 13). Alternatively, coupling (tagging) the reagent antibodies with various enzymes and observing the color change of the substrate at the site of the enzyme-antibody/antigen complex formation under a conventional microscope can be done. More than one antigen can be localized at the same time with this procedure by using additional antibodies coupled to different enzymes (see discussion of in situ hybridization in Chapter 15).

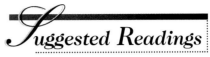

Suggested Readings

Schwartz MK: Tumor markers: what is their role? *Cancer Invest* 8:439-440, 1990.

Sell S: Cancer markers of the 1990s, *Clin Lab Med* 10:1-37, 1990.

Urban JL, Schreiber H: Tumor antigens, *Ann Rev Immunol* 10:617-644, 1992.

Review Questions

TERMINOLOGY

1. The ability of a stimulus (antigen) to induce a detectable immune response in a host is known as:
   a. immunotolerance
   b. immunogenicity
   c. antigenicity
   d. pathogenicity

2. From the factors listed following, select those factors that contribute to the immunogenicity of a molecule:
   a. size of the molecule
   b. accessibility to the immune system
   c. genetic dissimilarity with the host
   d. all of the above

3. A substance that is usually administered to a host together with an antigen to enhance an immune response defines which one of the following:
   a. hapten
   b. adjuvant
   c. vaccine
   d. toxoid

4. The term *allogeneic* refers to a relationship between:
   a. different species
   b. genetically dissimilar members of the same species
   c. different epitope sites in the same individual
   d. genetically identical members of the same species

TYPES OF ANTIGENS

5-9. Match the following statements with the appropriate class of MHC molecules (a and b may be used more than once):

    a. class I MHC
    b. class II MHC

    _____ found on surface of all nucleated cells
    _____ coded by genes of the HLA-A, -B, -C complex
    _____ involved in MHC-restricted antigen recognition by helper T (CD4+) cells
    _____ human HLA-D/DR complex
    _____ involved in MHC-restricted antigen recognition by the cytotoxic (CD8+) T cells

10. MHC restriction refers to self vs. non-self antigen recognition and activation of lym-

phocytes. The complex involved in these mechanisms is the:
a. MHC molecule/antigenic peptide
b. MHC molecule/antigen-presenting cell
c. MHC molecule/helper T cell
d. MHC molecule/B lymphocyte

11. Immunologic surveillance for the presence of tumor cells is thought to be a function of the natural immune response. Specific cells responsible for this function are the:
a. cytokines and natural killer (NK) cells
b. T lymphocytes and macrophages
c. B lymphocytes and NK cells
d. macrophages and NK cells

12. The occurrence of some tumors is limited by a mechanism of the immune system referred to as:
a. immune regulation
b. immune adherence
c. immune surveillance
d. all of the above

13-14. Tumor antigens are capable of triggering humoral and cell-mediated immune responses. Match the following tumor markers with the immune responses they induce:

____ tumor-specific markers
____ tumor-associated markers

a. humoral immune response
b. cell-mediated immune response
c. both a and b

15. Increased concentration of the tumor marker, carcinoembryonic antigen (CEA), may be seen in adults in association with the following malignancy (tumor):
a. breast
b. colon
c. prostate
d. lung

16. Transformation of a normal cell into a malignant cell may occur when a mutation occurs in the:
a. oncogene
b. regulatory gene
c. tumor suppressor gene
d. all of the above

17. The most reliable marker currently available for prostate cancer is:
a. CEA
b. PSA
c. AFP
d. CA 125

18. The first known tumor marker to be identified in patients with multiple myeloma (B lymphocyte malignancy) was the:
a. embryonic protein
b. Bence-Jones protein
c. beta-core fragment
d. alpha-fetoprotein

19. Peptides bound to class I MHC molecules may be referred to as all of the following, *except:*
a. antigenic peptides
b. degraded protein
c. intracellular antigens
d. genetically determined molecules

20. All of the following molecules can be immunogenic to a host, *except:*
a. polysaccharides
b. major histocompatibility complex (MHC)
c. macromolecules
d. proteins

21. A synthetic antigen usually consists of a known amino acid sequence (short peptide) that corresponds to a protein segment on an infectious organism. In order to be immunogenic, such an antigen may be linked with one of the following molecules:
a. haptens
b. carrier molecules
c. adjuvants
d. antigenic molecules

22. An antigen that may be able to induce B cells to differentiate into plasma cells and produce specific antibodies without the participation of T lymphocytes (some helper T cell "help" may be involved) is referred to as:
a. thymus-independent antigen
b. T cell–independent antigen
c. B cell–dependent antigen
d. tumor antigen

ANTIGEN CLASSIFICATION

23. Antigens displayed by an antigen-presenting cell (APC) for recognition by T lymphocytes (CD4+) are categorized as:
    a. extracellular antigens
    b. intracellular antigens
    c. T cell antigens
    d. none of the above

24. Viruses can alter the cell they invade, causing the cell to become abnormal. Recognition of the cell as foreign by the immune system triggers an immune response characterized by:
    a. generation of cytotoxic T cells
    b. production of antibodies
    c. induction of phagocytosis
    d. all of the above

FACTORS DETERMINING IMMUNOGENICITY

25. The immunogenicity of a foreign molecule can be affected by the:
    a. structure of the molecule
    b. size of the molecule
    c. genetic composition of the molecule
    d. all of the above

26. A specific antigen receptor (TCR), which recognizes an immunogenic molecule as foreign, is located on the surface of the:
    a. B lymphocyte
    b. immunogenic molecule
    c. CD4+ T lymphocyte
    d. all of the above

SITES OF ANTIGEN ELIMINATION

27. Which of the mechanisms listed following is involved in removal of antigens during the effector phase of an immune response?
    a. antigen/antibody formation
    b. cytotoxicity
    c. phagocytosis
    d. all of the above

28. All sites listed following are areas of antigen elimination in the host, *except:*
    a. skin
    b. tumor cells
    c. lymphoid tissue
    d. blood circulation

DETECTION OF ANTIGENS IN HOST

29. Antigen-specific monoclonal antibodies are most commonly used as reagents in detection of antigens in:
    a. plasma
    b. serum
    c. cells
    d. all of the above

30. Which of the following techniques can be used to detect antigens in cells
    a. fluorescent microscopy
    b. immunofluorescence assays
    c. enzyme immunoassays
    d. all of the above

31. Select the immunoassay or a molecular technique that can be used for detection of antigens in body fluids:
    a. labeled immunoassay
    b. hybridization assays
    c. immunoprecipitation
    d. all of the above

Cellular Components of the Immune System

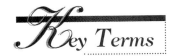

Learning Objectives

Upon completion of Chapter 3, the student will be prepared to:

LYMPHOID TISSUE
- Explain the organization of lymphoid tissue in terms of its functional division.
- Define the role of each of the components of the primary and secondary lymphoid tissue: bone marrow, lymph nodes, thymus, spleen, cutaneous and mucosa-associated lymphoid tissue.
- Identify the main site for the following:
   Origin of all the cells of the immune system
   Differentiation of T lymphocytes
   Clonal selection of T lymphocytes
   Acquisition of receptors for specific recognition of foreign antigens
   Primary response to antigens
   Immune response against blood-borne antigens
   "Clearing" of senescent (aging) cells
   Development of T and B memory cells
   Development of T cytotoxic/suppressor and helper lymphocytes
   Development of antibody-producing plasma cells (B cell lineage)
   Elaboration of soluble factors (i.e., cytokines, antibodies)
   Cell differentiation and proliferation

CELLULAR COMPONENTS
- Identify the subclass of lymphocytic cells capable of specific recognition of any antigen.
- Explain the mechanism of specific antigen recognition, including the participating cell surface receptors and markers.
- State the primary function of lymphocytic cells.
- Name the cells responsible for the specific recognition of non-self antigens and initiation of immune response.
- Describe the difference between the T cell and antibody recognition of antigen.
- Name the effector molecule elaborated by the B cell lineage in response to signals from T cells that have recognized a foreign antigen.
- State the main function of the following cells: helper T cells, cytotoxic T cells, B lympho-

cytes, natural killer cells (NK cells), granulocytes (neutrophils, eosinophils, basophils), mononuclear phagocytes.
- Describe the mechanism for target cell lysis, involving cytotoxic T cells.
- Associate the following cell surface receptors with specific cells or a subpopulation of cells of the immune system: Fc receptor, complement receptor (CR), class I major histocompatibility complex (MHC) molecule, class II MHC molecule, T cell receptor (TCR), CD3, CD4, CD8, and CD19, 20, 22 markers.
- Explain what is meant by MHC restriction.
- Name the phenotypic markers used to classify leukocyte antigens and to differentiate them from one another.
- Differentiate between the class I and II MHC in terms of: name of molecules in each class, cells bearing each class and function of each molecule.
- Identify the MHC class that reflects an individual's genetic make-up and may be used in tissue typing.

Key Terms

accessory cells - These cells are non-lymphoid cells, consisting of phagocytes, dendritic cells, and other cell populations. Accessory cells serve as antigen-presenting cells (APCs) and engage in phagocytosis. They show no specificity for any antigen.

antibodies - Antibodies are soluble molecules, secreted by plasma cells of the B cell lineage in response mainly to microbial antigens. They function as effector molecules in humoral immune response.

antigen receptors - Receptors present on surface of all cells of the immune system, except NK cells, for the recognition of antigens.

antigenic stimulant - Antigens may be foreign or self. Recognition of "non-self" stimulating antigen evokes an immune response (antibody production or cell-mediated cytotoxicity, etc.). The immune system normally does not respond to self antigens (i.e., histocompatibility antigens) because of clonal selection (tolerance).

clonal selection - Refers to elimination of T cell clones that may be capable of reacting against self-antigens (negative selection), thus conferring self-tolerance. Positive selection refers to selection of non-self–reacting lymphocytes (i.e., reacting only with foreign antigens). The process occurs in the thymus.

cluster of differentiation markers (CD) - A cell surface marker used to identify particular class of cells. CD markers are also known as *phenotypic markers* for lymphocytic cells.

complement receptors (CR) - Receptors located on the cell membrane of a variety of cells; mediate many biologic activities (e.g., CR for C3 fragment assists in clearance of immune complexes and enhances phagocytosis). They are named according to the complement molecule they can bind (e.g., C5b receptor binds C5b molecule).

cytolysis - Disruption (lysis) of a cell membrane, resulting in cell death. Usually refers to cell lysis, which involves complement components that are generated by activation of complement by antigen/antibody complexes.

cytotoxic T cells - Subpopulation of T lymphocytes whose function it is to lyse abnormal cells (usually virally infected) that elaborate foreign antigens on their surface.

cytotoxicity - Cytolysis is a function of cell-mediated immunity. T cytotoxic (CD8+) cells recognize an altered cell (virally infected or tumor cell) and destroy it by a process known as *cell lysis*.

effector cells or molecules - Cells, such as macrophages and other leukocytes, eliminate antigens by phagocytosis, thus serving as effector cells in a natural or specific immune response. Effector molecules (antibodies, cytokines) remove or inactivate foreign antigens by forming antigen/antibody complexes or by participating in a variety of mechanisms in a specific immune response.

Fc receptors - Receptors, expressed on monocytes and macrophages, that interact with the Fc domain of an antibody, triggering various biologic responses (e.g., phagocytosis, mediation of inflammation).

helper T cells - Cells developed in the thymus where they acquire surface markers (CD4). These cells are capable of recognizing foreign antigens and elaborating cytokines to promote activation, proliferation, and differentiation of T and B lymphocytes.

memory cells - When the T and B cells are stimulated by a specific antigen in the lymphoid tissue, they remain there as memory cells that respond to a subsequent but same antigenic stimulus (secondary immune response).

natural killer (NK) cells - Cells that have cytotoxic capability (similar to cytotoxic T cells) but are neither T or B cells because they lack the T cell antigen receptors (TCRs) and the surface immunoglobulins (Igs).

phenotypic markers - These markers serve to identify and differentiate cells within the lymphocyte population. CD markers specifically differentiate T cells as helper T cells (CD4+) or cytotoxic/suppressor T cells (CD8+). The sIg marker, recognized by specific monoclonal antibodies, identifies a B cell population.

plasma cells - Antibody-secreting cells of the B cell lineage, capable of producing all classes of antibodies in response to a variety of antigenic stimuli.

surface immunoglobulins (sIgs) - Antibody molecules located on the surface of B lymphocytes. These markers serve as antigen receptors for specific binding of antigens (mainly bacteria). The resulting antigen/antibody complex serves to inactivate or eliminate the stimulating antigen.

T cell receptors (TCRs) - TCRs are expressed exclusively on surface membrane of T cells. Specific antigen recognition through these receptors is closely associated with the CD3 molecule (TCR/CD3), also located on the surface of T cells. The TCR recognizes only processed antigen (antigenic peptides) bound to an MHC molecule and is an effective mechanism for eliminating intracellular antigens, such as viruses.

target cell - Cell that is the focus of activity for effector cells or molecules of the immune system. It is usually an altered cell (virally infected or opsonized), marked for destruction by cytolysis or phagocytosis, respectively.

The immune system consists of cells and their secretory products (soluble mediators) and the various lymphoid tissues and organs where these cells are organized and localized. Main components of the immune system, therefore, include:

- **Lymphoid tissue** (primary/secondary) (Figure 3-1)
- **Cellular components** (lymphocytes, accessory cells) (Figure 3-2)
- **Soluble components (mediators)** (cytokines, antibodies, complement components) (see Figure 3-2)

The primary function of cells of the immune system and the various mediators that they secrete during an immune response is their participation in (1) the recognition of the foreign antigen *(cognitive phase),* (2) the various responses of the immune system *(activation phase),* and (3) the resolution of the event by inactivating or eliminating the antigenic stimulus *(effector phase).*

An overview of key events that occur during an immune response and the involvement of the major cells and their products is presented in Figure 3-3.

LYMPHOID TISSUE

The cells of the immune system are organized and localized in many scattered lymphoid tissues or in various specialized organs (see Figure 3-1). The lymphoid tissues and organs also serve as reservoirs for foreign antigens, which are transported to and concentrated within the tissues.

Lymphoid tissue has been categorized into two divisions, according to their function (Figure 3-4):

- *Primary lymphoid tissue*
- *Secondary lymphoid tissue*

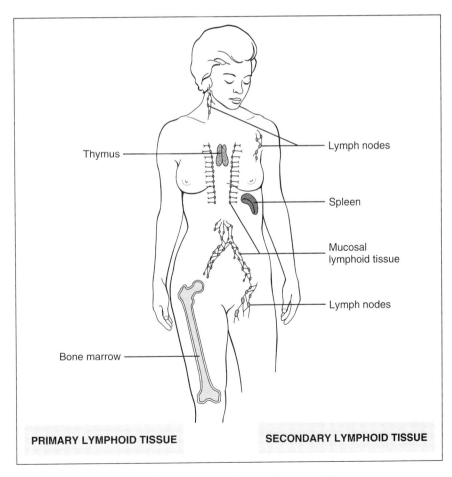

Thymus

Lymph nodes

Spleen

Mucosal lymphoid tissue

Lymph nodes

Bone marrow

PRIMARY LYMPHOID TISSUE   **SECONDARY LYMPHOID TISSUE**

FIGURE **3-1** Location of Major Lymphoid Tissue.

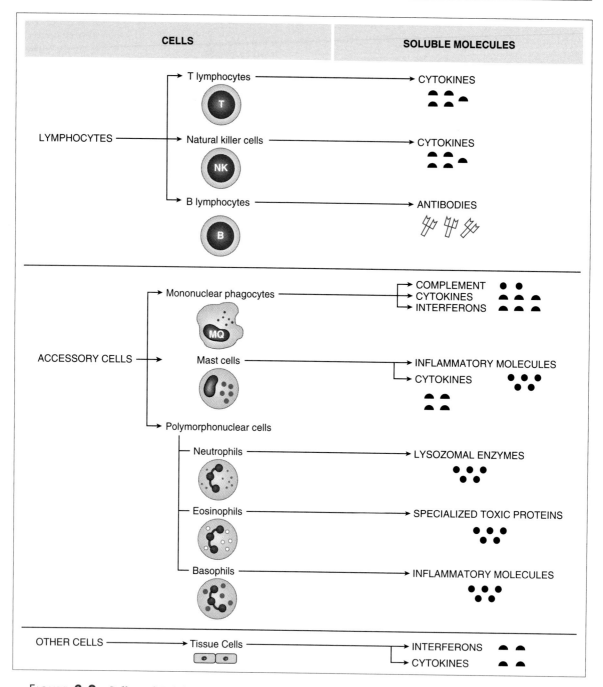

FIGURE **3-2** **Cells and Soluble Molecules of the Immune System.**   The soluble molecules are secreted by particular cells, as indicated. The soluble antibody molecules, however, are synthesized and secreted by plasma cells (activated B lymphocytes that have differentiated into antibody-secreting cells).

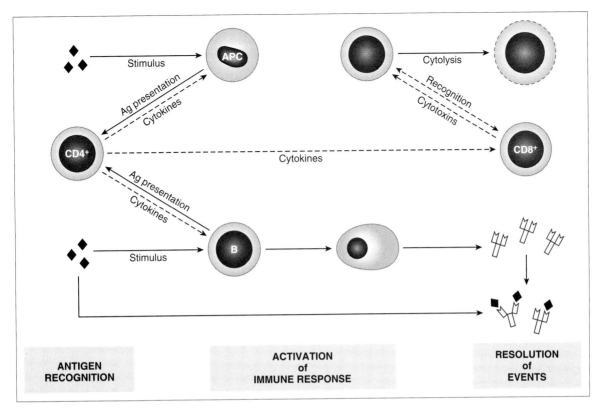

FIGURE **3-3** **Response of Major Components of the Immune System to a Foreign Stimulus.** APCs (mainly) and B cells present antigen to CD4+ cells, which release cytokines that activate CD8+ and B cells. CD8+ cytotoxic cells destroy altered target cells (cell-mediated immune response). Activated B cells differentiate into plasma cells, which secrete antibodies that bind with antigens to form antigen/antibody complexes (humoral immune response). During both immune responses, stimulating antigens are removed. *APCs,* antigen-presenting cells; *CD4+,* helper T cell; *CD8+,* cytotoxic T cell; *B,* B lymphocyte.

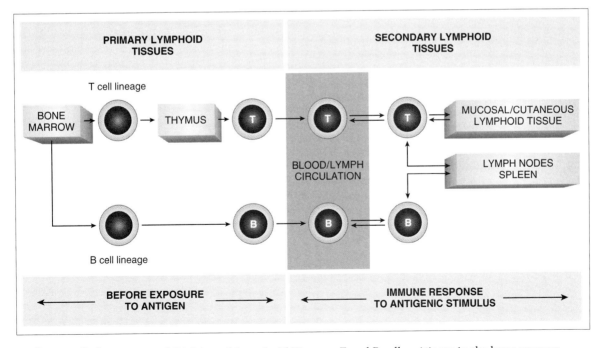

FIGURE **3-4** **Functional Division of Lymphoid Tissue.** T and B cells originate in the bone marrow, where B cells also mature. Cells committed to T cell lineage migrate from bone marrow to the thymus where they acquire antigen specificity. Both T and B cells circulate between blood and lymphoid tissue.

PRIMARY (GENERATIVE) LYMPHOID TISSUE

Two organs are designated as primary lymphoid tissue: *bone marrow* and the *thymus*. Both tissues are the site of maturation and differentiation of different types of lymphocytes.

Bone Marrow

All cells of the immune system are derived from an undifferentiated stem cell in the bone marrow, where they mature and differentiate by a process known as *hematopoiesis* (One Step Further Box 3-1).

Only the T lymphocytes, a subpopulation of lymphocytes, are unique in their development in that, although they originate in the bone marrow and are committed there to the lymphoid lineage, their proliferation and differentiation occurs in the thymus.

Thymus

Structure

The thymus gland is a bilobed structure, located in the thorax (see Figure 3-1). Each lobe contains lymphoid cells *(thymocytes)* that form a tightly packed outer cortex and an inner medulla. The cortex contains the immature and proliferating cells, while the medulla consists of the more mature cells, suggesting the existence of a maturation gradient from the cortex to the medulla.

The circulation of cells (traffic) in and out of the thymus is through the endothelial venules, a part of the thymic blood circulation. The cells have the ability to migrate via the circulation into the secondary lymphoid tissues (see Figure 3-4).

The thymus involutes (diminishes in size) with age, with only medullary remnants remaining. T cell production, however, continues throughout life. All conditions associated with an increase in steroids, such as stress, promote thymic atrophy (degeneration).

FUNCTION

Cell Differentiation   Entry of primitive cells from the bone marrow into the thymus is limited to the cells of lymphoid lineage that have been committed in the bone marrow to develop into T lymphocytes (Figure 3-5).

During the maturation process in the thymus, the T lymphocytes acquire many surface receptors, such as the T cell receptor (TCR) and others, important in antigen recognition and the T cell activation process as well as in identification of the cell's phenotype (One Step Further Box 3-2). The ability of the T cells to perform the various helper and cytolytic functions also develops in the thymus (Box 3-1) as the cells acquire the T cell surface markers, CD4+ and CD8+, respectively.

Box 3-1   ROLE OF THE THYMUS IN CELL-MEDIATED IMMUNITY

- T cell maturation and proliferation
- Development of various cell surface markers (e.g., T cell receptors, TCR phenotypic marker)
- Development of the ability of the T cell to recognize foreign antigens and initiate an immune response
- Development of helper (CD4+) and cytotoxic (CD8+) T cell function
- Elimination or inactivation of cells that may react to self-antigens (negative clonal selection)
- Development of self-tolerant T cells (positive clonal selection)
- Proliferation and "two-way" migration of T cells

Box 3-1

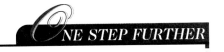

Hematopoiesis

Origin of Hematopoiesis

The site of hematopoiesis (growth and development of blood cells) during fetal life occurs within the blood islands of the yolk sac, liver, and eventually within the spleen. During childhood, however, the bone marrow of the flat bones takes over this function until puberty. At puberty and during adulthood, hematopoiesis occurs mostly in the sternum, vertebrae, iliac crest, and the ribs.

The pleuripotential stem cell, from which all cells originate, becomes committed to differentiating along two specific lineages or paths (Figure 3-5):

- *Lymphoid lineage:* Producing lymphocytes
- *Myeloid lineage:* Producing mononuclear phagocytes, granulocytes (neutrophils, eosinophils, basophils) and platelets

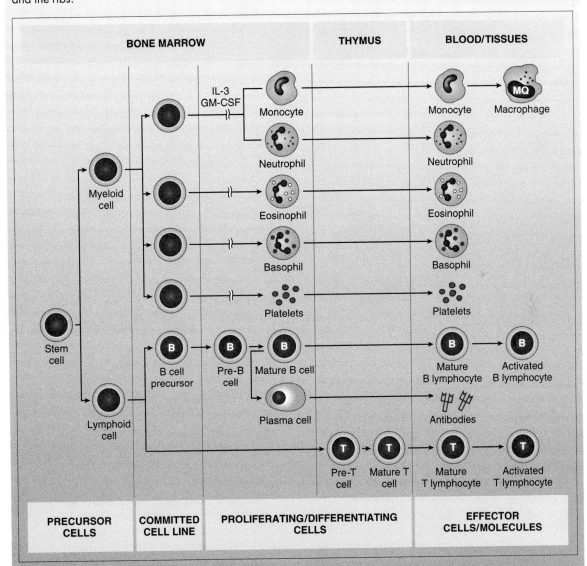

FIGURE 3-5 **Maturation of Cells of the Immune System (Hematopoiesis).** Maturation and proliferation of cells of a particular cell lineage are promoted by the various hematopoietic growth factors (see discussion in Chapter 4).

Continued

Box 3-1—cont'd

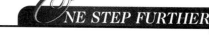

Growth-Stimulating Factors

Although little is known about the mechanism by which the stem cell becomes committed to the development of blood cells, cytokines (colony-stimulating factors [CSF]), produced by cells of the stroma (structural framework) of the bone marrow and by the macrophages present there, have been well defined. These CSF cytokines, specific for each functional lineage of precursor cells (see Figure 3-5), are responsible for stimulating the precursor cells to grow and differentiate into various cell lines. Other soluble products also participate in this process. For example, interleukin 6 (IL6), a broadly active factor, functions synergistically with other factors (e.g., IL3) to increase production of myeloid precursors.

The hematopoietic process is instrumental in replenishing cells consumed during an immune response, thus ensuring balance between production and destruction of cells.

Proliferation and Differentiation

All cells of the immune system, including the B lymphocytes (discussed in Chapter 5) originate in the bone marrow, where they proliferate and differentiate into mature cells. Only the T lymphocytes differ in this respect. Although the T lymphocytes originate in the bone marrow, they travel to the thymus where they acquire specific markers and become "committed" to specific T cell functions (i.e., helper [CD4+] and cytotoxic/suppressor [CD8+] T cells).

In Vitro Studies

T and B cells can also be induced to proliferate in vitro (in tissue cultures) in the absence of any antigen. When exposed to mitogenic lectins (mitogens) derived from various plants and bacteria, the cells can be induced to proliferate. Among the most studied mitogens capable of stimulating the T and B cells to proliferate are:

- Phytohemagglutinin (PHA): Stimulates T cells
- Concanavalin A (Con A): Stimulates T cells
- Lipopolysaccharide (LPS): Stimulates B cells to differentiate into antibody-secreting cells (plasma cells)
- Pokeweed mitogen (PWM): Stimulates both T and B cells

Clinical Application

The in vitro process involves stimulation of cells with a variety of antigens or mitogens in tissue culture (mixed lymphocyte culture [MLC]) and transformation of the stimulated cell into a blast form (blastogenesis or transformation) with subsequent DNA synthesis and cell replication (mitosis). This process can be used in a laboratory setting as an in vitro functional study to evaluate the magnitude of an immune response, by measuring the amount of DNA produced in response to the stimulating antigen or mitogen (diagnostic procedure).

It is believed that the in vitro response to an antigenic stimulus, although somewhat limited, shows a good correlation with events that occur in vivo.

Clonal Selection

The process of *clonal selection* (elimination of self-reactive T cell clones) occurs during initial antigen recognition by the T lymphocytes because of their ability to discriminate between the self and non-self antigens in the context of their MHC molecules, which they also acquire in the thymus. Thus the *T cell–MHC restriction originates in the thymus.*

Many of the cells entering the thymus with the ability to recognize self-antigens do not survive as a result of this clonal selection process.

Only those cells that have acquired specific receptors for recognizing foreign antigens are stimulated to mature in the thymus.

SECONDARY (PERIPHERAL) LYMPHOID TISSUE

Lymphocytes migrate from primary lymphoid tissue to the peripheral tissues, where they are either scattered or aggregated, forming secondary lymphoid tissues.

The secondary lymphoid tissues are present in two forms: (1) encapsulated tissue (*lymph nodes* and *spleen*) and (2) non-encapsulated tissue (*cutaneous-* and *mucosa-associated lymphoid tissue*).

The secondary lymphoid tissues are the primary site of humoral and cell-mediated responses to foreign antigens (see Chapter 1) that collect in the tissues from their sites of entry.

Box 3-2

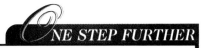

Cell Markers and Receptors

Receptors for Antigens

All cells of the immune system (except the natural killer [NK] cells) have molecular receptors for recognition of an antigen. These antigen receptors consist of two types of molecules capable of great diversity (through gene rearrangement) that permit recognition of an almost unlimited number of antigens. The receptors discussed following participate in antigen recognition.

T Cell Antigen Receptors (TCRs)

These T cell membrane receptors, consisting of alpha (α) and beta (β) chains that are linked by a disulfide bond and that contain a hypervariable region for antigen binding, are similar to the structure of immunoglobulin molecules (see Chapter 5, Figure 5-7).

TCRs are expressed exclusively on the surface membrane of the T lymphocytes. Recognition through these receptors, in association with the CD3 surface molecule, initiates immunologic events that include T cell helper and suppressor activity, cytotoxicity, and possibly NK cell activity.

CD3 Proteins

CD3 receptors are expressed on the cell surface of T cells in association with the TCR, forming a TCR/CD3 complex that allows the T cells to specifically recognize peptide antigens bound to MHC molecules (Figure 3-6). The current understanding is that the binding of an antigen to the TCR complex (TCR and associated CD3) sends signals to the T cell, resulting in cell activation.

The major function of the CD3 molecules in antigen recognition is to facilitate the expression of the TCR complex.

Immunoglobulin (Antibody) Molecules

These surface immunoglobulin (sIg) receptors, elaborated by a B cell and carried on its surface membrane, serve as antigen receptors for specific binding of native (unprocessed) antigens. The resulting antigen/antibody complex is an effective mechanism for inactivating or eliminating extracellular antigens, such as bacteria. The sIg receptors differ from the TCR in that the binding by sIg is an effector mechanism of the humoral immune response, whereas recognition of antigen by TCR initiates a humoral or cell-mediated immune response.

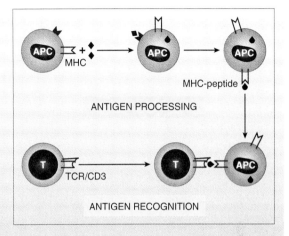

FIGURE **3-6** **MHC-Restricted Antigen Recognition.** Antigen is bound and processed by an antigen-presenting cell (APC) and expressed as a MHC-peptide complex on its surface. The antigen–MHC complex is presented to a T cell for recognition by its TCR/CD3 receptor as self or non-self (foreign). *APC,* antigen-presenting cell; *MHC,* major histocompatibility complex; *TCR,* T cell receptor (for antigen); *CD3,* accessory marker on all T cells.

These membrane immunoglobulins (Ig) differ from the secreted antibodies found in the blood and tissues in that they contain an additional amino acid sequence that spans the B cell membrane and ends in the cytoplasm near the carboxyl end of the spanning Ig molecule. The heavy chain isotypes (classes) of Ig expressed on the B cells differ according to the events that the B cells may have encountered.

Immature cells may express IgM, mature unstimulated cells may express IgM and IgD, and previously stimulated memory cells express surface Ig of the parent cell (see Chapter 5, Figure 5-4). Cross-linking of antigen with the membrane antibody through the determinants (idiotopes) of the Ig hypervariable region (antigen-binding site) may signal B cell activation and possibly production of anti-idiotypic antibodies that also bind to the Ig determinants, thus regulating the extent of the immune response (discussed in Chapter 5).

Continued

Box 3-2—cont'd

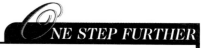
ONE STEP FURTHER

Major Histocompatibility Complex Molecules

The major histocompatibility complex (MHC) consists of structurally diverse (polymorphic) glycoproteins located on all nucleated cells of the body as transmembrane molecules (spanning the cell membrane). This structural diversity of the MHC enables it to bind to a variety of foreign antigenic peptides. The resulting MHC-peptide complex is presented on the surface of an antigen-presenting cell (APC) or virally infected cell for specific recognition by a T cell.

The specific recognition of the MHC-bound antigen is through the T cell receptors (TCR) and their associated CD3 receptors on the surface of the helper (CD4+) and cytotoxic (CD8+) T lymphocytes (see Figure 3-6). The events or responses that follow recognition are referred to as the *specific immune responses*.

The ability to differentiate between foreign and self-antigens in the context of the MHC is a vital step in determining if an immune response is appropriate or not.

Only MHC-bound antigenic peptides can be recognized by the T cells (CD4+ and CD8+ cells). This restriction in antigen recognition is referred to as **MHC restriction** and is discussed in One Step Further Box 3-3.

Phenotypic Markers

Each cell population of the lymphocytic series has a variety of cell surface markers, known as *phenotypic markers* (Table 3-1). These markers serve to identify and differentiate cells within the lymphocyte populations, using immunofluorescent cell surface labelling and detection usually by a fluorescence-activated cell sorter (FAC) (see flow cytometry in Chapter 14).

For example, phenotypic cell markers (sIg) on B lymphocytes can be recognized by class-specific monoclonal antibodies (reagent) directed against the surface immunoglobulins (sIg) on the B lymphocytes.

A CD system is used to classify human leukocyte antigens and antibodies that recognize them. *CD* refers to *cluster of differentiation,* a nomenclature established by the International Workshop on Human Leukocyte Differentiation Antigens. A database has been developed to assist with identifying and analyzing each molecule.

The CD designation is useful in:
- Differentiating cells from one another (i.e., helper T cells with a CD4+ marker from cytotoxic T cells [CTLs] expressing CD8+ phenotypic marker).
- Classifying lymphocytes according to the various CD markers present on a particular

cell. For example, CD3+CD4+CD8− markers are found on most helper T lymphocytes, while CD3+CD4−CD8+ markers are located on cytotoxic T lymphocytes.
- Identifying cells that participate in the various immune responses.

Fc Receptors

Three types of surface receptors for the Fc portion of an IgG molecule have been identified:
- FcγR I (CD64)
- FcγR II (CDW32)
- FcγR III (CD16)

These Fc (fragment, crystalline) receptors consist of a single transmembrane polypeptide with a varied affinity for the IgG subclasses. When the Fc receptor interacts with the Fc domain of an immunoglobulin (IgG) expressed on monocytes and macrophages, a variety of biologic responses (natural and specific immunity) are triggered, such as phagocytosis, endocytosis, release of inflammatory mediators, and enhancement of antigen presentation. Thus the Fc receptors serve as a link between natural and specific immunity.

In addition, binding of an antigen-antibody complex through its antibody molecule to the Fc receptor removes the stimulating antigen from any further stimulation of the immune system.

Complement Receptors

Binding of complement fragments to specific complement receptors on cell membranes of a variety of cells mediates many biologic activities. These receptors, which are protein in nature, may be categorized as:
- Receptors for fragments of C3, bound to activating surfaces
- Receptors for soluble C3a and C5a fragments, which have a regulatory effect on the inflammatory responses
- Receptors responsible for regulation of the complement cascades, by binding to and inhibiting certain complement proteins

Receptors for surface-bound C3 fragments have been characterized best and their functions defined. They participate in the clearance of circulating immune complexes (immune adherence) and enhancement of phagocytosis (opsonization).

Other Cell Markers

There are numerous other cell surface markers that are involved in a variety of cell functions and their identification that have not been included in this presentation.

Box 3-3

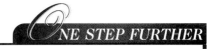
ONE STEP FURTHER

Major Histocompatibility Complex (MHC) Restriction

The major histocompatibility complex (MHC) is a large region of genes on chromosome 6 that codes for three types of gene products (proteins), known as the *MHC molecules* (see Figure 6-1). These molecules are expressed on the surface of a variety of nucleated cells as transmembrane (spanning cell membrane) proteins. The MHC gene products are identified as:

- Class I MHC: HLA-A, HLA-B, HLA-C molecules
- Class II MHC: HLA-D, HLA-DR, HLA-DP molecules

Although class III MHC molecules (PF or properdin factor, and C2, C4a, C4b complement components) are coded also by MHC region genes, they are not directly involved in antigen recognition as are the MHC class I and class II molecules (see major histocompatibility complex in Chapter 6).

Class I MHC (HLA-A, HLA-B, and HLA-C Molecules)

Class I molecules, also known as *human leukocyte antigens (HLA)* or *histocompatibility antigens,* are HLA-A, -B, and -C molecules (MHC gene products) that can bind endogenous proteins (expressed on altered target cells) and present the MHC-antigenic protein (peptide) complex to cytotoxic T cells for recognition and destruction. This type of antigen recognition in the context of the MHC molecule is referred to as **MHC-restricted antigen recognition.**

CLASS I MHC RESTRICTION

MHC restriction, also known as *MHC-restricted antigen recognition* or *antigen recognition within the MHC context,* refers to cytotoxic T cell (CD8+) recognition of target cells (virally infected or tumor cells) that bear class I MHC–antigenic peptide complex. The TCR/CD3 and CD8 receptors on cytotoxic T cells are responsible for the specific recognition of the MHC-antigen complex, which results in cytotoxicity (cell lysis) of a target cell (see Figure 1-12, Chapter 1).

Class II MHC (HLA-D, HLA-DR, HLA-DP Molecules)

HLA-D, -DR, and -DP molecules bind exogenous proteins, usually bacterial antigens that have been processed by an antigen-presenting cell (APC) and presented to helper T cells (CD4+) for recognition. Recognition of MHC-antigenic peptide complex by CD4+ cells triggers an immune reaction.

CLASS II MHC RESTRICTION

The initiation of an immune response depends on the recognition of a class II MHC–antigenic peptide complex on the surface of an antigen-presenting cell (APC) as foreign (see Figure 1-9, Chapter 1). This type of specific recognition of APC-processed antigen is a function of helper T lymphocytes (CD4+) and is referred to as MHC-restricted antigen recognition.

Table 3-1 | CHARACTERISTICS OF MAJOR LYMPHOCYTE POPULATIONS

Class	Antigen Receptor	Phenotype Markers	Cell Function
T lymphocytes			
Helper T cells	TCR/CD3	CD4+, CD8−	Stimulate B-cell growth/differentiation
			Macrophage activation through secreted cytokines (cell-mediated immunity)
Cytotoxic T cells	TCR/CD3	CD4−, CD8+	Lyse virally infected cells (antigen-bearing cells)
			Allograft rejection (cell-mediated immunity)
B lymphocytes	sIg	(CD19, CD20, CD22)*	Antibody (Ig) production (humoral immunity)
Natural killer (NK) cells	None	CD16, CD56	Lyse tumor cells (antibody-dependent cell-mediated cytotoxicity)

*Shared specificity with few T cells, granulocytes, and macrophages.
TCR, T cell receptor; *CD,* cluster of differentiation; *sIg,* surface immunoglobulin; *Ig,* immunoglobulin.

Lymph Nodes
Structure of Lymph Nodes
The lymph nodes are small aggregates of lymphoid tissue along the lymphatic channels throughout the body (see Figure 3-1). The structure of lymph nodes is not fixed but changes with the presence of antigen and regresses after its elimination.

Entry of any antigen into the lymph nodes is through the lymphatic capillaries that permeate tissues of the gastrointestinal or respiratory tract, connective tissue, and most organs and by subsequent transport of antigen by larger lymphatic vessels (lymphatic circulation) to the lymph nodes.

Function: Primary Immune Response
As antigen enters lymph nodes, it is recognized as foreign by the T and B lymphocytes present within the lymph nodes, triggering an immune response. These **primary immune responses** to the antigenic stimulus include:

- Production of soluble factors (e.g., cytokines) that create a cell-to-cell communication network
- Cell proliferation (transformation of lymphocytes)
- Development of effector cells
- Development of cytotoxic (CD8+) and helper (CD4+) T cells (cell-mediated immunity)
- Development of plasma cells that secrete antigen-specific antibodies (humoral immune response)
- Development of T or B memory cells

Function: Secondary Immune Response
Memory cells developed during the primary immune response remain in the lymphoid tissue where they are ready to respond with a greater intensity and efficiency to the same antigenic stimulus, which they previously encountered during a primary immune response (see secondary immune response, discussed in Chapter 1).

Spleen
Structure
The spleen is an organ containing lymphoid tissue, lymphocytes, and accessory cells. The antigens and lymphocytes enter the spleen through the vascular system.

Function
Although the immune responses occurring in the spleen are similar to those of the lymph nodes, *the immune responses occurring in the spleen are in response to antigens that are blood-borne (carried by blood), while immune responses in the lymph nodes are to antigens entering the lymph.*

The spleen has also the ability to "clear" the blood of foreign substances and senescent (aging) red blood cells by the process of phagocytosis by phagocytic cells present within the spleen. *This latter function of the spleen is independent of any specific immune response.*

Other Peripheral Lymphoid Tissues
The peripheral lymphoid tissues, found scattered or in aggregates within many mucosal and cutaneous tissues, promote contact between the cells that participate in the immune response. These tissues may also serve as a site for an immune response, as is seen in the synovium of the bone joints associated with rheumatoid arthritis.

CELLULAR COMPONENTS

Cells of the immune system that play a vital role in a variety of specific immune responses to a foreign configuration (antigen) are the **lymphocytes** and the **accessory cells** (mononuclear phagocytes, dendritic cells, and other cell populations) (see Figure 3-2). The **effector cells** (mononuclear phagocytes and various leukocytes) are active in eliminating or inactivating the antigenic stimulus, thereby preventing further immune responses. *The specificity for recognition of a multitude of foreign antigens (therefore the specificity of immune responses) is attributed to the lymphocytic cells.*

The maturation and development of cells of the immune system are presented in Figure 3-5, whereas their specific participation in variety of responses of the immune system to a foreign configuration is described in the sections that follow.

LYMPHOCYTIC CELLS

The lymphocytic cells (lymphocytes) are a class of leukocytes normally present in blood.

Their primary function is to survey the body and recognize any foreign material that may indicate the presence of virus, bacteria, parasites, or tumor cells. To optimize the detection of these foreign substances, the lymphocytes circulate throughout the body (i.e., blood, lymph, peripheral sites of entry, and lymphoid tissue).

There are three functionally distinct classes of lymphocytes that have been identified and which make up the lymphocyte repertoire (see Table 3-1):

- **T lymphocytes**
- **B lymphocytes**
- **Natural killer cells (NK cells)**

Unique Features of Lymphocytes
Antigen Recognition

Specific antigen recognition is attributed to only a small number of lymphocytes, namely, the T and B lymphocytes. The T and B cells have the unique ability to specifically recognize any antigen at the site of exposure and to trigger an appropriate immune response directed against the stimulating antigen.

An important differential feature in antigen recognition by these two lymphocyte populations is that *B cells recognize* **native antigen configuration** *and require helper T cell (CD4+) participation in order for the immune response to occur, whereas T cells (CD8+ and CD4+) recognize only a* **"processed" antigen and in the context of self-MHC molecule** (i.e., MHC-antigenic peptide complex). The recognition is **MHC-restricted** (One Step Further Box 3-3) and is followed by an immune response. The antigen processing and presentation to T cells for recognition is a function of **antigen-presenting cells (APCs).** Cells that function as APCs are the macrophages (phagocytes), dendritic cells, B cells, and epithelial cells.

Specific T cell recognition of processed (MHC-bound) antigen is through the genetically determined T cell receptors (TCR) and associated CD3 receptors on the T cell surface. The great diversity of these antigen receptors allows for the recognition of a multitude of foreign molecules in the context of the MHC molecule (Figure 3-7).

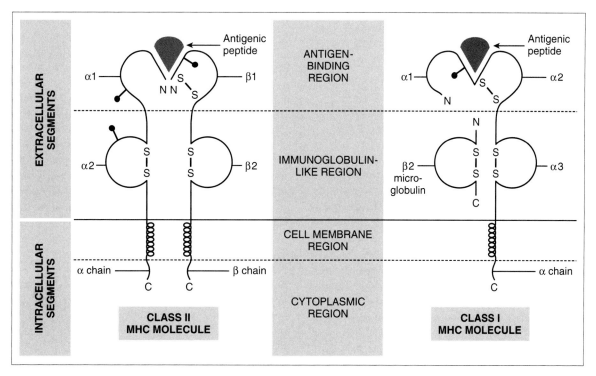

FIGURE **3-7** **Schematic Presentation of Class I and Class II MHC Molecules.** *S–S,* disulfide bonds; *C,* carboxyl terminal; *N,* amino terminal; *α,* alpha; *β,* beta. (See One Step Further Boxes 3-2 and 3-3.)

The T cell populations are most effective in recognizing intracellular antigens (virally infected cells, tumor cells) and are also able to recognize processed extracellular antigenic material. *Unbound antigens are not recognized by T cells.*

Specific recognition of unbound (native) antigen is the function of the B lymphocytes and their membrane immunoglobulin (Ig) receptors. Antigens need not be processed for recognition because recognition is not MHC restricted.

Lymphocyte Activation
Cell activation (stimulation) that follows specific recognition of an antigen depends on the nature of the antigenic stimulus:

- *Extracellular antigens (bacteria)* stimulate cell proliferation and differentiation of antibody-producing B lymphocyte lineage, also known as **plasma cells** (effector cells of humoral immune response).
- *Intracellular antigens (viruses, intracellular bacteria)* stimulate differentiation of **T cells** into specific effector cells, such as helper and cytotoxic T cells, thus triggering the cell-mediated immune responses.

Lymphocytes may also be activated by several **plant mitogens,** which show specificity in their ability to stimulate a particular cell lineage. For example, *phytohemagglutinins (PHA) and Concanavalin A (Con A) stimulate T lymphocytes to proliferate, while lipopolysaccharide (LPS) mitogen is an effective stimulant of B lymphocytes. Pokeweed mitogen (PWM) can stimulate both the T and B cells.*

Lymphocyte Populations
T Lymphocytes
The precursors of T lymphocytes originate in the bone marrow, then migrate to the thymus and mature there. The "T" refers to "thymus-derived" lymphocytes.

T cells are normally found in the blood, lymphoid organs, and scattered in all tissues (except the central nervous system) and have the ability to circulate and exchange between the blood and the various lymph tissues (see Figure 3-4). This is an important protective feature in that these cells may quickly be recruited to any site within the body where recognition and response to an antigen is required.

T cell–based functions. Specificity of the immune response, *recognition* of a foreign antigen (processed antigenic peptides), and *self-tolerance* (see Chapter 1) are typically attributed to the T lymphocyte population, although B cells can recognize unprocessed antigens (usually microbes), a concept discussed later in the chapter. The T cell–based specificity of the immune system depends on the ability of the T cells to:

- Recognize non-self configuration
- Specifically recognize antigenic peptides
- Distinguish a variety of antigenic determinants
- Initiate specific humoral and cell-mediated immune responses

Further, *T lymphocytes are the only cells of the immune system that are capable of a specific recognition of a foreign antigen in the context of the MHC restriction* (see One Step Further Box 3-3). Recognition of foreign antigen by the B cells is not MHC restricted.

T lymphocyte subpopulations. The mature T lymphocytes are further categorized into subsets or subpopulations (see Table 3-1) that are functionally different. The two best described T cell subsets, which originate and mature in the bone marrow, and are "selected" in the thymus are:

- **Helper T lymphocytes (CD4+ CD8−)**
- **Cytotoxic/suppressor T lymphocytes (CD8+ CD4−)**

The subsets of T cells, CD4+ and CD8+, are not related to each other and are mutually exclusive. Approximately two thirds of T cells found in the peripheral blood are CD4+ (express CD4 antigen), whereas the remaining one third of peripheral cells express the CD8 antigen and are CD8+. They are structurally similar to the antibody molecules, being members of the same immunoglobulin (Ig) superfamily (see structural characteristics of immunoglobulin molecules and Figure 5-3 in Chapter 5).

T cells have a distinct pattern of MHC restriction in specific antigen recognition. *CD4+ T cells are class II MHC restricted, whereas CD8+ T cells are class I MHC restricted* (see Figure 3-7 and One Step Further Box 3-3).

helper T lymphocytes
- *Structure:* Helper T cells, a subset of T lymphocytes, can be identified by their

CD4+ markers, known as a *transmembrane receptors* (glycoprotein structures that span the cell membrane). The CD4 (and CD8) membrane receptors have a specificity for antigens bound to the MHC molecule and are structurally related to the antibody molecules (see Figure 5-3).

Two groups of helper T cells, TH1 and TH2, have been more recently described according to their cytokine secretion pattern and the functions that they mediate. For example, TH1 cells mediate cytotoxicity and local inflammatory reactions (IL-2 cytokine and IFNγ, respectively), while TH2 cells stimulate B cells to proliferate and secrete immunoglobulins (IL-4, -5, -6, and -10 cytokines), thus affecting the humoral immune responses.

- *Function:* The function of the CD4 transmembrane receptors in the activation of T cells—in a weak association with the T cell receptor (TCR/CD3 membrane receptor)—is to specifically recognize and respond to an antigen (polypeptides) present in association with the major histocompatibility complex (see Figure 3-6) on an antigen-presenting cell (APC). This is referred to as the MHC restriction (see One Step Further Box 3-3). *Because the CD4+ cells are class II MHC restricted and have a specificity for antigens that are bound to the MHC, the T cells will only recognize and respond to cell surface–associated antigens and not to an unbound, soluble antigen.*

In addition, the CD4+ cells, when stimulated by an antigen, also have the ability to secrete cytokines (see Chapter 4, One Step Further Box 4-1), which promote activation, proliferation, and differentiation of T cells and other cells (B cells and macrophages). The elaborated cytokines also recruit and activate inflammatory leukocytes (macrophages and granulocytes), thus serving as a link between natural and cell-mediated immunity.

cytotoxic T lymphocytes
- *Structure:* The cytotoxic T lymphocytes (CTLs) originate and mature in bone marrow and are selected in the thymus. They are identified by their CD8+ marker.

Two functional subsets have been identified, some of which produce IL-2 in response to activation signals and others which do not. The CTLs are activated by cross-linking of the T cell receptor (TCR) and the CD3 receptor on their cell surface, a mechanism also associated with the helper T cells, discussed in subsequent chapters.

- *Function:* The primary function of CTLs is to recognize and destroy target cells that express the class I MHC–associated antigen complex (see Cell-Mediated Immune Response and Figure 1-13 in Chapter 1). Because target cell lysis is antigen specific, antigen recognition in the context of the MHC is essential for CTL effectiveness in the elimination of any intracellular viral infection (virally infected cells). Lysing of the target cell (cytolysis) by the CTL may be through one of the following mechanisms:
  1. Secretion of toxins from their granules in the area of the target cell that results in blocking of ions and water from the cell, which causes swelling and cell lysis
  2. Activation of target cell intracellular enzymes, resulting in degradation of the cell's DNA and subsequent cell lysis

The CTLs are not destroyed during target cell lysis and are capable of destroying other target cells (Figure 3-8). In addition to cytolysis, the CTLs may also participate in the following situations as *effector cells:*
  1. Allograft rejections (destruction of incompatible cells/tissues)
  2. Rejection of tumors (destruction of cells expressing foreign antigenic peptides)

suppressor cells. Originally these were thought to be another subset of T cells, which secrete antigen-specific "suppressor" factors and which were identified as CD8+ lymphocytes (distinct form of CTLs and helper T cells). However, attempts to isolate and characterize these "suppressor" cells or the "suppressor" factors have been unsuccessful. It is now believed that this population of T cells may not exist and that many T cells may block (sup-

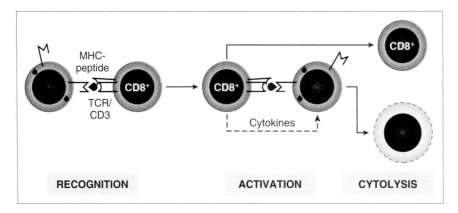

FIGURE **3-8**   **CTL-Mediated Cytolysis.**   CD8+ T cell is activated by class I MHC–antigenic peptide complex, which is expressed on the surface of altered (target) cell. Activated CD8+ cell (cytotoxic T cell) releases cytokines (cytotoxins), causing lysis of target cell without damage to itself. Unaltered CD8+ cell is able to continue its function as a cytotoxic cell. *MHC,* major histocompatibility complex; *TCR,* T cell receptor (for antigen); *CD,* cluster of differentiation; *CD3+,* accessory receptor to TCR.

press) various immune responses by secreting inhibitory cytokines.

B Lymphocytes

structure of B lymphocytes. B lymphocytes are named after the organ in birds known as the bursa of Fabricius, which has no equivalent in humans. Also, because the initial stages of maturation of B lymphocytes in humans occur in the bone marrow, the "B" may refer to bone marrow–derived lymphocyte. Unlike T lymphocytes, which mature and acquire various receptors in the thymus, during their maturation, B cells secrete immunoglobulin molecules (antibodies), which are inserted into their surface membrane. *These surface antibodies serve as specific antigen receptors and phenotypic markers, identifying the cell as a B lymphocyte.*

B lymphocyte maturation. B cells develop through the following stages (Figure 3-9):
- *Pre-B lymphocyte,* which has no ability to recognize or respond to antigens
- *Immature B lymphocyte,* with immunoglobulin molecules (IgM) on its surface but with no ability to proliferate or differentiate in response to antigens; this is the stage during which tolerance to self-antigens is developed
- *Mature B cell,* expressing both the IgM and IgD membrane molecules responsible for specificity and having the ability to respond to antigens

- *Activated B cell (blast),* transformed cell after stimulation with an antigen, also expressing IgM and IgD molecules on its surface
- *Plasma cell,* differentiated B cell, or an antibody-secreting cell capable of elaborating various classes of antibodies (not membrane bound) in response to an antigenic stimulus (primary immune response)
- *Memory B cell,* expressing surface immunoglobulin (sIg) molecules and producing the same but having a more rapid and magnified antibody response to previously encountered antigenic stimulus (secondary immune responses)

The mature B lymphocytes migrate out of the bone marrow into the circulation and the lymphoid tissue, where they continue to mature and function. It is believed that a B cell will die within a few weeks if it does not encounter an antigenic stimulus.

B lymphocyte function. After stimulation with an antigen, the B cell becomes an activated B lymphocyte, capable of proliferating and differentiating into an antibody-secreting cell (plasma cell).

B lymphocytes are the only cells that produce antibodies.

B lymphocytes may also function as *antigen-presenting cells.* This function is possible because B cells can specifically bind an antigen to

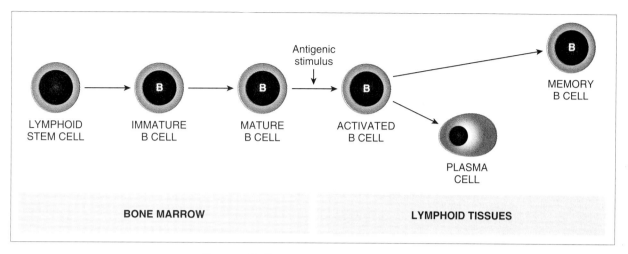

FIGURE **3-9** B Lymphocyte Maturation.

their cell surface immunoglobulins (Ig), which function as antigen receptors (see Box 3-2). The bound antigen is more easily endocytosed, degraded into antigenic peptides, bound to the class II MHC complex on the B cell membrane, and presented to the T helper (CD4+) cells for recognition (see Chapter 1, Figure 1-9). The antigen presentation by B lymphocytes is also an important mechanism in helper T cell–dependent antibody production.

Natural Killer Cells

structure of natural killer cells. The natural killer cells (NK cells) are a third population of lymphocytes. They express the CD2 marker, the Fc receptor for IgG molecule (CD16), the IL-2 receptor, and elaborate tissue necrosis factor (TNF). *These cells are neither T nor B lymphocytes because they lack both the immunoglobulin (Ig) receptors normally present on a B lymphocyte surface and the specific T cell receptors (TCR) for antigen recognition also normally present on the mature, thymus-derived T lymphocytes (CD4+ helper; CD8+ cytotoxic).*

function of natural killer cells. The NK cells are similar in their function to cytotoxic T lymphocytes (CTLs); however, because they lack the TCR present on the CTL, the similarity to the CTL is limited to the cytolytic (cytotoxic) function of the NK cells.

NK cells are activated by the CD4+ helper T cells and differentiate in response to IL-2 stimulation. They differentiate into cells that are capable of lysing or "killing" target cells through a mechanism referred to as *antibody-dependent cell-mediated cytotoxicity (ADCC), which is not MHC restricted. NK cells do not require prior contact with an antigen to develop this cytolytic function,* a characteristic observed in natural (non-specific) immunity (see Chapter 1).

Target cells for NK cell cytolytic activity are certain tumor cells and most cells infected with a virus; thus, the role of NK cells is to eliminate altered or "abnormal" cells.

ACCESSORY CELLS

Accessory cells do not express receptors for antigen recognition but do participate in the initiation of an immune response, described following.

Mononuclear Phagocytes

The mononuclear phagocytes originate in the bone marrow, where they develop into partially differentiated cells (immature macrophages), known as *monocytes* before entry into the blood circulation and subsequently into distant tissues. Within the tissues, monocytes acquire surface receptors for antibodies (FcR) and for certain complement components (CR) and become both fixed and free (mobile) tissue macrophages (MQ), also known as *phagocytes.*

In general, tissue macrophages are named after the tissue where they remain (i.e., Kupffer cells in the liver and alveolar macrophages in the lungs, among others).

Functional Characteristics of Phagocytes

The participation of mononuclear phagocytes in natural and specific immunity has been well defined (Box 3-2). They function mainly as:

- *Effector cells and phagocytes* in both the natural and specific immune responses
- *Accessory cells* (antigen-presenting cells [APCs]) in the specific immune response

---

Box 3-2 FUNCTION OF MONONUCLEAR PHAGOCYTES IN NATURAL AND SPECIFIC IMMUNE RESPONSES

Natural Immunity
- Phagocytosis and antigen degradation
- Elaboration of mediators (prostaglandins)
- Elaboration of enzymes
- Production of cytokines
- Production of growth factor

Specific Immunity
- Amplification of immune response of foreign particles
- Acting as antigen-presenting cells (APCs)
- Elaboration of soluble and membrane molecules for T cell activation
- Phagocytosis of opsonized (antibody-coated) particles

---

effector cells. Mononuclear phagocytes may function as effectors cells because of their ability to *elaborate such substances as complement, prostaglandin, and other mediators* that help control infection. These soluble mediators may also provide a communication network between the macrophages and stimulated lymphocytes, thus serving as effector cells in a variety of immune responses.

phagocytic cells. The mononuclear phagocytes also function as body "scavengers," phagocytosing not only foreign substances they encounter but also injured or dead self tissue, such as aged (senescent) red blood cells. The phagocytosed material is degraded within the cell by lysosomal enzymes during a process of antigen elimination that takes place in natural immunity.

Phagocytosis is the principal mechanism by which the body is protected from various microbes and antigenic substances (Figure 3-10; see also Chapter 1, Figure 1-4). Recently, it has been speculated that the spread of cancer (metastasis) may be halted by a greater degree of tissue infiltration with macrophages; however, the data is not conclusive.

Another important function of phagocytic cells is the presentation of degraded antigenic material to the T lymphocyte for recognition (see discussion following).

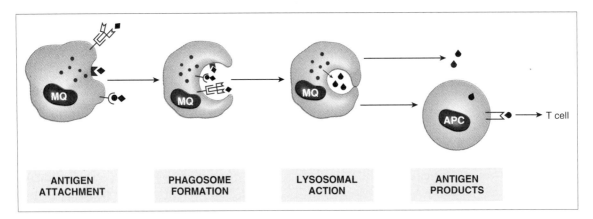

| ANTIGEN ATTACHMENT | PHAGOSOME FORMATION | LYSOSOMAL ACTION | ANTIGEN PRODUCTS |

FIGURE **3-10** **Phagocytosis.** Extracellular antigen attaches to receptors on phagocytic cells (macrophages) and is engulfed and processed (degraded) by lysosomal action within the formed phagosome. The degraded product (peptides) is expressed bound to surface MHC on the phagocytic (serving also as APC) cell surface as MHC-peptide complex for recognition by T cells (cell-mediated immunity). Free degraded antigen (peptides) and unaltered (unprocessed) antigen may also bind with B cell receptors (humoral immunity). *MQ*, macrophage.

antigen-presenting cells. There are two types of antigen-presenting cells.

- *Mononuclear phagocytes:* As antigen-presenting cells (APCs), mononuclear phagocytes have the ability to phagocytose a variety of foreign antigens, process them, and display the degraded foreign antigens on their surface for recognition by antigen-specific T lymphocytes (CD4+ and CD8+ T cells). *The recognition and response occurs only if the antigen is complexed to a MHC molecule on an APC that the T cells recognize as self-MHC.* This recognition mechanism is known as *MHC restriction* (see One Step Further Box 3-3). *The self-MHC refers to the MHC present on the APC not on the T lymphocyte.*
- *Dendritic cells:* Another type of antigen-presenting cell (APC) located in the spleen and lymph nodes are the dendritic cells. These cells are derived from the bone marrow and may be related to the mononuclear phagocytic lineage.

  Dendritic cells participate in immune reactions through the presentation of protein antigen to the helper T cells, thus serving as APCs. It is possible that they may also be involved in T cell responses to foreign MHC in tissue transplants.

Granulocytes

Granulocytes have the ability to participate both in natural and specific immune responses as effector cells, "inflammatory" cells, and phagocytic cells.

Three types of granulocytes that have been identified in the blood according to the staining characteristics of their granules and the morphology of their nuclei are (1) **neutrophils,** (2) **eosinophils,** and (3) **basophils** (Box 3-3).

Neutrophils (Polymorphonuclear Leukocytes)

Neutrophils express surface receptors (FcR) for antibodies and for complement components (CR). This is an important feature in phagocytosis of opsonized particles and in complement activation (see Figure 4-1, Chapter 4).

As part of humoral immunity, the neutrophils function as "effector cells."

Eosinophils

These cells are most effective in eliminating such foreign agents as helminths. In response to the parasitic stimulus, the immune system produces antibodies (IgE) that can bind to Fc receptors for IgE on the surface of the eosinophil and cause degranulation of its cytoplasmic content. The released substances adversely affect the parasite. This mechanism is observed when the stimulating antigen, such as a parasite, is too large to be phagocytosed. The eosinophils are also capable of directly binding to the parasite at the site of infection through their Fc receptors for antibodies coating the parasite.

As effector cells in an immune response, eosinophils are present at the site of *immediate hypersensitivity* ("allergic reaction"), where

---

MAJOR FUNCTIONAL CHARACTERISTICS OF POLYMORPHONUCLEAR LEUKOCYTES

Box **3-3**

Neutrophils
- Effector cells in humoral immunity
- Respond to chemotactic stimuli
- React to cytokines produced by mononuclear phagocytes
- Major cell population in inflammatory response
- Phagocytose opsonized particles
- Have major cell receptors: Fc and complement

Eosinophils
- Effector cells in immune response to parasites and "allergic reactions" (immediate hypersensitivity)
- Abundant at site of immediate hypersensitivity reaction
- Their growth and differentiation stimulated by T cell–derived cytokines
- Have Fc receptors for IgE molecules

Basophils
- Effector cells in IgE-mediated immediate hypersensitivity
- Have high-affinity receptors for IgE; bind IgE molecules
- Stimulated by IgE to release mediators of immediate hypersensitivity

they contribute to the inflammatory reaction and tissue damage (discussed in Chapter 1).

Basophils

Basophils are found in a small number in the blood and have membrane-enclosed granules, containing heparin and other anaphylactic substances that cause symptoms of allergy. Mast cells, it is believed, are the tissue counterparts of basophils, although their relationship has not been well defined. Both cells express high-affinity receptors for IgE molecules, binding free IgE found in blood.

Stimulation with an antigen (usually allergen) attracts IgE molecules to the IgE receptor on the basophil, where they form clusters and cause the basophil or mast cell to degranulate. The released inflammatory and vasoactive mediators such as histamines, stored in these granules, cause a vascular and inflammatory response *(immediate hypersensitivity)*.

The response is referred to as an *allergic reaction* (discussed in Chapter 7), resulting in tissue injury and inflammation (see Chapter 1).

Suggested Readings

Abbas AK, Lichtman AH, Pober JS: Cells and tissues of the immune system. In *Cellular and molecular immunology,* Philadelphia, 2000, WB Saunders.

Ada G: Twenty years into the saga of MHC-restriction, *Immunol Biol* 72:447-454, 1994.

Bodmer JG, Marsh SGE, Parham P, et al: Nomenclature for factors of the HLA system, *Tiss Antig* 51:214, 1997.

Caruso I, Caruso EM, Signo P: Laboratory tests in immunology, *JIFCC* 6:124-130, 1994.

Ikuta K, Uchida N, Friedman J, Weissmen IL: Lymphocyte development from stem cells, *Annu Rev Immunol* 10:759-783, 1992.

Julius M, Maroun CR, Haugn L: Distinct roles for CD4 and CD8 as co-receptors in antigen receptor signalling, *Immunol Today* 14:177-181, 1993.

Mackay CR: Immunological memory, *Advan Immunol* 53:217-265, 1993.

Schlossman SF, Boumsell L, Gilks W, et al: CD antigens, *Immunol Today* 15:98-99, 1994.

Review Questions

LYMPHOID TISSUE

1. All of the following are main components of the immune response *except:*
   a. lymphoid tissue
   b. lymphocytes and accessory cells
   c. cytokines
   d. leukocytes and red blood cells

2. Cells of the immune system are localized in a variety of lymphoid tissues and organs. Select an organ that is *not* a component of lymphoid tissue *in an adult:*
   a. thymus
   b. spleen
   c. bone marrow
   d. liver

3. T lymphocytes mature in one of the following lymphoid tissues:
   a. thymus
   b. bone marrow
   c. lymph nodes
   d. circulating blood

4. T cell surface receptors (TCRs), used to identify the phenotype of a T lymphocytes, are acquired in the:
   a. spleen
   b. thymus
   c. thyroid
   d. bone marrow

5. Elimination of cells capable of reacting with self-antigens is referred to as:
   a. self-clone rejection
   b. self-discrimination
   c. clonal rejection
   d. clonal selection

6. Select the site where recognition of a "foreign" antigen occurs in a primary immune response:
   a. thymus
   b. bone marrow
   c. spleen
   d. lymph nodes

7. All of the following immune responses occur in the lymph nodes *except:*
   a. development of antibody-producing plasma cells
   b. secretion of cytokines
   c. development of T or B memory cells
   d. development of helper T cells
   e. "clearing" the blood of aging blood cells

8. T and B memory cells are stored in the following site, where they are ready to respond to a previously encountered antigenic stimulus:
   a. spleen
   b. bone marrow
   c. lymph nodes
   d. thymus
   e. mucosal tissue

9. Select the location of an immune response directed against blood-borne antigens:
   a. peripheral lymphoid tissue
   b. spleen
   c. thymus
   d. blood

CELLULAR COMPONENTS

10. The primary function(s) of cells and/or various mediators of the immune response is (are):
    a. recognition of foreign antigens
    b. inactivation or elimination of an antigenic stimulus
    c. secretion of antibodies
    d. production of effector cells and mediators
    e. all of the above

11-13. Match the following cells of the immune system with their function:

    ____ basophils
    ____ eosinophils
    ____ neutrophils

    a. act as effector cells in immune response to parasites
    b. phagocytose opsonized particles
    c. release mediators of immediate hypersensitivity
    d. act as antigen-presenting cells

14. Lymphocytes may be stimulated to proliferate by antigenic products and by which of the following:
    a. complement
    b. mitogens
    c. opsonins
    d. cytokines

15-18. Match the following classes of lymphocytes with their specific phenotypic cell markers:

    ____ cytotoxic T   a. CD8+
         cells   b. CD16 and
    ____ B lymphocytes   CD56
    ____ helper T cells   c. CD19+
    ____ natural killer   d. CD4+
         cells

19. CD system is used to classify human leukocytes. Define the abbreviation *CD:*
    _____.

20. Select receptors are involved in the *specific* recognition of foreign antigens. Select all that apply:
    a. T cell receptors (TCRs)
    b. major histocompatibility complex (MHC)
    c. surface immunoglobulins (sIg)
    d. Fc receptors

21. All of the following are accessory cells of the immune system *except*:
    a. plasma cells
    b. mononuclear phagocytes
    c. neutrophils
    d. basophils

22. Certain cells of the immune system are capable of *specific recognition* of any antigen. Select all that apply:
    a. B cells
    b. T cells
    c. mononuclear phagocytes
    d. NK cells

23-32. Match the following subsets of T cells with their specific characteristics. Select all that apply:

    a. helper T cell
    b. cytotoxic T cell

    ____ CD8+, CD4−
    ____ class II MHC restricted
    ____ T cell receptor (TCR)
    ____ CD3 receptor
    ____ involved in graft rejections
    ____ CD4+, CD8−
    ____ class I MHC restricted
    ____ mature in bone marrow
    ____ destroy target cells
    ____ promote antibody secretion

33. The major histocompatibility complex (MHC) binds a variety of foreign antigenic peptides and presents them for specific recognition. Select the cells that display the MHC-peptide complex:
    a. antigen-presenting cells
    b. mononuclear phagocytes
    c. virally infected cells
    d. all of the above

34. T cells are capable of circulating between the blood and the various tissues of the immune system *except*:
    a. lymphoid organs
    b. blood circulation
    c. central nervous system
    d. mucosal lymphoid tissue

35. Mononuclear cells are non-lymphoid cells that participate both in natural and acquired (specific) immune responses. In both responses they:
    a. show specificity for any antigen
    b. do not show specificity for any antigen
    c. play the same role
    d. function as antigen-presenting cells

36. The only cells with the ability to produce antibodies are the:
    a. B cell lineage
    b. T cell lineage
    c. mononuclear phagocytes
    d. helper T cells

37. Mononuclear phagocytes participate in immune responses through all the following mechanisms *except*:
    a. phagocytosis
    b. elaboration of mediators
    c. secretion of antibody molecules
    d. antigen presentation for recognition

38. Natural killer (NK) cells have all the following characteristics *except:*
    a. are neither T or B cells
    b. have specific T cell receptors
    c. are cytotoxic (cytolytic)
    d. eliminate tumor and virally infected cells

39. Receptors for surface-bound C3 fragments are best characterized as including the following functions:
    a. clearance of immune complexes
    b. enhancement of phagocytosis
    c. opsonization
    d. all of the above

40. Select the membrane receptor that is expressed on monocytes and macrophages and that has the ability to bind with an antibody to produce or enhance a variety of biologic responses:
    a. Fc receptor (FcR)
    b. T cell receptor (TCR)
    c. surface immunoglobulin (sIg)
    d. major histocompatibility complex (MHC)

41. Mononuclear phagocytes have the ability to phagocytose foreign antigens and display them for recognition by helper T cells. The phagocytes performing this function are referred to as:
    a. macrocytes
    b. antigen-presenting cells
    c. inflammatory cells
    d. antigen-processing cells

Soluble Components of the Immune System

Upon completion of Chapter 4, the student will be prepared to:

CYTOKINES
- List three cytokines involved in specific immune response that regulate lymphocyte growth and differentiation.
- Describe three ways in which cytokines function as signals in host defense against an antigen.

ANTIBODIES
- Describe three functions of an antibody molecule.

COMPLEMENT SYSTEM
- Describe the similarities between the classical and alternative complement activation pathways.
- Identify the activation pathway involved in the following: cell lysis, initiation of complement cascade by antigen/antibody complex, and formation of membrane attack complex (MAC).
- Name two biologic effects of complement fragments.
- Describe the events in each complement activation pathway, indicating the point of convergence and complement components involved in the final lytic sequence (MAC).
- Explain the mechanism of cell lysis.

Key Terms

antibodies - Also known as *immunoglobulins (Igs)*. They are a group of serum proteins (globulins), secreted in a "soluble" form by B lymphocyte lineage in response to antigenic stimuli. These antigen-specific antibodies bind with the stimulating antigen, thus inactivating it.

complement components - Complement components are a group of plasma proteins produced by sequential activation of complement. They function as effector molecules in the body's defense mechanisms (i.e., natural and specific immune responses), causing such biologic effects as cell lysis and chemotaxis.

complement pathway - Sequential activation and assembly of a series of complement components in plasma, which leads to binding of terminal components of the pathway to form the membrane attack complex (MAC) that causes cell lysis. Two complement activation pathways are operable in plasma, the *classical* and *alternative*.

cytokines - Soluble protein molecules secreted by cells of the immune system in response to an antigenic stimulation. They serve mainly as signals and mediators in cell-to-cell communication during humoral and cell-mediated immune responses.

cytolysis - Lysis or destruction of target cells.

opsonization - A process of attaching an opsonin (e.g., antibody or complement fragment) to the surface of an antigen to enhance phagocytosis.

soluble mediators - Protein molecules (cytokines, antibodies, and complement components) secreted by cells of the immune system. They serve as specific signals and/or components that promote interactions occurring during an immune response.

---·-•-•-•-·---

Soluble components of the immune system, involved in both non-specific (natural) and specific (acquired) immunity, consist of a diverse group of soluble molecules secreted by a variety of cells. The following soluble molecules are included:
- **Cytokines:** soluble mediators of immune responses
- **Immunoglobulins (antibody molecules):** effector molecules of humoral immunity
- **Complement components:** effector molecules of natural and specific immunity

Detection of the listed soluble molecules in the clinical immunology laboratory has been limited mainly to serum *immunoglobulins* and *complement* (see Indications for Laboratory Testing in Chapter 8 and Complement Assays in Chapter 14).

Box 4-1

Cytokines

Nomenclature

Originally, cytokines were known as *lymphokines* (mediators released by lymphocytes) and *interleukins* (mediators released by leukocytes [e.g., T cells and macrophages] and interacting with other leukocytes). In an attempt to standardize the nomenclature, interleukins were assigned an IL number. The term **cytokines** evolved with the understanding that these mediators act as signals or chemical messengers between leukocytes and other cells.

Mechanism of Action

The stimulating cytokines are synthesized by a variety of cells in response to an antigen. The secretion of cytokines is brief and self-limiting. They exert their effect either at the site of the stimulus ("autocrine" action), where they bind to cytokine receptors on the surface of a target cell that secreted them, or they may enter the circulatory system and act at a distant site ("endocrine" action). The signal from the bound cytokine is transferred to the interior of the target cell (nucleus), changing the gene expression. This may result in expression of new functions, proliferation of the target cell, or increased expression of cytokine receptors.

Functions

Cytokines function primarily as signals, communicating information between the various cells involved in an immune response, producing effects that include:

- Regulation of B and T cells and their responses by affecting their activation, growth, and differentiation
- Production of memory cells
- Switching of Ig classes in B cells
- Enhancement of destruction of virally infected or tumor cells
- Activation of inflammatory leukocytes and placement under T cell regulation
- Stimulation of bone marrow progenitor cells (colony-stimulating factors) to grow and their differentiation into specific cell lineage, thus increasing the cell pool
- Providing amplification mechanisms that enable a small number of cells to respond to any one antigen

These functional characteristics have been determined primarily through in vitro studies (tissue cultures).

Discussion of cytokines, antibodies, and complement in this chapter is for completeness and is intended to provide an overview of these components of the immune system. For a more detailed discussion of cytokines and complement (beyond the scope of this book) refer to suggested readings (end of chapter). Discussion of immunoglobulins (antibodies) is contained in Chapter 5.

CYTOKINES

Cytokines are a group of proteins (polypeptides) that are produced (upon recognition of an antigen by the immune system) by different cell populations and affect different target cells (One Step Further Box 4-1). However, their biologic action may overlap so that the functional classification of cytokines is not absolute (see discussion following).

Cytokines have been classified into three main functional groups according to their principal action during an immune response:

- *Mediators and regulators of non-specific immune responses* (e.g., TNFα, IL-1, IL-12, IFN-γ): The major physiologic function of these cytokines is mediation of non-specific immune responses and inflammation (local and systemic).
- *Mediators and regulators of specific immune responses* (e.g., IL-2, IL-4, IL-5, IFN-γ): These cytokines regulate lymphocyte growth/differentiation and activation of effector cells (macrophages, eosinophils, mast cells).
- *Regulators of hematopoiesis* (e.g., IL-3, IL-7, and colony-stimulating factors [CSF]: GM-CSF and M-CSF): See One Step Further Box 3-1.

These soluble molecules exert their effect (i.e., promotion or inhibition of proliferation of specific target cells) in conjunction with other

Table 4-1	SELECTED CYTOKINES OF THE IMMUNE SYSTEM		
Cytokine	Origin	Target Cell	Effect on Immune Response
IL-2	T cell	T cell, NK cell	Proliferation of antigen-specific cells and other immature cells (e.g., NK)
IL-3 (CSF)	T cell (CD4+)	Progenitor cells (BM)	Growth/differentiation of all cell types
IL-4	T cell (CD4+)	B cell	Stimulation of Ig heavy chain switching to IgE isotype
		T cell	Development and differentiation of T cells
IL-5	T cell	B cell	Growth and differentiation of eosinophils
		Eosinophil	Activation of mature eosinophils
IL-7	Stroma cell (BM)	Lymphocyte	Growth factor (generate pre-B and pre-T cells)
IL-10	MQ, T cell	MQ, T cell	Inhibition of MQ function, control of immune response
IL-15	MQ, others	NK cell, T cell	Proliferation
Type 1 IFN-α	MQ	All cells	Anti-viral interferes with viral replication
Type 1 IFN-γ	Fibroblasts	NK cell	Activation
TNF	MQ, T cell	Leukocyte, endothelial cells	Activation/inflammatory process
TGF-β	T cell, MQ, other cells	T cell	Inhibit activation and proliferation of lymphocytes, inhibit activation of MQs
		Other	
		MQ	

IL, interleukin; *NK,* natural killer; *CSF,* colony-stimulating factor; *IFN,* interferon; *MQ,* macrophage; *TNF,* tumor necrosis factor; *TGF-β,* transforming growth factor; *BM,* bone marrow; *Ig,* immunoglobulin.

signals and mediators (Table 4-1). Based on their previous encounter, the target cells receiving the signal translate the information provided and respond accordingly through the cell-mediated or humoral immune system (see One Step Further Box 4-1).

ANTIBODIES

Antibodies, also known as *immunoglobulins (Igs),* are a group of proteins (globulins) found on the B cell surface and in serum and other body fluids. Thus the immunoglobulin (Ig) molecules that are secreted by B cells and that are attached to their surface serve as the Ig surface receptors and B cell markers. The soluble (free) immunoglobulins are secreted by plasma cells (antibody-secreting cells of the B cell lineage [i.e., differentiated B lymphocyte]) into body fluids where they can bind with an antigen with the same specificity. The structure and function of these immunoglobulin molecules are briefly discussed following and in greater detail in Chapter 5.

STRUCTURE

The immunoglobulin molecule has two distinct regions, one of which (Fab) contains an antigen-binding site that binds to an antigen, whereas the other (Fc) contains receptors that interact with a variety of components of the immune system such as complement and phagocytes (see Chapter 5, Figure 5-8) and is responsible for the various biologic functions.

The various classes of immunoglobulin molecules are similar in their basic structure but have a large diversity in their antigen-binding region and biologic functions. This diversity in antigen specificity accounts for their almost limitless ability to distinguish between various antigenic substances (see Generation of Antibody Diversity, Chapter 5).

FUNCTION

The main function of soluble antibodies (immunoglobulins [Igs]) is to bind foreign antigens showing the same specificity, thereby inactivating or removing the antigenic stimulus.

Antibodies may also bind with the Fc surface receptor on the various cells of the immune system (e.g., MQs and neutrophils) through their Fc region of the molecule (see Figure 5-8, Chapter 5), thus directly interacting with these cells. And, finally, antibodies may serve as opsonins (Figure 4-1), enhancing phagocytosis of the opsonized antigen (see discussion following).

Binding of Antigens by Antibodies

Antibodies that are bound to the membrane of a B lymphocyte (*known as surface immunoglobulin (sIg) receptors*) serve as B cell receptors (BCRs) that may specifically bind with various antigens (see One Step Further Box 3-2).

Binding of antigens to these surface antibodies on a B cell and recognition of B cell–bound antigen by CD4+ T cells triggers a specific humoral immune response.

Free (circulating) antibodies have the ability to bind with an unprocessed (intact) antigen that exhibits the same specificity as the antibody (see Antigen Recognition and Binding, Chapter 5). This results in formation of antigen-antibody (Ag/Ab) complexes and removal or inactivation of the antibody-bound antigen. The formed Ag/Ab complexes can be detected and the antigen and/or antibody identified by methods available in the clinical immunology laboratory (described in Chapters 11 to 14).

Opsonization

Opsonins are molecules that attach to an organism (microbe) and promote or enhance phago-cytosis (see Figure 3-10, Chapter 3). This process is known as *opsonization* (Figure 4-1). Opsonins can be recognized by surface receptors on a phagocytic cell (e.g., macrophage or neutrophil). The most efficient opsonin is the immunoglobulin G (IgG), which is recognized by the Fcγ receptor on the phagocyte and which greatly increases phagocytosis. Other potent opsonins are the components of the complement system, particularly C3 fragments, which are recognized by the CR1 (CD35) receptor on the phagocytic cell. Complement fragments are produced during activation of either the classical or alternative pathways (discussed following).

COMPLEMENT SYSTEM

The *complement system* is defined as a group of plasma and membrane proteins (complement fractions) that, when activated, produce several effects associated with humoral immune responses. These effects include immune adherence, opsonization, chemotaxis, kinin activation, cell lysis, and inflammation (anaphylatoxis).

Because the complement system lacks specificity, it has the capability of participating in both the natural and specific immune responses.

STRUCTURE

Complement components (C), found in plasma and as membrane proteins, can be identified

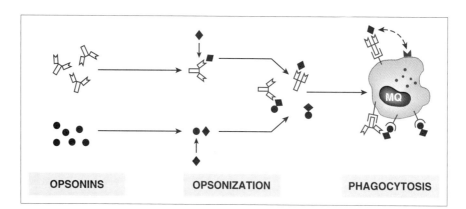

OPSONINS   **OPSONIZATION**   **PHAGOCYTOSIS**

FIGURE **4-1**   **Opsonization.**   Antibodies and/or complement fragments (C3b, C4b) may serve as opsonins by binding to antigens independently or together. This process of opsonization (coating) enhances binding of opsonized antigen to Fc and/or complement receptors on the surface of a macrophage (MQ), thus enhancing phagocytosis.

within the major fraction of the β1 and β2 globulin region of the plasma proteins by electrophoretic technique (see Chapters 5 and 11,
Figure 5-9).

The complement components are normally
present in blood in an *inactive form (zymo-
gens)*. When the complement system is activated through a series of steps of the classical
pathway or the alternative pathway (One Step
Further Box 4-2), the inactive protein molecules are converted by proteolysis (protein
hydrolysis) to *active enzymes,* known as *pro-
teases.* An active enzyme is then capable of
cleaving and activating the next protein in
the activation pathway and so on, thus creating a cascade or "waterfall" effect (see Figure
4-2).

Complement Activation

There are two interrelated enzyme cascades
(pathways) involved in the activation of complement (see One Step Further Box 4-2):
- **Classical pathway**
- **Alternative pathway**

*The activation of either of these two path-
ways leads to events that produce biologically
active fractions of complement (Table 4-2),
which serve as effector molecules in the
various defense mechanisms of the natural
and specific immune system* (discussed in
Chapter 1).

Destruction of Complement In Vitro

Complement components are heat labile (sensitive to heat) because of their protein composition. Thus, when exposed to heat, their biologic activity is inhibited. Substances that
function as anticoagulants (e.g., EDTA) may
also serve as complement inhibitors.

*In both situations, the complement is pre-
vented from (1) being activated, (2) exerting
its lytic effect, and (3) exerting other biologic
effects.*

FUNCTION

Two categories of defense mechanisms in
which the complement components participate
in are:
- **Biologic effects (opsonization, chemotaxis)**
- **Cell lysis**

Biologic Effects of Complement Fragments

The effect of the biologically active fragments
(Table 4-3) is through their binding to specific complement receptors (CR) on various
cell surfaces. These major effects include the
following mechanisms.

Bacterial Opsonization

A process of coating surface of bacteria by opsonins (C3b and/or IgG) for more effective
phagocytosis. The opsonization occurs when:
- C3b binds to the bacteria through its C3b
receptor
- Antibodies (IgG) bind to the Fc receptor
on a phagocyte
- Both the C3b and antibodies bind to the
bacteria and/or phagocyte

The most effective opsonization processes
occur when both the C3b and the antibodies
are involved (see Figure 4-1).

Chemotaxis

During inflammation, accompanied by tissue
damage and complement activation by an infectious agent, certain chemotactic substances
(peptides) are also released at the site of inflammation (see Chapter 1 and One Step Further
Box 1-1). *The most important of these chemotactic peptides is the C5a complement component.* C5a attracts both neutrophils and monocytes (inflammatory cells) from capillaries
to the site of inflammation. These inflammatory cells migrate by diapedesis (mobility by
pseudopodia) to the site of inflammation, where
they participate in phagocytosis and other
immune reactions. The process of attracting
"inflammatory" cells to the site of inflammation
is referred to as *chemotaxis* (Figure 4-4).

Cell Lysis

Cell lysis is an important defense mechanism
developed by the humoral immune system
against microbes (extracellular antigens). Production of specific antibodies during a humoral
immune response to a microbial antigen results
in binding of the antigen and forming an
antigen/antibody complex on its surface (cell
surface). The antigen/antibody complex, in
turn, activates the classical complement pathway (see One Step Further Box 4-2), thus
producing a variety of biologically active

Box 4-2

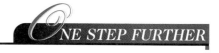

Complement Activation

The activation of complement may proceed through either of two enzymatic pathways, also known as *cascades* (Figure 4-2):

- The **classical pathway,** first to be discovered, is activated by immune complexes (antigen/antibody complex)
- The **alternative pathway** is primarily activated by polysaccharide (microbial) structures

Both pathways lead to cleavage of C5 and converge in a common assembly of the membrane attack complex (MAC), a C5b to C9 sequence, responsible for cell lysis (Figure 4-3).

The Classical Pathway of Complement Activation

The sequence of activation is as follows: C1→ C4→ C2→ C3→ C5→ C6→ C7→ C8→ C9.

The initiation of the classical pathway occurs when C1q of the C1 complex (C1q, C1r, C1s), an interlocking enzyme system, binds to the IgG or IgM of the antigen/antibody complex (immune complex).

A **cascade sequence** follows binding of antibody to the C1 complex,

1. C1 binds to the antibody of the immune complex and cleaves C4 and C2 components, producing C4a, C4b, C2a, C2b, respectively (C2b and C4a are unstable molecules and are lost).
2. C4b fragment acts as a binding site for the C2a molecule.
3. C4b, C2a complex is formed, serving as the enzyme C3 convertase.
4. C3 convertase cleaves the C3 component to the C3b fragment (C3a fragment is lost).
5. C3 convertase becomes C5 convertase (C4b, C2a, C3b) when C3b fragment is added.

Alternative Pathway of Complement Activation

The alternative pathway is activated by C3b binding to various activating surfaces, such as the microbial membrane polysaccharides, as follows:

1. C3 molecule, normally present in blood plasma, is the first molecule to be activated through spontaneous hydrolysis, resulting in the C3b fragment (C3a is lost).
2. The activated C3b molecule binds to the surface of a microorganism and leads to the subsequent binding of Factor B, in the presence of Factor D, resulting in formation of C3 convertase (C3b, Bb).
3. The C3 convertase enzyme cleaves more C3 molecules, producing additional C3b fragments.
4. C3b binds to C3 convertase enzymes (C3b, Bb complex), changing them to C5 convertases (C3b, Bb, C3b).

Convergence of Pathways

The C5 convertases (C4b, C2a, C3b complex) emerging from the two separate complement activation pathways catalyze the proteolytic cleavage of the C5 protein producing C5b fragment.

Production of the C5b is the point at which both pathways converge and share the same final steps.

The final sequence of the complement activation cascade does not involve enzymatic events but a sequential and consecutive binding of soluble complement proteins (C6, C7, C8, and C9) to the activating surface of the initiating stimulus. The **resulting membrane attack complex (MAC), consisting of complement fragments C5b through C9,** forms at the cell membrane of a target cell that displays the initiating stimulus (immune complexes or microbial polysaccharides). MAC is responsible for creating pores in the cell membrane of the target cell that cause cell lysis (see Figure 4-3).

Regulation of Pathways

The regulation or inhibition of the complement activation events is through naturally occurring proteins (inhibitors) in serum. For example, C1 INH inhibits the action of C1 by binding to C1s and C1r, thereby dissociating them from the C1 complex (C1q, C1r, C1s). Most studied inhibitors include: C1INH (C1 inhibitor), factor I (C3b inactivator), factor H (binds C3 band, displaces Bb), C4bp (C4 binding protein).

Box 4-2—cont'd

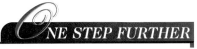

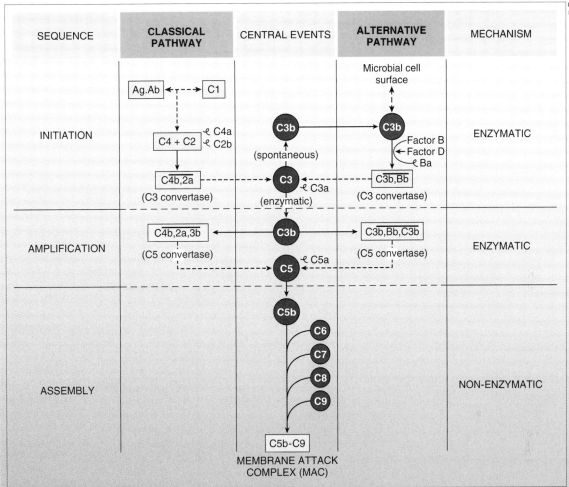

FIGURE **4-2** **Activation of Complement.** The complement activation process, referred to as a "cascade," may proceed through two separate pathways that consist of several steps involving sequential enzymatic action by generated complement (C) fragments. Assembly (non-enzymatic) of these fragments (C5b, C6, C7, C8, and polymerized C9) form a membrane attack complex (MAC) that produces cell destruction (lysis, see also Figure 4-3). *Initiation: Classical pathway* activation occurs when C1 (C1q, C1r, C1s) binds to an antibody (IgG or IgM) of an antigen-antibody complex. *Alternative pathway* is initiated by binding of C3b to the microbial surface and production of C3 convertase. *Amplification:* In both pathways, C3b becomes C5 convertase that binds to the target cell membrane (microbe), with production of additional C3b molecules (C3b is amplified). C5 convertase splits C5 to produce C5b, a point where the two pathways converge. *Assembly:* C5b binds C6, C7, C8, and C9, thus generating the membrane attack complex (MAC). Central events occur in both activation pathways.

Continued

Box 4-2—cont'd

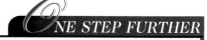

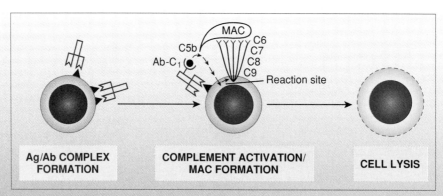

| Ag/Ab COMPLEX FORMATION | COMPLEMENT ACTIVATION/ MAC FORMATION | CELL LYSIS |

FIGURE **4-3**   Cell Lysis.   Antibody attaches to the target cell surface antigen to form an antigen/antibody complex. This complex can activate complement by a series of enzymatic actions (see Figure 4-2) that produce C5b fragments. C5b fragments bind C6 and C7 to form C5b, C6, C7 complex, which attaches to the target cell membrane (at the site of activity). C8 attaches to the complex, penetrates the membrane, and polymerizes C9. These events produce the membrane attack complex (MAC) (C5b to C9) that forms pores in the cell membrane, causing its destruction (cell lysis).

Table 4-2 COMPARISON OF COMPLEMENT ACTIVATION PATHWAYS

	Classical Pathway	Alternative Pathway
Initiation (activation)	Antigen/antibody complex	Microbial surface polysaccharide
Recognition of antigen	C3b fragment	C3b fragment
C3 cleavage (in plasma)	C3 convertase	C3 convertase
C3 convertase	C4b, C2a	C3b, Bb
C5 cleavage (in plasma)	C5 convertase	C5 convertase
C5 convertase	C4b, C2a, C3b	C3b, Bb, C3b
Membrane attack (on cell surface)	C5 through C9	C5 through C9

complement fragments. These fragments produce cell lysis as well as other biologic effects, discussed in this section.

Cell lysis or destruction of the target microorganism occurs when the classical complement pathway is activated by an antigen/antibody complex on the cell surface of a target cell.

The final sequence of the activated classical pathway produces complement components (C5 through C9) known as the *membrane attack complex (MAC)*. MAC inserts into the surface membrane of the target cell or organism that contains the antigen/antibody complex, causing cell lysis (cytolysis) and its destruction (see Figure 4-3).

Mechanism of Osmotic Cell Lysis

The mechanism involved in osmotic cell lysis of the target cell is as follows: when MAC inserts into the cell surface membrane of the target cell, pores form that allow passage of water and small molecules (e.g., Ca++ ions) out of the cytoplasm of the target cell. The large molecules remain, creating a concentration gradient that results in an entry of water molecules into the cytoplasm to maintain an equilibrium between the interior and exterior of the cell. The entry of water molecules into cytoplasm causes swelling and cell lysis.

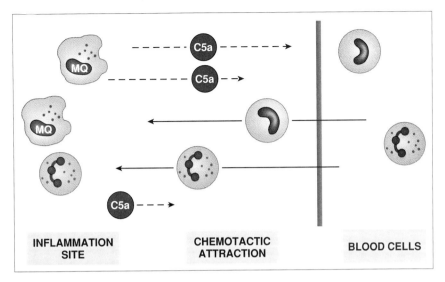

FIGURE **4-4**   **Chemotaxis.**   Release of chemotactic peptides (C5a is most effective) attracts phagocytes (monocytes and neutrophils [PMN]) from blood into the site of inflammation. PMNs remain at the site. The monocytes become macrophages (MQ) and may leave the site by entering secondary lymphoid tissue to function as antigen-presenting cells (APCs). *PMN*, polymorphonuclear neutrophil.

Table 4-3	MAJOR FUNCTIONS OF SELECTED COMPLEMENT COMPONENTS
Components	Function
C5 through C9 (MAC)	Cell lysis (MAC forms membrane pores)
C3b, iC3b, or C4b	Bacterial opsonization and phagocytosis (C binding to CR on neutrophils/macrophages)
C5a	Chemotaxis (attraction of "inflammatory" cells)
C3b	B cell activation, removal of immune complexes (complex-bound C binds to CR on RBC, cleared by liver/spleen)

MAC, membrane attack complex; *C*, complement component; *CR*, complement receptor; *RBC*, red blood cell (erythrocyte).

NOMENCLATURE

The names of the various complement components have been designated and categorized according to the complement activation pathway in which they take part.

Classical Pathway and Membrane Attack Complex

Protein molecules of the classical pathway and membrane attack complex are identified by numbers and include:
- Fragments cleaved from the original components, designated by *small letters* (e.g., C3a, small fragment; C3b, large fragment).
- Enzymatically active components (activated) with a *bar designation above the numeral* ($\overline{C1r}$)
- Hemolytically inactive components with a *suffix "i"* (C3bi)

Alternative Pathway

Protein molecules of the alternative pathway are assigned a letter that is preceded by the word *"factor"* or *"F"* (e.g., factor H).

Complement Receptors

These receptors are designated according to the complement molecule they can bind (e.g., C5b receptor binds C5b molecule) (see Chapter 3 and One Step Further Box 3-2).

LABORATORY EVALUATION OF COMPLEMENT

Detection of complement activity and the concentration of its components is performed to establish clinical diagnosis and is discussed in Chapter 14.

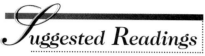
Suggested Readings

Abbas AK, Lichtman AH, Pober JS: Cytokines (pp 235-269) and the complement system (pp 316-331). In *Cellular and molecular immunology,* Philadelphia, 2000, WB Saunders.

Arai K, Lee FA, Miyajima AS, et al: Cytokines: coordinator of immune and inflammatory response, *Annu Rev Biochem* 59:783-836, 1990.

Balkwill F: Cytokines in health and disease, *Immunol Today* 14:149-150, 1993.

Review Questions

CYTOKINES

1. Cytokines are molecules that serve as mediators in the cell-to-cell communication that occurs during an immune response. Select the cells that *do not* secrete these molecules:
   a. B cells
   b. T cells
   c. plasma cells
   d. NK cells

2. Select a mediator of natural immunity that has an anti-viral effect on cells:
   a. gamma interferon
   b. interferon, type 1
   c. tumor necrosis factor
   d. interleukin-2

3. All principal functions listed following can be attributed to cytokine molecules, *except:*
   a. mediators of specific immune response
   b. regulators of hematopoiesis
   c. mediators of non-specific immune responses
   d. regulators of complement activation

4. The effects of cytokines on various cells involved in an immune response include:
   a. activation, growth, and differentiation of T and B cells
   b. switching of Ig classes in B cells
   c. stimulation of progenitor cells to grow and differentiate into a specific cell lineage
   d. all of the above

ANTIBODIES

5. Select the soluble effector molecules of humoral immunity:
   a. cytokines
   b. interleukins
   c. immunoglobulins
   d. complement components

6. Interaction of antibodies with other cells of the immune system occurs through binding of antibodies to the cell surface receptors on these cells. The cell surface receptors are known as:
   a. Il receptors
   b. Fc receptors
   c. Ig receptors
   d. all of the above

7. Select the main function(s) of antibodies:
   a. enhancement of phagocytosis by opsonization
   b. activation of complement

c. removal of antigen by formation of antigen-antibody complexes
d. all of the above

8-10. Match the following functions with the appropriate complement fraction(s). Select *all* that apply:

____ C3b	a. cell lysis
____ C5a	b. bacterial
____ C5b through	opsonization and
C9	phagocytosis
	c. chemotaxis

COMPLEMENT SYSTEM

11. The C3 and C5 complement components are normally present in blood in an inactive form. Select their cleaved products in the classical and alternative activation pathways:
    a. C3a and C5a
    b. C3b and C5b
    c. C3a and C5b
    d. C3b and C5a

12. Both activation pathways converge at the C3b fragment, from which they share the same final steps that culminate in:

a. recognition of C3b
b. membrane attack complex
c. immune complexes
d. recognition of microbial polysaccharides

13. Initiating stimuli in the activation of complement through the classical pathway are the:
    a. repeating microbial polysaccharides
    b. IgG or IgM molecules bound to antigen
    c. C5b binding to antibody
    d. C1q binding to antigen

14. The complement components may be destroyed through all the following in vitro processes, *except:*
    a. removal of Ca++
    b. treatment with heparin
    c. treatment with antibiotics
    d. heating plasma to 56° C for 20 minutes

15. The following functions are associated with the activated complement (select *all* that apply):
    a. chemotactic attraction of phagocytic cells
    b. promotion of phagocytosis
    c. cell lysis
    d. bacterial opsonization

CHAPTER 5

Immunoglobulin Molecules

Learning Objectives

Upon completion of Chapter 5, the student will be prepared to:

HUMORAL IMMUNE RESPONSE

- Describe each event associated with humoral immune response (antibody response), identifying cells and their receptors and the soluble molecules involved in each event.
- List in chronological order, B cell maturation events and differentiation into plasma cells, including anatomic location, class of surface Igs expressed at each stage, point at which gene rearrangement stops, and the stage when class-switching may occur.
- Indicate three ways in which B lymphocytes participate in the humoral immune response.
- Compare the mechanisms used by B cells and T cells to recognize antigens.
- Describe events that occur during B cell–T cell interaction.
- Compare and contrast primary with secondary humoral immune response in terms of class of antibodies produced, extent of response (serum antibody levels), and constant region gene rearrangement (class-switching).

IMMUNOGLOBULIN MOLECULES

- Describe differences in structural and functional characteristics of surface immunoglobulins (sIgs) and the secreted form of immunoglobulins, known as *antibodies.*
- Given a diagram of an immunoglobulin molecule, identify the following components: light and heavy polypeptide chains, constant and variable regions, hypervariable regions, disulfide bonds, carbohydrate units, amino and carboxyl terminals, site of antigen binding, and region associated with biologic activity.
- Describe the structural and functional differences between B lymphocyte surface immunoglobulins (sIgs) and immunoglobulins (antibodies) found in body fluids, such as plasma or serum.
- Explain the difference between immunoglobulin diversity and specificity.
- Describe immunoglobulin heavy chain class-switching in production of different classes of immunoglobulins.

- Discuss the current use of monoclonal antibodies in diagnostic laboratory procedures.
- Define the following key terms: *epitope, exon, gene, genetic coding, isotype.*

FUNCTIONAL CHARACTERISTICS OF IMMUNOGLOBULINS

- List the functions of variable and constant regions of immunoglobulin molecules.
- State biologic (effector) functions for each of the five immunoglobulin classes.
- Describe characteristics of in vitro methods for production of monoclonal antibodies (i.e., hybridization technology and recombinant DNA and PCR method) that make each procedure unique.
- Discuss the use of antibodies as reagents in laboratory procedures for detection of antibodies in serum, detection of antigens within tissues or cells, and identification of surface markers (molecules) in studies of cell populations.
- Explain the importance of pre-transfusion testing for IgM and IgG in blood banking.

Key Terms

allotype - Inherited polymorphic (allelic) variation between individuals of the same species in the heavy chain constant region of an immunoglobulin. For example, different alleles at a particular gene locus are responsible for the expression of several allelic forms of one immunoglobulin isotype (class).

antibodies - Term commonly used to designate soluble effector molecules known as *immunoglobulins (Igs).* Antibodies are produced by plasma cells (B cell lineage) during a humoral immune response to an antigenic stimulation.

antibody diversity - Genetically determined ability of antibodies to specifically bind with an almost limitless variety of antigens.

antibody specificity - Refers to the exact fit or complementarity between an antigen and antibody, which permits their binding to produce an antigen/antibody complex.

antigen-binding site - Located within the heavy and light chain variable region and composed of highly variable amino acid stretches. This variable region is responsible for the immunoglobulin specificity and diversity in specifically binding a variety of antigens.

classes (isotypes) - Five immunoglobulin classes (IgM, IgG, IgA, IgD, IgE) have been defined by their functional (biologic activity) and structural (genetically coded) differences in the constant (C) region of a heavy chain.

clone - Genetically identical lineage of cells, originating from a single cell.

coding (genetic) - Transfer and transcription of information from genetic material (functional genes) by mRNA that determines the sequence of amino acids in a protein (e.g., immunoglobulin) to be synthesized.

constant (C) region - Carboxyl (C) terminal portion of each polypeptide chain. The heavy (H) chain constant region is responsible for biologic activities associated with an antibody molecule.

domain - Globular region of a polypeptide chain within the variable and constant regions of the heavy and light chains of an Ig molecule, resulting from folding of amino acid sequences held together by disulfide bonds (-S-S-).

effectors - Usually refers to cells (e.g., lymphocytes, phagocytes) or soluble molecules (e.g., antibodies) produced during an immune response, which participate in elimination or inactivation of the stimulating antigen (resolution or effector phase of immune response).

epitope - A part of an antigen, also known as an *antigenic determinant,* that binds with a specific antibody.

heterogeneity - Genetic variability, expressed within the structure of an immunoglobulin. The variability is classified as *isotypic, allotypic,* or *idiotypic.*

hinge region - Flexible area of the H chains, located between the first (C_H1) and the second (C_H2) constant region of an Ig molecule, that facilitates its binding with an antigen. Papain enzyme cleaves antibody into Fab and Fc fragments at this area.

hypervariable region - Highly variable area, known as *complementarity-determining region [CDR],* located within the variable region of L and H chains of an immunoglobulin molecule. This is an area of the immunoglobulin molecule where antigen binding actually occurs, sometimes referred to as the "hot spot."

idiotype - Variability within the variable (V) region of an Ig molecule. Idiotypes are unique for each Ig molecule.

immunoglobulin gene - Refers to DNA-encoding polypeptides of the complete heavy (H) and light (L) chains. The two separate genes (H and L) consist of multiple gene segments (exons) that code for the variable (V) and constant (C) regions; other regions are separated by stretches of non-coding DNA (introns).

isotype - Genetically expressed differences (variations) in the constant regions of heavy and light chain Ig classes and subclasses. Genes for these isotypic variants (species-specific variation) are present and may be expressed in all individuals.

J chain - Sequence of polypeptide chains present in polymeric forms of immunoglobulins.

monoclonal antibodies - Homogenous Igs (showing specificity for one antigenic determinant or epitope) derived from a single clone of antibody-secreting cells (B cell line). These homogenous antibodies may be produced (in vitro) by hybridoma technique (defined in Chapter 14, Box 14-1) or molecular cloning.

monomer - Basic structural unit (four polypeptide chains) found in all Ig molecules. Every normal antibody contains at least one monomer within its structure (e.g., IgG class is a monomer).

polyclonal antibodies - Mixture of antibodies (heterogenous antibodies), each antibody showing unique specificity for antigens. These antibodies originate from different clones of antibody-secreting cells (B cell line).

polymeric forms - Consist of more than one basic (monomeric) structural unit of an antibody. For example, the IgM class consists of five monomers (basic structural units) and is known as a *pentamer.* Secretory IgA class is a *dimer* (two monomeric units).

secretory component - Additional polypeptide sequence found only within the secretory immunoglobulin (sIgA), which possibly transports the molecule into body secretions, such as saliva and mucosal secretions.

serology - Diagnostic area of clinical immunology that includes the detection, identification, and quantification of antibodies or antigens in serum.

specificity - Refers to complementarity of an antibody molecule for a particular antigen, which allows the binding of antigen and antibody to occur.

variable (V) region - Amino (N) terminal domain of each light (L) and heavy (H) polypeptide chain of an antibody molecule, showing variation in amino acid sequence that is responsible for antibody diversity in antigen recognition and binding.

– –·–•–●–•–·– –

*I*mmunoglobulins (Igs) and *antibody molecules* are terms that are often used interchangeably. However, for consistency and clarity where possible, the terms will be used as follows:

- *Immunoglobulins (Igs):* Generic designation that refers to all forms of Ig molecules (i.e., secreted antibodies and antigen receptors that are known as *B cell surface immunoglobulins [sIgs]* or *B cell receptors [BCRs]*).
- *Antibodies or antibody molecules:* Refers to secreted forms of Igs that are produced by plasma cells (B cell lineage) and secreted into body fluids, such as blood.

With the understanding that antibodies are specific for an antigen that induced their production and therefore bind only with an antigen that shows the same specificity, new methods employing this concept (specificity in antigen/antibody binding) have become available for the diagnosis of various infections.

It is now possible to identify and quantitate antigen-specific antibodies by using specific antibody/antigen reactions, thus establishing the existence of an infection and monitoring its progress and treatment. Also, in the absence of an overt (manifested) infection, presence of antigen-specific antibodies may be indicative of the presence of immunity, caused by either a previous infection or immunization with a specific antigen.

The focus of this chapter is on a specific response of the immune system (antibody or humoral immune response) to an antigen.

Newer concepts presented include such topics as the role of immunoglobulins in the initiation of an antibody response, the interaction between T and B lymphocytes, use of monoclonal antibodies, antigen-specificity of immunoglobulins, and the basis for antibody diversity.

HUMORAL IMMUNE RESPONSE

We have seen in previous discussions that the ability of the immune system to trigger cell-mediated and humoral immune responses to a foreign antigen depends on its ability to recognize an antigenic configuration as foreign. This function of the immune system is attributed to the T lymphocytes (CD4+ and CD8+ T cells).

In a humoral immune response, helper (CD4+) T cells are required for specific recognition of antigens as foreign or non-self. Antigen recognition is a function of the antigen receptors on T cells, known as *T cell receptors (TCRs)*, and depends on the presence of self-major histocompatibility complex (MHC) located on certain cells of the immune system that function as antigen-presenting cells (APCs).

Macrophages and B lymphocytes are the main APCs in the humoral immune response. These cells first process an antigen and display it on their cell surface as a MHC-peptide complex in order that recognition by the T cells may occur (see also Chapter 1). This type of MHC-restricted antigen recognition by T cells allows the immune system to differentiate between self and non-self molecules, thereby responding only to non-self antigens (see One Step Further Box 3-3).

The sequence of events occurring in the humoral immune response has been previously described in Chapter 1. Briefly, as the CD4+ T cells recognize the antigen and become activated, they elaborate cytokines that activate B cells and induce them to differentiate into antibody-secreting plasma cells. The antibodies that are produced show specificity for the antigen that induced their production.

Thus activation of the humoral immune response and production of antibodies requires B cell activation and differentiation into antibody-secreting cells (plasma cells) by helper T cells (Figure 5-1). Various cytokines and cell receptors participate in these events (i.e., B cell–T cell interaction, see discussion following).

ROLE OF B LYMPHOCYTES IN IMMUNE RESPONSE

As previously described in Chapter 1, B lymphocytes participate in a **humoral immune response** also known as an **antibody response,** as follows:

- By serving as **antigen-presenting cells (APCs)**
- By producing two forms of **immunoglobulin (Ig) molecules** (B cell surface immunoglobulins and secreted immunoglobulins or antibodies)

Antigen Recognition and Binding

Antigen recognition and induction of a humoral immune response is a function of B lymphocytes, helper (CD4+) T lymphocytes, and various cytokines and accessory cells.

B cells participate in the response by specifically binding antigens (unprocessed) by their cell surface immunoglobulin (sIg) receptors, known as **B cell receptors (BCRs),** which show the same specificity as the antigen. The specificity in antigen binding by the BCR may be considered as a form of antigen "recognition."

This antigen "recognition" by BCRs, however, is not MHC restricted and does not trigger an immune response because BCRs do not have the ability to discriminate between self and foreign (non-self) antigens and require "assistance" from CD4+ (helper) T cells. Therefore antigen recognition by B cells is unlike antigen recognition by T cells, which have TCRs located on their surface, with the unique function of specifically recognizing processed foreign (non-self) antigens (MHC-antigenic peptide complex) and triggering an immune response.

B Cell–T Cell Interaction

B cell–T cell interaction is essential for antigen recognition by the immune system and its response to the antigenic stimulus by production of antibodies.

The principal and most sensitive interaction between B and T lymphocytes (see Figure 5-1) is through the B cell surface class II MHC-antigenic peptide complex (Table 5-1) and the

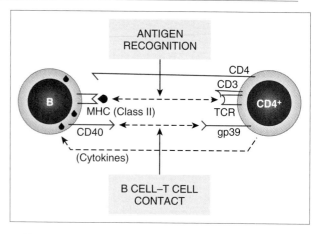

FIGURE 5-1 B Cell–T Cell Interaction. The most specific event during B cell–T cell interaction is the contact between the class II MHC–antigenic peptide complex expressed on the surface of the B cell and the antigen-specific receptor (TCR) on the helper T cell surface. This contact induces a T cell to secrete B cell–activating signals (IL-2, IL-4 cytokines). Other cell surface molecules on B and T cells also exchange information. The most potent signal (independent of MHC-peptide complex) is the cell-to-cell contact through the CD40 B cell surface molecule, which links with gp39 (complementary ligand or linking molecule) on the surface of activated CD4+ T cell, thus initiating B cell proliferation. *MHC,* major histocompatibility complex; *CD,* cluster of differentiation receptors; *TCR,* T cell receptors.

helper T cell surface receptor for antigens (TCR). This interaction is amplified by cytokines and receptor molecules associated with B and T cells.

In this process of cell interaction, B cells (serving as antigen-presenting cells [APCs]) interact with T lymphocytes by presenting **T cell–dependent antigen** to helper T cells for recognition. The MHC–antigen complex (T cell–dependent antigen) is displayed on the surface of a B cell (APC) and is recognized by helper T cells as foreign. This triggers secretion of various cytokines that induce B cells to proliferate, differentiate, and secrete antigen-specific antibodies (Figure 5-2).

Although most antigens are T cell dependent (i.e., require B cell–T cell interaction), certain other antigens (e.g., lipopolysaccharides [LPS]) can activate B cells without helper T cells by a reaction not completely understood. These antigens, known as **T cell–independent antigens,**

Table 5-1	SELECTED SURFACE MOLECULES ON B LYMPHOCYTES
Surface Molecules	Description
sIg or BCR	Surface immunoglobulin or B cell receptor complex (mainly IgM and IgD; few cells express IgG, IgA, IgE)
Class II MHC (HLA-D)	Most specific B cell–T cell interaction in antigen recognition (TCR/CD3 on CD4+ T cell with MHC-antigenic peptide on B cell)
CD35, CR1	Complement receptors for C3b
CD21, CR2	Complement receptors for C3d
CD19, CD20, CD22	Markers used to identify B cells
CD40	Most potent signal in initiating B cell growth (links with gp39 on CD4+ cell) during B-T cell contact

Ig, immunoglobulin; *MHC*, major histocompatibility complex; *HLA*, human leukocyte antigen; *TCR*, T cell receptor (for antigen); *CD*, cluster of differentiation (leukocyte differentiation antigens); *CR*, complement receptor; *C*, complement.

are mainly products of bacteria and can induce an immune response without helper T cells. Instead, they induce macrophages to secrete cytokines (IL-1, IL-6, TNFα). However, because of the lack of T cell cytokines (IL-2, IL-4, IL-5), the immune response to T cell–independent antigens is short-lived and lacks production of IgG (no class-switching occurs), even after secondary stimulation (see discussion following). Thus antibodies produced in response to T cell–independent antigens are only of the IgM class (see Figure 5-2).

Production of Immunoglobulins

Humoral immune response, also referred to as *antibody response*, is initiated by antigen recognition and activation of mature or memory B cells by CD4+ T cells. This culminates in the appearance of plasma cells (antibody-secreting transformed B cells) that synthesize and secrete

antigen-specific immunoglobulin (Ig) molecules (see Figure 5-2).

Antigen-specific immunoglobulin molecules are synthesized in two structurally similar forms (Figure 5-3):

- *B cell receptors (BCRs) (also known as surface immunoglobulins [sIgs]):* These immunoglobulins are secreted by B lymphocytes and bound to their surface where they function as antigen receptors (binding antigens at the variable region of the sIg).
- *Antibody molecules or antibodies (referred to as secreted immunoglobulins [soluble effector molecules]):* These are synthesized and secreted into body fluids by plasma cells of the B cell lineage.

The specificity of an antigen-binding site for an antigen in both forms of immunoglobulin molecules is located within their variable regions. The specific binding between immunoglobulins (BCRs or antibody molecules) and antigens produces antigen/antibody complexes on the surface of B cells or "free" complexes within the body fluids.

The antibody molecules (secreted form of Igs) are **bifunctional,** each of their functions reside in two separate regions (i.e., the variable and the constant regions) of the Ig molecule. Thus antibodies have the ability to:

- *Specifically bind with antigens through the variable region of the Ig molecule (a function exhibited also by the B cell surface Igs)*
- *Trigger various class-specific biologic activities, a function unique to the constant region of the antibody molecules*

Factors Affecting Antibody Production
The nature and the extent of immunoglobulin production during an antibody response depends mainly on the following factors:

- *Function of the immune system* (e.g., presence of various cytokines and accessory cells, class-switching, function of helper T cells and their cytokines)
- *Nature of the antigen* (e.g., quantity or dose and site of entry)
- *First or second exposure of the host to the particular antigen* (inducing primary or secondary antibody response, discussed following)

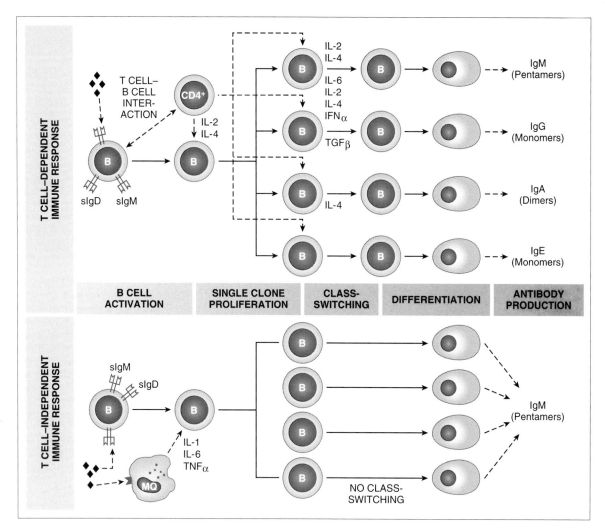

FIGURE **5-2**   **Events During Production of Antibodies.**   **T cell–dependent responses** are humoral (antibody) and are initiated by an antigen but require B cell–T cell interaction (see Figure 5-1) and various signals (cytokines) from helper T cells for activation, growth, class-switching (e.g., sIgM/sIgD to other classes of sIgs), and differentiation into antibody-secreting plasma cells (differentiated B cells) or into memory cells. Production of any class of antibodies may occur and is genetically determined (see text). In **T cell–independent** responses, certain antigens bypass T cell help and stimulate macrophages to secrete cytokines that induce B cells to produce antibodies. No class-switching occurs in T cell–independent immune response, so that only the IgM class is secreted in these events. Memory cells are not produced. *Ig,* immunoglobulin; *IL,* interleukin; *sIg,* surface immunoglobulin; *IFN$_\alpha$,* interferon; *TNF$_\alpha$,* tissue necrosis factor; *TGF$_\beta$,* T cell growth factor.

Development of B Lymphocytes

All members of a particular B cell clone arise from a single cell committed to the B cell lineage and have the ability to perform various biologic activities, such as production of immunoglobulins, class-switching, and generation of diversity. These processes are regulated by rearrangement (changes in organization)

of the Ig genes and transcription and translation of these genes. Development of B cell progeny (descendants) originates from various single B cell clones and proceeds as follows (Figure 5-4):

- *Stem cells:* B cells develop from bone marrow stem cells, which become committed to the B cell lineage.

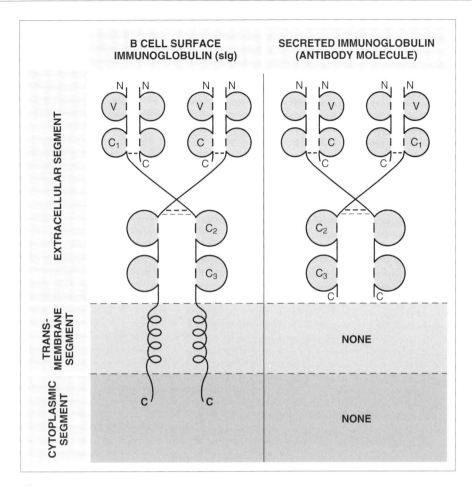

FIGURE 5-3 Two Forms of Immunoglobulin (Ig) Molecules. Surface immunoglobulins (sIgs) and the secreted forms of Ig molecules are structurally exactly the same (coded by the same gene segments), i.e., both contain the extracellular segment, except for an extra tail piece within the constant (C) region of the sIg. This extra amino acid sequence (tail piece) of the sIg is coded by additional gene segments (see text) and extends through the B cell membrane into the cytoplasm, thus anchoring the sIg molecule to the B cell. *N*, amine (NH_2); *C*, carboxyl; *V*, variable region; C_1, C_2, C_3, constant regions.

- *Pre-B lymphocytes:* First cell of the B cell lineage shows cytoplasmic μ heavy chain polypeptide (Ig gene product), containing the variable and constant regions. Pre-B lymphocytes are found only in the bone marrow (and fetal liver) and *do not express functional (assembled) surface IgM and therefore cannot bind or respond to antigens.*

- *Immature B lymphocytes:* Next cells in the maturation sequence are the immature B cells, which express assembled (complete) IgM molecules on their surface and function as receptors for antigens and show antigen specificity. *Immature B cells are not activated by antigens.* Contact with self-antigens may result in tolerance or B cell death (see Chapter 1).

- *Mature B lymphocytes:* Once immature B cells acquire antigen specificity, they migrate to blood and lymphoid tissues, where they continue to mature and express B cell surface IgD in addition to the surface IgM molecules. Thus the majority of mature B cells found in blood and lymphoid tissues are IgM+ or IgM+IgD+. *Because both classes of surface Igs (IgM and IgD) contain structurally the same V region, their antigen specificity is also the same.*

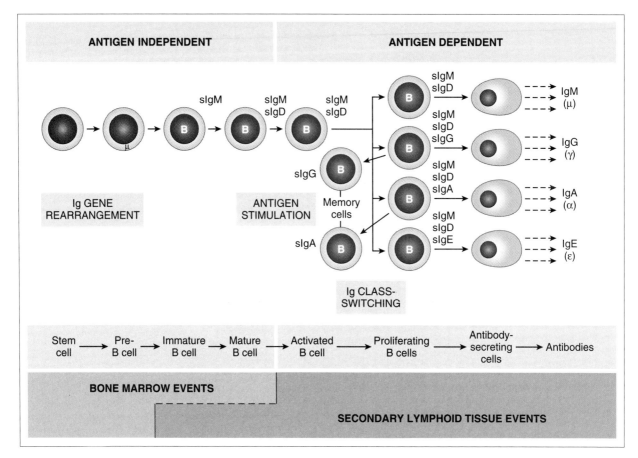

FIGURE **5-4**   **B Lymphocyte Maturation and Differentiation.**   Schematic representation of B cell development, before antigen stimulation, in the bone marrow and in secondary (peripheral) lymphoid tissues upon encountering an antigen. Genes that code for immunoglobulins (Igs) are rearranged before pre-B stage of development, after which B cells begin to synthesize surface IgM (sIgM). No further gene rearrangement occurs. Upon maturation, B cells may express other classes of sIgs (in addition to sIgM and sIgD) and switch classes in response to a particular antigen and stimulation with various cytokines. Thus activated mature B cells, expressing a particular class sIg, can develop into plasma cells and synthesize a secreted form of Igs (antibodies). B cells expressing sIgG or sIgA may also develop into antigen-specific memory cells (see text).

- *Activated B lymphocytes:* Mature cells that come in contact with a specific antigen become activated, proliferate, and differentiate into effector cells (antibody-secreting plasma cells). *Heavy chain class-switching (isotype) may occur in some of the progeny (cells derived from a single cell) of activated B cells, resulting in production of heavy chain classes (IgG, IgA, IgE) in addition to the IgM and IgD classes (see following).*

- *Antibody-secreting B cells (plasma cells):* Activated B cells proliferate and differentiate into plasma cells (morphologically identified) that produce secreted forms of IgM and IgD antibodies but less membrane-bound Igs of the same Ig classes. Through class-switching by activated B cells, other Ig classes may also be synthesized and secreted.

- *Memory B lymphocytes:* Certain antigen-activated B cells may persist for weeks or months as *memory B cells expressing their surface Igs but not secreting antibodies.* These memory cells circulate between the blood, lymph, and lymphoid organs. Contact with an antigen having the same specificity as their surface Igs (antigen receptors) results in **secondary antibody response** (described following).

Memory cells show higher affinity (specific attraction) for antigens than the precursor cells (resting or unstimulated lymphocytes) that have not been activated. This accounts for the greater secondary immune (antibody response) observed after activated B cells are again stimulated with antigen showing the same specificity.

With the availability of molecular techniques, studies of B cell maturation and differentiation (see Figure 5-4) and analysis of different immunoglobulin molecules has led to the following findings:

- All cells of the same B cell clone show the same antigen specificity because of the presence of the same V gene (variable region gene) within each cell.
- Each B cell clone and the cells derived from it (its progeny) has specificity for only one epitope (antigenic determinant), thus always expressing only one set of light and heavy chain V genes (see discussion of antibody diversity following and One Step Further Box 5-1).
- Clones are capable of showing specificity for a different epitope.
- Heavy chain class-switching occurs after B cell activation but light chains always remain the same (either kappa [κ] or lambda [λ], not both).

Primary Antibody Response
This is a form of humoral immune response characterized by a production of antibodies on first exposure to a particular antigen (immunization or active infection).

Antibody specificity for a variety of antigens, referred to as an *antibody repertoire,* exists before exposure to antigens and is determined by the number of B cell clones (more than 10^9 are available) that express surface Igs with definite specificities for antigens. These antigen-specific lymphocyte clones develop in the bone marrow without any exposure to antigens (see Clonal Selection, Chapter 1).

The information required to produce such a highly diverse antibody repertoire is located within the DNA of each individual and is expressed through a genetic mechanism that is present within each B lymphocyte (see One Step Further Box 5-1).

As a B lymphocyte encounters an antigen in the lymphoid tissue, it becomes activated and may either differentiate into an effector cell (antibody-secreting cell) or become a B memory cell (see Figure 5-4).

The **effector B cells** in a primary immune response synthesize mainly IgM molecules (antibodies) that show specificity for the stimulating antigen. Their function as effector molecules depends on their ability to participate in resolving the events of an immune response, either by inactivating or eliminating the stimulating antigen.

B memory cells also participate in an immune response in the lymphoid tissue, where they respond to an antigen with the same specificity as the antigen that stimulated their production, thus initiating a secondary immune response (see discussion following).

Secondary Antibody Response
A second encounter with an antigen showing the same specificity as the B cell receptor (BCR) on the surface of a B memory cell triggers a *secondary antibody response,* known as the *secondary immune response.*

The main events that occur during the primary antibody response also occur during the secondary antibody response (previously referred to as *anamnestic response*). However, the responses differ as follows (see Figure 5-6):

- Antibodies produced in the secondary antibody response are mainly of the IgG class (also a small number of the IgM class) whereas in the primary antibody response IgM is the predominant antibody class.
- The secondary response is much greater than the primary response and shows higher antibody affinity (known as *affinity maturation*) toward the stimulating antigen.
- Heavy chain switching is characteristic of secondary immune response and involves helper T cells and their cytokines.

affinity maturation. An increase in antibody affinity (attraction) to an antigenic stimulus during a second contact with the same T cell–dependent antigen (requiring helper T cells) results in a heightened secondary antibody response. No such affinity is associated with the primary immune response.

Box 5-1

Genetic Basis for Immunoglobulin Diversity

It is a fact that the chromosomes that we inherit do not have immunoglobulin genes but contain "building blocks" (multiple coding segments) from which the immunoglobulin (Ig) genes are assembled by a developing B lymphocyte. These multiple coding segments (**exons**) contain information that codes for immunoglobulin molecules (Figure 5-5). Exons are distributed along the DNA strand and are separated by non-coding DNA segments (**introns**).

The Ig gene assembly involves a complex enzymatic process that is responsible for the cutting (removal), rearrangement, and rejoining (recombination) of the gene segments on the chromosomal DNA strands. The **recombination of coding gene segments** is a key feature in this process because Ig genes are not intact (they are non-functional) and must be assembled into functional genes before activated B cells can synthesize immunoglobulins (Figure 5-6):

- *Genes coding for variable (V) and constant (C) regions:* The assembly of the two separate functional Ig genes, which code for the V and C regions, involves joining of exons that code for the heavy (H) and light (L) chains of the immunoglobulin molecule.
- *Genes coding for light (L) and heavy (H) chains:* Each light (L) and heavy (H) chain of the various classes (idiotypes) of Ig molecules is coded by the **V** and **J** gene segments

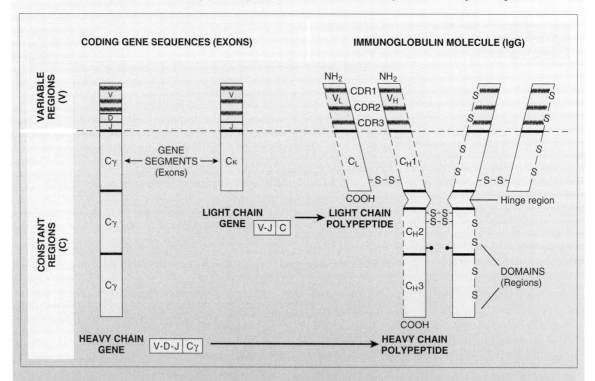

FIGURE **5-5** Genes Coding for Production of Immunoglobulins.   Separate genes code for complete heavy (H) and light (L) chain peptides, comprising all immunoglobulin (Ig) classes. Each H and L gene consists of multiple gene segments (exons) that code for each variable (V) and constant (C) region and are separated from each other by DNA stretches (non-coding segments) that are not transcribed. After rearrangement of DNA coding segments (recombination), the V-D-J/C (heavy chain gene) and V-J/C (light chain gene) is transcribed by mRNA and translated into polypeptides (gene product), comprising heavy and light chains of Ig molecule, respectively. This process occurs within the antigen-activated B cell and results in production and expression of immunoglobulin molecules. NH_2, amine terminal; *COOH*, carboxyl terminal; *S*, disulfide bond, C_H, constant region of heavy chain; *CDR*, complementarity-determining region (hypervariable region); V_L, variable region of light chain; V_H, variable region of heavy chain.

Box 5-1—cont'd

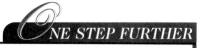

(exons). However, an additional **D** (diversity) gene segment is required for coding the heavy chain. Thus the light chain is coded by two joined gene segments **(assembled V/J gene),** while the **assembled V/D/J gene** (three joined segments) codes for the heavy chain.

As the rearranged (assembled) immunoglobulin genes—containing variable (V) region segments, non-coding sequences (introns), joining segment (J), and a constant (C) region—are transcribed by a primary RNA, the non-coding regions are removed. The V-J/C gene (coding for light chain) or V-D-J/C (coding for heavy chain) is thus assembled into a single messenger RNA molecule (mRNA). The mRNA is then translated within the B cell cytoplasm

into a light or heavy chain protein, and the B cell capability for rearrangement of V-J and V-D-J segments is discontinued (see Figure 5-6).

It is important to note that once either a L or H chain gene is assembled and becomes a functional gene, other gene rearrangements of the same type are prevented from occurring within the same B cell.

The proliferating (multiplying) B cell passes the rearranged functional genes to its progeny (descendants), which continue to express these genes without further rearrangement of the V-J and V-D-J. It is because of this fact that all immunoglobulins synthesized by a particular B cell and its progeny show identical antigen specificity and L chain type (kappa or lambda).

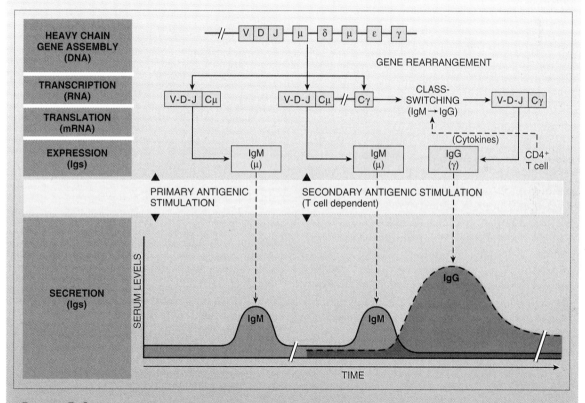

FIGURE **5-6** **Immune Response to Primary and Secondary Antigenic Stimulation.** Diagrammatic representation of B cell response through a genetic mechanism (gene assembly), coding for class-specificity and for synthesis of immunoglobulins. Synthesis of class-specific immunoglobulins (Igs) is induced by exposure to a primary antigenic stimulus, resulting in an increased secretion of IgM molecules that are detectable in serum. Upon secondary stimulation with the same antigen, IgM secretion reaches the same level as in primary immune response. However, because of class-switching and the presence of B memory cells with sIgG (produced during primary immune response), serum levels of IgG are much greater than IgM levels. Note the gene rearrangement and transcription of the heavy chain during coding for IgM (V-D-J/Cμ exon), class-switching to IgG (V-D-J/Cγ exon) that occurs upon second stimulation, and the T cell cytokine "help" that occurs during class-switching. (See also text.)

Continued

Box 5-1—cont'd

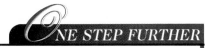

However, this is not the case with the H chain. There are situations when through a class or isotype switching (rearrangement of H chain) during clonal B cell proliferation, a new trait can be passed to the progeny, resulting in production of different class of antibodies (see Figure 5-6).

Moreover, slight changes in C_H gene sequence (exon), which codes for the tail piece of the surface immunoglobulin that anchors sIg to B cell membrane, determine whether the Ig will be expressed in a surface-bound (B cell receptor) or a secreted form (antibody molecule). In a mature B lymphocyte that differentiates into a plasma cell, the H chain mRNA lacks the exon that codes for the Ig anchoring piece, thus producing only the secreted form (see Figure 5-3).

IMMUNOGLOBULIN MOLECULES

There are possibly as many as a million (10^9) different immunoglobulin (Ig) molecules present in every individual. Each immunoglobulin molecule, depending on the number of available antigen-binding sites, is able to specifically bind one or more antigens because of the unique amino acid arrangement (sequence) within its variable (V) regions of the paired heavy (H) and light (L) chains (Figure 5-7). These amino acid sequences, which are characteristic for each Ig molecule, form the antigen-binding sites that determine immunoglobulin specificity for an antigen.

The diversity (variability) in amino acid sequences and immunoglobulin specificity for antigens within the V region (fit or complementarity between antigen and Ig molecule) results from the capability of the immune system to produce a variety of amino acid sequences within the V regions. This capability of the immune system allows immunoglobulins to bind with different antigens that are encountered and is the result of gene rearrangement within B cells that synthesize Igs (see following discussion).

Each immunoglobulin is also capable of initiating a variety of biologic activities that are characteristic for each class of immunoglobulins (e.g., activation of complement) but do not depend on antibody specificity for a particular antigen. These biologic activities are attributed to the constant (C) region of the Ig molecule and are the same in all Igs of the same class (Figure 5-8).

It is important to note that specificity is a characteristic required for binding of antigens but that the initiation of various (class-specific) biologic activities is not antigen specific.

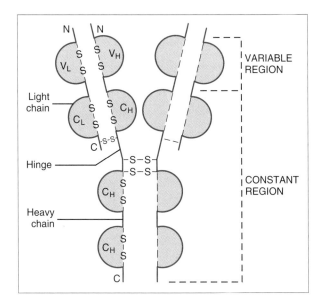

FIGURE **5-7**   **Basic Structure of the Immunoglobulin Molecule.**   Representation of a unit or core structure that is present in all immunoglobulins (Igs), which also represents an IgG molecule. The molecule consists of four polypeptide chains (two identical heavy [H] and two identical light [L] chains held together by disulfide [-S-S-] bonds [as indicated]). Note the location of C (carboxyl, COOH) and N (amine, NH_2) terminals shown at each end of the chain and the location of the variable (V) and constant (C) globular regions within each chain.

FORM

Each B cell has the ability to synthesize and secrete two forms of Igs within each of the five immunoglobulin classes or isotypes (IgM, IgG, IgD, IgE, IgA). The two forms are:

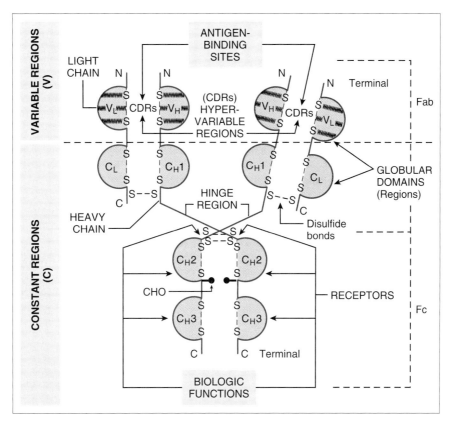

FIGURE **5-8** **Functional Sites of Antibody Molecule.** Each single unit structure (monomer) of an immunoglobulin is bifunctional (i.e., exhibits two separate functional sites): (1) an antigen-binding site (a hypervariable amino acid sequence within the variable region, known as *CDR,* that binds complementary antigenic configuration) and (2) a site of induction of biologic activities (receptors located on the heavy chain constant region that bind various cells and soluble molecules [e.g., macrophages and complement]). *N,* NH_2 terminal; *C,* COOH terminal; *V,* variable; *C,* constant; *H,* heavy; *L,* light; *-S-S-,* disulfide bonds holding the molecule (chains) together; *CHO,* carbohydrate unit; *CDR,* complementarity-determining region (hypervariable region) within variable regions; *Fab,* antigen-binding fragment; *Fc,* fragment, crystallizable.

- *Cell surface (membrane-bound) immunoglobulins*
- *Secreted immunoglobulins (antibodies)*

Both forms of immunoglobulins are structurally similar (see Figure 5-3) and show antigen specificity. The membrane-bound (surface) immunoglobulin molecule, however, has an additional segment of amino acid residues (sequences) at the carboxyl terminal of the heavy chain, which is responsible for anchoring the Ig molecule to the B cell membrane. The additional segment consists of a transmembrane segment (spanning the cell membrane and anchoring the heavy chain to the B cell) and a cytoplasmic segment.

When this additional segment is absent, the

immunoglobulin molecule contains only the tail piece. Not being able to anchor to the B cell, the Ig is secreted into body fluids (e.g., blood) and is detectable by various laboratory methods.

The change (transition) from a membrane to a secreted immunoglobulin occurs at the messenger RNA (mRNA) transcription level during encoding for amino acid sequences within the heavy chains of the Ig molecule (see One Step Further Box 5-1 and Figure 5-5). The transition depends on whether or not the transmembrane and cytoplasmic exons encoding for these amino acid segments are included (transcribed) in the mRNA. If the exons are not included, a secreted form of immunoglobulin (antibody) is synthesized.

Surface (Membrane-Bound) Immunoglobulins (sIgs)

These are known as *B cell receptors (BCRs)* or *membrane-bound immunoglobulins* (see Figure 5-3). Because sIg molecules are expressed only on B cells, they serve as *specific B cell markers (identifying B cells). They also serve as receptors for antigens and are capable of binding antigens.*

The predominant surface immunoglobulins that function as BCRs for antigens are class IgM and IgD. However, only the IgM molecules are expressed on the surface of immature B cells (see Figure 5-4).

Secreted Immunoglobulins

The "free" or soluble immunoglobulins are most frequently referred to as *antibody* or *antibody molecules* (see Figure 5-3).

Secreted immunoglobulins are soluble molecules produced and secreted into body fluids by plasma cells (B cell lineage) during a humoral immune response to an antigen (see Figure 5-2).

Presence of antigen-specific antibodies indicates previous exposure (immunity) to that particular antigen or existence of an active infection. Thus antibodies that specifically react (bind) with the etiologic agent (infection-causing antigen) are referred to as *serum markers* for a particular infection. The characteristic that makes this antibody function possible is their *specificity* for the antigen that induced their production.

The binding of antigen by a specific antibody occurs during an antigen/antibody reaction, which in vitro forms a complex known as *antigen/antibody complex.* In vivo, these antigen-antibody complexes are known as *immune complexes.*

Antigen/antibody reactions serve as a foundation for immunologic procedures used for the detection of specific antibodies or antigens (see Section II).

Monoclonal Antibodies (MAbs)

Blood of healthy individuals contains antibodies produced in response to exposure to many different antigens, either through actual infection or through immunization (vaccination). These antibodies, known as *polyclonal* or *heterogeneous antibodies,* contain many different antigen specificities.

Although each specific antibody originates from a single clone of B cells and has a unique structure and specificity for the stimulating antigen, there is a basic structural similarity among all of the antibodies (see Figure 5-7).

With the development of a technique for production of *homogeneous* or *monoclonal antibodies* (see Chapter 14, Box 14-1), a complete determination of the amino acid sequence of an individual antibody molecule and the detection of previously selected specificity, affinity for specific antigens, and immunoglobulin class (isotype) became possible.

The following experimental monoclonal antibodies have also been developed using genetic engineering.

"designer" monoclonal antibodies. It is now possible to alter antibody genes and construct novel (designer) genes, using molecular techniques to produce monoclonal antibodies. For example, genetically engineered chimeric monoclonal antibodies (mouse variable regions attached to human constant regions) have been produced against several antigens and have been used in clinical trials (testing according to FDA regulations).

"humanized" monoclonal antibodies. These genetically engineered monoclonal antibodies are produced by grafting mouse CDR (complementarity-determining region or the hypervariable region of an Ig molecule) into a human variable (V) region to produce humanized monoclonal antibodies. The technique has been successful in producing certain mouse monoclonal antibodies that show reduced human anti-mouse antibody (HAMA) response in clinical trials.

Heterophil Antibodies

In clinical laboratory practice, heterophil antibodies are typically associated with infectious mononucleosis (infection with Epstein-Barr virus) although they may also be present in low concentration (titer less than 1:56) in healthy individuals. These heterophil antibodies are non-specific (i.e., produced by an individual in response to one antigen [undefined]), but they have the capability to react with another antigen on the surface of cells from other species, such as sheep or horse erythrocytes.

Reactivity (antigen/antibody reaction) of heterophil antibodies with sheep red blood cells was first observed in patients with infectious mononucleosis by Paul and Bunnell (1932). They used this observation to develop a test that detected heterophil antibodies present in most individuals showing clinical symptoms of infectious mononucleosis (80% to 90%).

The Paul-Bunnell Screening Test, later modified by Davidsohn (Differential Test) and now replaced with various Rapid Slide Tests, had been used in screening and differential testing before the availability of procedures that detect antibodies with specificity for the Epstein-Barr virus (EBV).

Anti-Idiotypic Antibodies

These antibodies are produced against specific idiotypes (unique amino acid sequences) located within the antigen-binding site (hypervariable regions) of an antibody molecule. These idiotypes serve as antigenic determinants or epitopes and are characteristic for every immunoglobulin molecule.

Therefore *idiotypes are immunogenic or can serve as antigens, capable of inducing an immune response.* The anti-idiotypic antibodies develop because of the variability of the idiotype (rearrangement of amino acid sequences) that prevents the immune system from developing tolerance to them. Tolerance to the constant region of the immunoglobulin molecule, how-ever, is possible because of the stability (constancy) of this region of the Ig molecule.

STRUCTURAL CHARACTERISTICS

Immunoglobulins (Igs) are glycoproteins synthesized by B cells in two forms (see Figure 5-3), as discussed previously: (1) B cell receptors (BCRs) that bind extracellular (non-processed) antigens and serve as B cell markers and (2) the secreted form, generally known as *antibodies*. The latter are synthesized and secreted into body fluids by plasma cells of the B cell lineage. The secreted Igs constitute approximately 20% of serum proteins.

Each immunoglobulin molecule shows heterogeneity (variability) that is expressed as difference in size, charge, carbohydrate content, and amino acid composition. These differences are genetically determined (see discussion following) and form the basis for the characteristic electrophoretic patterns (bands or zones) that are produced by separation of serum proteins by electrophoresis (Figure 5-9) (described in Chapter 11). These bands appear as albu-

min, alpha$_1$ globulins, alpha$_2$ globulins, beta globulins, and gamma globulins, in the order of the fastest to the slowest moving fraction in an electrical field. The characteristic patterns of Ig molecules are located mainly within the gamma through beta regions. Identification of these various immunoglobulin classes is possible by immunoelectrophoresis or an immuno-fixation procedure (see Chapter 11).

All immunoglobulins (Igs) share the same basic, four-chain polypeptide structure (see Figure 5-7). This basic structural similarity allows isolation of antibodies from blood and other body fluids.

Minor differences observed in certain immunoglobulin characteristics, such as size, charge, and solubility, are the basis for separation and categorization of immunoglobulins into several classes (isotypes) and subclasses (subtypes), shown in Figure 5-9 and discussed following.

Basic Immunoglobulin Molecule

At least one basic immunoglobulin (Ig) unit has been identified in every class of immunoglobulins. This basic structural unit (see Figure 5-7) is a **monomer,** which consists of *four polypeptide chains* of repeating amino acid sequences or units that are linked together by covalent bonds and non-covalent forces (discussed in Chapter 10).

The four polypeptide chains making up the basic Ig unit consist of two *identical* **light (L) chains** and two *identical* **heavy (H) chains.** The heavy chains are attached to the light chains by covalent (interchain) *disulfide bonds (-S-S-).* H chains are also attached to each other by disulfide (intrachain) bonds and by non-covalent forces. *The disulfide bonds are essential in maintaining the three-dimensional structure of the Ig molecule (Figure 5-10).*

Light Chains

Each of the two smaller light (L) chains has a molecular weight of approximately 25,000. L chains are identified as *kappa (κ)* or *lambda (λ)* and occur in all immunoglobulin classes.

Each of the L chains is folded independently into several regions, referred to as the **variable (V)** and **constant (C) regions** (see following). The V and C regions end in an *amino (N) terminus* and a *carboxyl (C) terminus,* respectively.

Although structural differences are present in

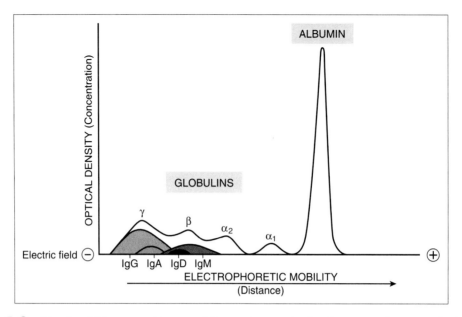

FIGURE **5-9**   **Simulated Movement Pattern of Serum Protein Molecules in an Electric Field (Electrophoretic Mobility).**   Separation of protein molecules by electrophoresis depends on their mobility in an electric field, according to their charge and weight. Note albumin mobility (smallest and fastest moving serum protein molecule). The separated protein fractions (see peak patterns on electrophoretogram) can be quantified with a densitometer (a modified spectrophotometer), which determines intensity (density) of the area under each peak. Note the heterogeneity of immunoglobulins (Igs) as shown by their four separate class locations (IgG, IgA, IgD, IgM) within the globulin fractions of serum proteins (γ, β, α2, α1). IgE *(not shown)* and IgD have a similar electrophoretic mobility.

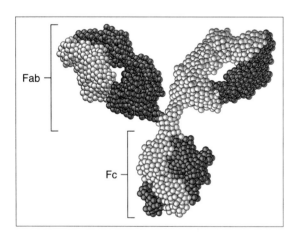

FIGURE **5-10**   **Three-Dimensional Immunoglobulin Structure (Computer-Generated IgG Molecule).** Shown are two Fab pieces, consisting of two light (L) and two heavy (H) chains, bound together by disulfide bonds and one Fc piece, consisting of two H chains.

the constant region of the κ and λ L chains, thus showing antigenic differences, *no functional differences exist between the two types of L chains.*

A particular immunoglobulin molecule always contains identical κ or λ chains but not a combination of the two classes.

Heavy Chains

Heavy (H) chains are the larger chains of the immunoglobulin molecule (molecular weight of 50,000 to 70,000) and fold into **variable (V)** and **constant (C) regions,** in the same way as do the light chains.

*The H chains are structurally distinct (specific) for each immunoglobulin class or subclass and are designated as **gamma (γ), alpha (α), mu (μ), delta (δ), and epsilon (ε).** The name of each class corresponds to the particular H chain (i.e., IgG, IgA, IgM, IgD, and IgE), respectively. Each immunoglobulin class or subclass is associated with characteristic biologic functions (see discussion of biologic [effector] functions following).*

Regions of the Immunoglobulin Molecule

The four polypeptide chains (linear sequences of amino acids) of the Ig molecule have the ability to fold independently into *two structurally and functionally distinct* **regions** or **domains** *(globular forms)* within the light (L) and heavy (H) polypeptide chains (see Figures 5-8 and 5-10).

Each immunoglobulin domain is approximately 110 amino acids long and has a central portion of a peptide loop that is held by a disulfide bond (see Figure 5-8). These regions are designated as:

- **Variable (V) region** (antigen-binding region)
- **Constant (C) region** (region associated with biologic activity)

Within the **variable (V) regions** are highly variable amino acid sequences—comprising the **hypervariable region** (antigen-binding site)—that are associated with the binding of antigens. The **constant (C) regions** participate in various biologic activities (Table 5-2).

variable (V) regions. The first domain of the polypeptide chains is the variable (V) region (at the amino-terminal of the Ig molecule), which is characterized by the variability (heterogeneity) observed in its amino acid sequences. There are four variable regions—two variable regions of the light chains (V_L regions) and two variable regions of the heavy chain (V_H regions).

The four variable regions (one region within each of the four polypeptide chains) form two separate **antigen-binding sites** at the amino (N) terminal of the immunoglobulin molecule and are designated as **hypervariable regions.**

hypervariable regions. The antigen-binding sites within each variable region of the light and heavy chain constitute the hypervariable regions (see Figure 5-8).

Each hypervariable region contains three highly variable amino acid sections (stretches or sequences), known as the **complementarity-determining regions,** or **CDR1** (beginning at the N terminus), **CDR2,** and **CDR3** (showing most variability).

As the variable regions fold into globular domains in a three-dimensional configuration (see Figure 5-10), the CDRs form protruding loops on the surface of the domain that are complementary to the configuration of the antigen with which the immunoglobulin can bind.

Table **5-2**	FUNCTIONS ASSOCIATED WITH THE IMMUNOGLOBULIN MOLECULE
Antibody Domain	Function
V_H/V_L	Antigen binding
C_H1	Complement binding (C4b fragment)
C_H2	Interaction with C1q fragment
C_H3	Binding to Fc receptors on macrophages and monocytes

V, variable region; *H,* heavy chain; *L,* light chain; *C,* constant region; *C4b* and *C1q,* complement fragments; *Fc,* fragment, crystallizable.

These protruding amino acid sequences of the CDRs vary with different antibody molecules, thus exposing a different and unique chemical structure at the surface of each antibody molecule that determines the **specificity of an antibody for an antigen.**

It is now a well-established fact that immunoglobulin specificity for antigens and the differences observed in antigen binding by the immunoglobulins reside within these hypervariable regions of the heavy and light chains.

constant (C) regions. The constant (C) regions are located at the carboxyl-terminal of the Ig molecule and show consistency of their amino acid sequences, which provides for the stability of this region.

The constant regions of the heavy chains (C_H) are responsible for the biologic activity (effector functions) attributed to each class of immunoglobulins.

Bound covalently to amino acids within the polypeptide chains of the H chain constant region are carbohydrate chains (see Figure 5-8), which may play a role in the secretion of immunoglobulins and in biologic functions associated with this region.

Various receptors for certain cells and molecules (e.g., macrophages, complement fractions) are also located within the constant region (see Figure 5-8).

hinge region. Between the first and second constant region (C_H1 and C_H2) is the hinge region, which provides the Ig molecule with

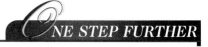

Box 5-2

Fragmentation of Immunoglobulin Molecule

Although the structure of antibodies (immunoglobulins) has been studied for over 50 years, it was not until 1962 that Rodney Porter and his colleagues proposed a basic four-chain model for an antibody molecule, based on two distinct types of polypeptide chains. Their structural model for the immunoglobulin (Ig) molecule is now accepted as a single unit structure (monomer) that is present in all classes of antibodies (see Figure 5-7).

The Classic Experiment

In his classic experiment, Porter was able to generate antibody fragments by cleaving rabbit IgG antibody (monomer) with proteolytic enzymes (papain, pepsin) under controlled conditions of time and enzyme concentration. These fragments have been extremely useful in defining the structure and function of an antibody molecule.

FRAGMENTATION OF IMMUNOGLOBULIN MOLECULE

The fragmentation of an IgG molecule by papain and pepsin occurs because of cleavage of certain peptide bonds within the hinge region of the Ig molecule, which is the most susceptible region of the antibody molecule to enzyme treatment (Figure 5-11). This susceptibility of the hinge region to enzymes results from its extended configuration (form), which has greater flexibility than the more enzyme-resistant globular domains (folded polypeptides). Fragmentation of the immunoglobulin molecule by the two enzymes occurs as described following.

FRAGMENTATION WITH PAPAIN

Papain cleaves rabbit IgG at the hinge region (between C_H1 and C_H2 domains) into three fragments or pieces:

- *Two identical Fab fragments (fragment, antigen-binding):* The two cleaved Fab pieces consist of identical fragments of light (L) chains (V_L, C_L domains) that are bound by disulfide bonds to the V_H-C_H1 fragment of the heavy (H) chain. Each Fab fragment includes the antigen-binding region, consisting of the V_L and V_H domains.
- *One Fc fragment (fragment, crystalline):* The Fc piece contains identical fragments of the heavy (H) chain (C_H2 and C_H3 domains) that associate with each other and crystallize into a lattice, showing that both domains contain a

common amino acid sequence in the same subtype (Ig class). The Fc fragment is responsible for mediating the effector functions (biologic activities) of the antibody molecule (e.g., activation of complement, binding to Fc receptors on various cells).

After a prolonged digestion with papain, a secondary enzymatic cleavage of the Fc fragment produces another fragment of the C_H3 region, referred to as the *Fc' fragment.*

FRAGMENTATION WITH PEPSIN

Cleaving rabbit IgG molecule with this proteolytic enzyme produces different results than those observed during proteolysis with papain. Pepsin cleaves the heavy (H) chain of the antibody molecule at two sites to form:

- *F(ab')$_2$ fragment:* Fragmentation of the Ig molecule at the hinge region near the C_H2 domain produces two Fab' fragments that retain the heavy chain hinge region. The two Fab' pieces are held together by interchain disulfide bonds and comprise an antigen-binding fragment, known as the *F(ab')$_2$,* which contains two separate antigen-binding sites.
- *pFc' fragments:* The central fragment of the pFc' portion is further degraded by pepsin to low molecular weight peptides.

EXPERIMENTAL OUTCOMES

Based on these classic experiments and the proposed model for the basic structure of an immunoglobulin molecule, the following observations contribute to the current understanding of the basic immunoglobulin (molecule) structure (see Figures 5-7 and 5-8):

- All basic (monomeric) Ig molecules, such as IgG, have two separate antigen-binding sites, each site consisting of a V_L V_H pair
- Each V_L V_H pair serves as an independent antigen-binding site
- The secreted (free) form of IgM molecules contain five monomeric units (ten separate antigen-binding sites) (see Figure 5-12)
- The hinge region of an Ig molecule provides flexibility that determines the number of its antigen-binding sites that will simultaneously bind with different antigenic determinants (epitopes) on a particular antigen
- The location and functions of the Fc region of the Ig molecule are separate from that of the Fab region (antigen-binding sites)

Box 5-2—cont'd   *O*NE STEP FURTHER

- Biologic (effector) functions that are activated by Fc regions during an immune response are not antigen specific
- The type of effector functions that occur during an immune response are class-specific (determined by the isotype or class of immunoglobulin molecule)

With the availability of newer technology, such as x-ray crystallography, electron microscopy, genetic engineering, and computers (generation of atomic Ig models), information on the complete structure of an immunoglobulin molecule (see Figure 5-8) and association of its function with specific amino acid sequences on the molecule (Table 5-3) is now available.

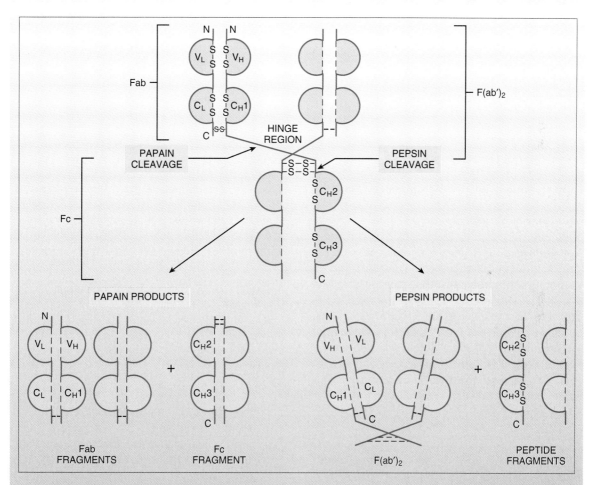

FIGURE **5-11** **Cleavage of IgG Molecule.** Diagrammatic presentation of various polypeptide fragments or cleavage products, resulting from degradation (fragmentation) of IgG molecule by action of two proteolytic enzymes (papain and pepsin) at specific cleavage points. In both types of enzymatic fragmentation, the Fab fragments retain their antigen-binding activity (see also text). *N*, NH$_2$ terminus; *C*, carboxyl terminus; *Fab*, antigen-binding fragment; *Fc*, fragment, crystallizable; *V$_L$*, light chain variable region; *V$_H$*, heavy chain variable region; *C$_L$*, light chain constant region; *C$_H$*, heavy chain constant region; *-S-S*, intrachain and interchain disulfide bonds; *F(ab')$_2$*, Fab unit with hinge region and intact interchain disulfide bonds.

flexibility (bending) necessary for binding with antigens. It is also an area that is more accessible to chemicals and enzymes. For example, the enzyme papain splits an IgG molecule at the hinge region into two Fab (antigen-binding) and one Fc (fragment, crystallizable) fragments (One Step Further Box 5-2).

J Chain

The J chain is present in all polymeric forms of immunoglobulins that contain two or more basic monomeric Ig units. It is a small polypeptide that is synthesized by cells genetically coded for the secretion of polymeric (more than one monomer) immunoglobulins, such as IgM (pentamer) and IgA (dimer). *Only one J chain is present in each of the polymeric Ig molecules and is covalently bonded to the μ and the α chains of the IgM and IgA molecule, respectively* (Figures 5-12 and 5-13).

The presence of the J chain on a polymeric molecule may be responsible for facilitating polymerization (combining) of the basic Ig units of these molecules, but its function is still debatable.

Secretory Component

Typically, IgA can be detected in serum as a monomeric unit (four-chain molecule) but is able to polymerize to form a **dimer** (two Ig monomers joined by disulfide bonds) that has *one J chain and one secretory component* in addition to the two basic Ig units (see Figure 5-13).

This polymerized form (secretory IgA) is the largest form of IgA and is detectable in body secretions such as saliva and sweat. The secretory component protects the secretory IgA from being degraded by enzymatic action.

CLASSES

As previously described, an immunoglobulin molecule consists of two regions (variable and constant), which exhibit two separate functions (Ig is a **bifunctional** molecule, see Figure 5-8):

- *Antigen-binding:* This is a characteristic of the variable region, which shows variability in its amino acid sequences. The same specificity for a particular antigen remains in all Ig classes, even after class-switching occurs (see discussion of generation of antibody diversity following).
- *Biologic (effector) activities:* These are a

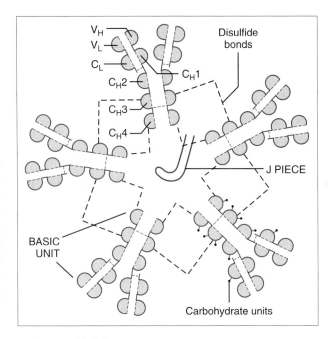

FIGURE **5-12** **Pentameric Immunoglobulin Molecule.** This IgM molecule consists of five monomeric Ig units (basis units), which are held together by cross-linking disulfide bonds (-S-S-); it is known as a *pentamer*. The molecule is stabilized by a joining polypeptide chain (J piece) that is present only in polymeric Ig molecules (i.e., IgM and IgA), possibly attached to the carboxyl end of two adjacent monomers. Note the absence of a hinge region within each monomer and the presence of an additional constant region (C_H2 domain), which allows some flexibility. Each of the IgM monomers shows numerous carbohydrate units. V_H, variable region of heavy chain; V_L, variable region of light chain; C_L, constant region of light chain; C_H, constant region of heavy chain.

function of the constant region. The constant region shows no variability in its amino acid sequences (remains constant) but has the ability to change to a different class (isotype) of immunoglobulins as it responds to an antigenic stimulation. This capability is genetically based (see discussion of class-switching following and Figure 5-6). *The biologic activity described following is unique for each class of immunoglobulins.*

The name of each immunoglobulin (Ig) class, also known as **immunoglobulin isotype,** corresponds to the name of the heavy chain constant region in the particular immunoglobulin molecule. For example, the IgG class (monomer) consists of two gamma (γ) heavy chains with either two kappa (κ) or two lambda (λ) light chains (see Figure 5-7), whereas two mu (μ) heavy chains and two light chains form one of five basic units of an IgM molecule (pentamer) (see Figure 5-12).

Immunoglobulin Subclasses

Immunoglobulin classes are further divided into subclasses according to their type of heavy (H) chain, showing serologic and chemical differences within the constant regions. Structural differences have also been observed among the heavy chain subclasses, including the number and location of disulfide bonds (interchain S-S bonds) (see Figure 5-12).

Four heavy chain subclasses of IgG (IgG1, IgG2, IgG3, and IgG4) and two subclasses of IgA (IgA1 and IgA2) have been identified. These heavy chain subclasses are more closely related to each other than to other immunoglobulin classes. No subclasses of IgM, IgD, and IgE classes have been described (Table 5-4).

Characteristics of Immunoglobulin Classes

Structural differences of the heavy chains account for the differences in size, charge, amino acid composition, and carbohydrate content observed within each of the five immunoglobulin classes (isotypes): IgG, IgA, IgM, IgD, IgE (see Table 5-4). These differences in the structural characteristics permit separation of each of the Ig classes by laboratory methods discussed in Chapter 13 and are responsible for the differences in biologic activities attributed to each immunoglobulin class (see Table 5-3).

Immunoglobulins may be expressed in two forms (i.e., as cell surface immunoglobulins [sIgs] and as secreted immunoglobulin molecules [antibodies]).

Immunoglobulin M (IgM)

In normal adults, IgM is a large complex that is produced in two forms (antibodies detectable in serum and B cell antigen receptors, see Figure 5-3) and consists of five monomeric immunoglobulin units or molecules (pentamer, see Figure 5-12). Each monomer contains two

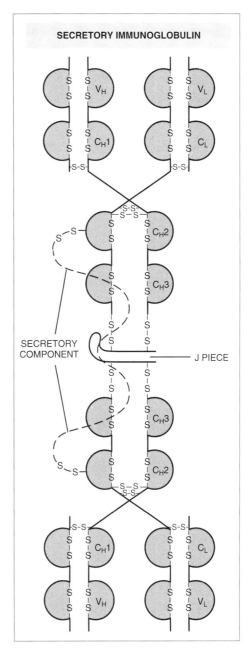

FIGURE **5-13** Secretory Immunoglobulin A (sIgA). Representation of a dimeric immunoglobulin structure (sIgA molecule), which consists of two monomers (basic Ig units), joined by J chain (piece). A secretory component (present only in this Ig class) that winds around the molecule and attaches to the C_H2 domain of each IgA unit, possibly facilitates transport of the molecule into body secretions. -S-S-, disulfide bonds; V_L, variable region of light chain, C_L, constant region of light chain; V_H, variable region of heavy chain; C_H1, C_H2, C_H3, constant regions (domains) of heavy chain.

Table **5-3**	SELECTED FUNCTIONAL CHARACTERISTICS OF IMMUNOGLOBULIN CLASSES					
Functions	IgG	IgA	sIgA	IgD	IgM	IgE
VARIABLE REGION (ANTIGEN-BINDING SITES)						
Specificity in binding antigens	+	+	+	+	+	+
CONSTANT REGION (BIOLOGIC ACTIVITY)						
Activation of complement	+	−	−	−	+	−
Placental crossing	+	−	−	−	−	−
Binding to Fc receptors on:						
Mononuclear phagocytes	+	−	−	−	−	−
Neutrophils	+	+	−	−	−	−
Basophils/mast cells	−	−	−	−	−	+
Enhancement of phagocytosis (opsonization)	+	−	−	−	−	−
Antibody-dependent cell-mediated cytotoxicity	+	+	−	−	−	+
Mucosal immunity (secretory piece)	−	−	+	−	−	−
Allergic reactions	−	−	−	−	−	+
Neonatal immunity (maternal Igs)	+	+*	−	−	−	−
Placental crossing in fetus	+	−	−	−	−	−

*Ig, immunoglobulin; Fc, fragment, crystallizable; * in maternal breast milk.*

Table **5-4**	STRUCTURAL CHARACTERISTICS OF IMMUNOGLOBULIN CLASSES (ISOTYPES)*						
Class	Number of Monomers	H Chain Domains	M.Wt. H Chains $(\times 10^3)$ (mg/ml)	Subclasses	J/S Piece	Serum Concentration	Isotype
IgG	1	4 (1V, 3C)	150	Gamma (γ)	IgG1, IgG2, IgG3, IgG4	− −	9.0, 3.0 1.0, 0.5
IgA	1	4 (1V, 1C)	150	Alpha (α)	IgA1, IgA2	−	3.0, 0.5
	2		300		sIgA	J,S	0.05
IgM	5	5 (1V, 1C)	950	Mu (μ)	−	J	1.5
IgD	−		180	Delta (δ)	−	−	0.03
IgE	1	5 (1V, 4C)	190	Epsilon (ε)	−	−	Trace

*The characteristics of each immunoglobulin (Ig) class presented refer to the secreted (free) form of immunoglobulins (antibodies). The two characteristic heavy (H) chains of each Ig class are responsible for the different properties exhibited. Secretory Ig (sIgA) occurs as a dimer (two basic Ig units with a J and S piece), while IgM is a five basic unit with a J piece.
Ig, immunoglobulin; M.Wt., molecular weight; J, joining segment; S, secretory segment; V, variable domain (region) on each H chain; C, constant domain (region) on each H chain.

heavy (mu) chains and two light (lambda or kappa) chains that are held together by a J chain (see previous discussion) but which lack the hinge regions and hence the flexibility. *IgM constitutes approximately 10% of serum immunoglobulins and is the major immunoglobulin class expressed on the surface of B lymphocytes (see Figure 5-2) serving as a B cell* receptor (BCR) for antigens having the same specificity.

Immunoglobulin G (IgG)

IgG is the predominant class of immunoglobulins in serum (75% of total serum Igs). It is a monomer with each side of the molecule reflecting the other side (mirror image). *The IgG*

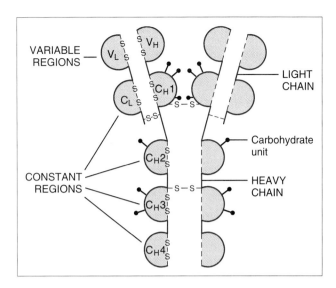

FIGURE **5-14** **Structural Organization of Immunoglobulin E (IgE).** Representation of globular variable (V) and constant (C) regions within the heavy (H) and light (L) chains of an IgE molecule, held together by disulfide bonds (-S-S-). Note absence of a hinge region and presence of an additional region (C_H4) within the heavy chain structure.

molecule is the basic unit (monomer) that is found in all classes of immunoglobulins (see Figure 5-7).

Four subclasses of IgG have been identified: IgG_1 constituting the highest concentration (60% to 70%), IgG_2 (14% to 20%), IgG_3 (4% to 8%), and IgG_4 (2% to 6%). IgG comprises 10% to 20% of total serum proteins.

Immunoglobulin A (IgA)

IgA is produced in two forms:

- *Secretory IgA:* A major class of immunoglobulins (antibodies) found in secretions (saliva, tears, bronchial secretions, prostatic fluid, vaginal secretions, mucosal secretion of nose and small intestine, and in colostrum and breast milk). Secretory IgA is a dimer (two basic Ig units, see Figure 5-13) that is linked by J chains and contains a secretory component (SC), but lacks a hinge region. The secretory component protects the molecule from degradation by proteolytic enzymes and possibly facilitates transport of the molecule into body secretions.
- *Monomeric IgA:* Present in serum as a monomer (one basic Ig unit) antibody molecule. Both forms of IgA (monomer and dimer) are detectable in serum and

make up approximately 15% of the total serum immunoglobulins.

Immunoglobulin D (IgD)

IgD is also produced in two forms:

- *IgD class antibodies:* These secreted forms of immunoglobulins (antibodies) are detectable in serum as monomeric Ig molecules (one Ig unit) in trace amounts (0.2% of total immunoglobulins).
- *IgD class surface immunoglobulins (sIgs) or B cell receptors (BCRs):* sIgD molecules also appear on the surface of B cells as the major receptors for antigens (see Figures 5-3 and 5-4).

Immunoglobulin E (IgE)

The majority of class E immunoglobulins (50%) are present in the intravascular system (blood) in a monomeric form (Figure 5-14) but may also be detected in the respiratory and gastrointestinal mucous membranes. IgE molecules constitute only 0.004% of total serum immunoglobulins, but the levels may vary because of genetic factors and environmental (antigenic) stimulation.

IgE molecules show high affinity for binding to Fc receptors on mast cells through a site located on the Fc region of the IgE molecule (see Figure 5-8). This affinity plays a major role in hypersensitivity reaction. The reaction occurs when mast cell–bound IgE molecules bind to an antigen, mast cells release their mediators (e.g., histamines) and the typical clinical symptoms of allergy are produced (see discussion of immediate hypersensitivity in Chapter 7).

GENERATION OF ANTIBODY DIVERSITY

The immune system of every healthy individual has the ability to produce an almost limitless number of immunoglobulins (Igs), each showing specificity for a singular antigen within the vast number of antigens that are encountered throughout a lifetime and each capable of inducing a variety of biologic activities.

These superb capabilities can be attributed to the organization of the Ig loci on the B lymphocyte chromosomal DNA and to the ability of each B cell precursor to independently and in different combinations rearrange its Ig genes to produce a large variety of B cell clones (see One Step Further Box 5-1 and Figure 5-6). The resulting diversity among the various immunoglobulins is both structural and functional.

The gene rearrangement responsible for this diversity involves recombinations of the V, D, and J regions; diversification of variable regions; variations in joining site; and the existence of multiple D regions within the two separate Ig genes that code for the variable (V) and constant (C) regions of the immunoglobulin molecule.

Availability of recombinant DNA techniques for study of Ig genes have made these observations possible.

Diversity in Immunoglobulin Specificity for Antigens

Each B cell originating from a bone marrow stem cell is able to produce only one type of antigen-specific antibody. B cell maturation and development of antigen specificity occurs in the bone marrow without any exposure to a specific antigen (see clonal selection). Therefore many B cells with different antigen-specific Ig receptors on their surface must be produced from the stem cells to be available for binding with the many antigenic determinants (epitopes) that they will encounter.

Acquired immunoglobulin specificity for antigens is located within the variable region of the light (V_L) and heavy (V_H) chains of an Ig molecule. It is made possible by genetically determined variability in amino acid sequences within the variable region and occurs following B cell maturation. This variability in amino acid sequences is responsible for the Ig specificity.

The diversity in Ig specificity is observed only after antigen activation of B lymphocytes, which then produce antigen-specific antibodies (see antibody specificity discussion following).

Diversity in Biologic Functions (Immunoglobulin Class-Switching)

The immune response is triggered by the interaction of an antigen and an IgM and/or IgD antigen receptor (BCR) on a mature B lymphocyte that shows specificity for that particular antigen.

It is now a well-established fact that during exposure to a specific antigen (immunization or active infection), B cells that initially express either IgM and/or IgD antigen receptors are able to switch to expression of IgE class (isotype) or one of the subclasses of IgG or IgA. This class-switching phenomenon is genetically determined (see One Step Further Box 5-1).

The current view is that T cell and non-T cell–derived cytokines act as "switch factors" by selectively activating RNA transcription of the constant region of heavy chain (C_H) genes, which code for the immunoglobulin class to be expressed.

Activation of C_H gene makes the DNA accessible to the "switch" recombinase. The cytokines, however, do not independently induce the resting B cells to switch immunoglobulin class by recombination of DNA without participation of a B cell activator such as an activated antigen-specific T cell (CD4+). *Thus T cells are essential in isotype switching.*

In addition to the genetically determined class-switching, the site at which a humoral immune response takes place may also determine antibody class (e.g., production of IgA in mucosal lymphoid tissue).

As a particular immunoglobulin class switches to another class during B cell differentiation into an antibody-secreting plasma cell, the antibodies produced by the plasma cells reflect the new (switched) immunoglobulin class (isotype).

Each secreted class of immunoglobulins has a different effector region that determines the biologic activity of the molecule; thus, as the Ig class is switched, so is its effector function (biologic activity) (see Table 5-3).

The antigen-binding site (variable region of each Ig class) remains unchanged during class-switching and shows the same structural and antigen-binding characteristics (i.e., antigen specificity and structural diversity in antigen binding). This occurs because all variable regions of the various Ig isotypes (classes) are coded by the same variable region genes (see One Step Further Box 5-1).

IMMUNOGLOBULIN VARIANTS

The mRNA for an immunoglobulin polypeptide chain is produced by a B lymphocyte in response to an antigenic stimulus by splicing together sections of mRNA that code for different sections of the chain, thus producing a different polypeptide chain from the various genes (discussed previously). The resulting immunoglobulin molecules that are secreted express these structural differences or variability (heterogeneity). These Ig molecules are referred to as *immunoglobulin variants* and are designated as *isotypic, allotypic,* and *idiotypic variants.*

Isotypic Variations (Isotypes)
Variations observed among heavy chains of different classes and subclasses of immunoglobulins are known as *isotypic variations.* Each **isotype** has a distinct locus in the individual's genome (complete set of hereditary factors) that codes for its expression.

The genes that code for these variations (isotypes) are present in all individuals of the same species and are expressed as various immunoglobulin isotypes, also known as *classes* and *subclasses* or *subtypes of immunoglobulins.* These isotypic variants are named according to the type of immunoglobulin chain that is expressed (i.e., mu, alpha [1,2], gamma [1,2,3,4], delta, epsilon, kappa, or lambda chains).

Allotypic Variations
Allotypic variations are genetic variations in individuals of the same species that reflect the presence of different alleles (alternative genes) at the same locus of a particular gene. Allotypes appear as *variants of heavy chain constant*

regions, so that a particular immunoglobulin class (isotype) may show alternative (allelic) forms. A particular variant or allelic immunoglobulin class is known as an **allotype.** Because an allotype is a genetic variation in the particular individual, it is not present in all individuals of the same species.

Idiotypic Variations
Idiotypic variations **(idiotypes)** determine antigen specificity of the antigen-binding site within the V region of an immunoglobulin molecule.

These variations are located within the variable (V) region, particularly in its highly variable amino acid sequences (hypervariable region), and are *specific for each immunoglobulin molecule (each B cell clone).* However, the genetic basis for the variations has not been fully defined.

FUNCTIONAL CHARACTERISTICS OF IMMUNOGLOBULINS

The primary function of immunoglobulins is to eliminate or inactivate an antigen that has passed the individual's natural barriers (natural immunity) and induced the immune system to respond through a specific humoral immune response.

There are two ways by which immunoglobulins (antibodies) participate in this function, thus terminating (resolving) events to which the immune system responds:
- *Binding of the stimulating antigen*
- *Inducing various class-specific biologic activities that facilitate antigen removal*

BINDING OF ANTIGENS

With the availability of more advanced laboratory techniques to study immunoglobulins, a better understanding of their structure and function is now possible. For example, initial research findings associated binding of antigens by antibodies with the Fab fragment of the molecule (see One Step Further Box 5-2). However, subsequent studies were able to provide more precise information, such as the location of the antigen-binding site and specificity for antigens on the immunoglobulin molecule.

Basis for Antigen Binding

The current view is that binding of antigen occurs at the three hypervariable segments, located within the variable (V) regions of the light (L) and heavy (H) chains of the immunoglobulin molecule. It is proposed that the V_L and V_H chains fold into immunoglobulin domains, bringing together (in a three-dimensional space) the three hypervariable regions, known as **complementarity-determining regions CDR1, CDR2, and CDR3,** of both chains (L and H) to form protruding loops on the surface of the domains (see Figure 5-8).

The protruding complementarity-determining regions (CDRs) within the variable regions differ in amino acid sequence of the various immunoglobulin molecules, thus exposing a different and unique structure at each immunoglobulin surface. These protruding CDR surfaces create an **antigen-binding site** (paratope), which is complementary to the three-dimensional configuration of the particular antigen, thus allowing the immunoglobulin molecule to specifically bind with the particular antigen.

This structural variability (different amino acid sequences) accounts for the ability of immunoglobulins to bind with the vast numbers of antigenic structures in our environment (see previous discussion).

Antibody Specificity

Immunoglobulins (Igs) are able to distinguish ("recognize") small differences in amino acid sequence of antigenic proteins as well as difference in charge, optical configuration, and steric conformation, thus demonstrating a high degree of specificity.

It is believed that this specificity in antigen "recognition" and binding does not depend on the antigen's fit within the clefts of an antibody molecule (as previously believed) but rather that the **Ig molecule "recognizes" the general configuration of the particular antigen (epitope) that is complementary to its binding site (see discussion following).**

This type of antibody "specificity" in antigen binding accounts for the fact that antibodies have the ability to bind with an intact (unprocessed or native) antigen that shows tertiary or globular structure (three-dimensional configuration) as discussed in Chapter 2. This is unlike the antigen recognition by T lymphocytes that can only recognize processed (degraded) antigens in the context of self-MHC molecules but can induce an immune response. Antibodies require helper T cells for induction of humoral immune response.

bond formation. Binding of antigen with an antibody produces an antigen/antibody complex that is held together by various non-covalent bonds (e.g., hydrogen bonds) (see Chapter 10 and Figure 10-1). These bonds form between the specific antigen (epitope) and the amino acids that constitute the antigen-binding site within the variable region of an antibody molecule. Although each bond is weaker than any covalent bond, the total energy (intermolecular attractive force) that binds antigen to antibody is stronger.

A further discussion relating to factors that affect antigen/antibody binding is presented in Chapter 10.

Antibody Affinity and Avidity

Both *antibody affinity* and *avidity* refer to the strength of a bond or bonds formed between an antigen and an antibody molecule. Because the bond is non-covalent, the antibody and antigen may dissociate, thus showing reversibility in antigen/antibody reaction (binding). The reaction can be measured by the Law of Mass Action and by the *antibody affinity constant,* also known as *equilibrium constant (K),* that can be mathematically calculated (see Chapter 10).

affinity. **Affinity** of an antibody refers to the strength of a non-covalent bond that forms between a single combining site on an Ig molecule and a single epitope (or a monovalent antigen). High affinity antibodies are more effective than low affinity antibodies in such biologic activities as hemagglutination, hemolysis, complement fixation, and cell membrane damage.

avidity. **Avidity** is the strength of the bonds that form between a multivalent antigen and a multivalent antibody. Because each Ig molecule has at least two antigen-combining sites (IgG, see Figure 5-8) and as many as ten binding sites (IgM, see Figure 5-12), it is able to bind with more than one epitope (antigenic determinant). However, the binding is competitive so that binding of one epitope excludes the binding of another epitope.

Avidity (functional affinity) refers to a combined (overall) strength of interaction between an antigen and an antibody.

cross-reactivity. As a B cell is stimulated by a particular antigen (with T cell help), it responds by producing antigen-specific antibodies. In situations in which the stimulating antigen shares the same epitope with another antigen, the antibody (antigen-binding site) showing specificity for an antigen that induced its production may also bind with another antigen that contains an epitope common to both antigens.

This type of antibody binding with antigens that share a common epitope is known as **cross-reactivity.**

CLASS-SPECIFIC FUNCTIONS

As previously stated, the primary function of immunoglobulins is to bind with antigens that have stimulated their production for the purpose of eliminating them. Except for few situations where antigen binding by an antibody is effective alone (e.g., preventing viruses from infecting cells and neutralizing bacterial toxins), antibody effector functions are also required for elimination of the antigen (see Table 5-3).

Biologic (Effector) Functions

Biologic activities that contribute to the elimination of an antigen are associated with different sites on the constant (C) region of Ig heavy (H) chains (Fc segment) and are class-specific (i.e., dependent on the Ig class showing the characteristic biologic function).

IgM Class Function

IgM molecules are able to directly cross-link or bind to cellular (cell surface) and particulate (bacterial) antigens, thus forming antigen/antibody aggregates (complexes). IgM molecules are also the most efficient complement binders (one IgM molecule can activate the complement cascade).

IgM is the first class of immunoglobulins to appear when the immune system responds to an antigenic stimulation. Typically, as IgG molecules are subsequently produced, the IgM level (concentration) falls and remains at a low level (see Figure 5-6).

IgM is the first immunoglobulin class that is synthesized by a newborn and is the first class to appear on the surface of B cells as receptors for antigens (see Figure 5-4).

Also the presence of these large IgM molecules (see Figure 5-12) is responsible for an *increase in blood viscosity* and *decrease in blood flow* (e.g., Waldenstrom's macroglobulinemia).

IgG Class Function

All IgG subclasses, except IgG_4, are capable of binding (fixing) serum complement at the CH_2 domain of the molecule (binding site for C1q fragment), thus initiating the classic complement cascade (see Chapter 4, One Step Further Box 4-2). Also *IgG is the only immunoglobulin that is capable of crossing the placenta,* thereby serving as a defense mechanism against infections in infants (maternal IgG is present in the infant's blood until it is replaced with the infant's own immunoglobulins at 6 months, reaching adult levels at 6 years).

IgG is an important body defense against infections, so that decreased levels of IgG are associated with recurrent infections (particularly pyogenic or pus forming), while an increase in IgG levels is seen in many autoimmune diseases. Autoantibodies, such as anti-nuclear and anti-basement membrane antibodies, are of the IgG class.

The IgG molecule can bind to surface Fc receptors on macrophages, thus serving as an opsonin that facilitates phagocytosis (see Chapter 1, Figure 1-4) and is involved in antibody-dependent cytotoxicity. The site at which the IgG (IgG_1, IgG_3) molecule binds to the Fc receptor on the macrophage is possibly the C_H3 domain within the Fc region.

IgG is the major class of antibodies that is produced during secondary antibody response (see Figure 5-6) and is the only immunoglobulin class with antitoxin activity.

sIgA Class Function

The major function of secretory IgA is to provide primary protection against local infections. The presence of IgA in colostrum and breast milk may be an important mechanism for preventing gastrointestinal infections in infants.

The specific function of IgA class molecules (antibodies detectable in serum) is not apparent.

IgD Class Function

No function has been assigned to this class of antibodies, detectable as soluble molecules in serum. However, as B cell surface immunoglobulins, *IgD molecules serve as the major receptors for antigens.*

IgE Class Function

The importance of IgE molecules (antibodies) is their mediation of immediate hypersensitivity, produced in response to a specific allergen (antigen). This type of an immune response is known as an *allergic reaction* or *allergy (*discussed in Chapter 7).

USE OF ANTIBODIES IN DIAGNOSTIC PROCEDURES AND THERAPY

Therapeutic use of monoclonal antibodies is a newly emerging area of clinical therapy in immunosuppression, infectious diseases, and cancer, all of which are not responsive to currently available chemical drugs. The safety and efficacy (efficiency) of this form of clinical therapy is under careful scrutiny by the FDA (Food and Drug Administration) as are all other pharmaceuticals.

The use of monoclonal antibodies (MAbs) is preferable to the use of polyclonal antibodies (serum or intravenous gammaglobulins) in clinical therapy because their specificity and affinity can be selected and their dose is lower. MAbs can also be more easily standardized by using the same hybridoma (see One Step Further Box 14-1).

Reagent Antibodies in Laboratory Procedures

The use of monoclonal antibodies as reagents in a variety of clinical laboratory procedures (described in Section II of this text) has been shown to be an invaluable tool for quantifying, identifying, and characterizing various antigens in diagnostic and research studies.

Production of Reagent Antibodies

In the past, the fact that antigens could stimulate an antibody response in vivo created new possibilities for the production of antibodies in animals (usually rabbits) through immunization (administration of selected antigens).

These antibodies (known as **polyclonal antibodies**) originating from different cell clones and showing specificity for various antigens, allowed a reaction to occur between different epitopes on a particular antigen.

The availability of newer methods for production of **monoclonal antibodies** (somatic cell hybridization) (see Box 14-1), as well as recombinant DNA methods that produce a genetically stable source of antibodies (known as the human antibody library) and PCR (polymerase chain reaction) technology that allows production of immunoglobulins through amplification, make production of large quantities of antibodies with predetermined specificity readily available.

Use of Reagent Antibodies

Most laboratory procedures using antibodies depend on the ability of the antibody to bind with an antigen showing the same specificity, thus forming an antigen/antibody complex that can be detected by various methods (discussed in Section II of this text).

It is possible for an Ig molecule to also function as an antigen, thus inducing an immune response. The resulting antibodies, directed against the antibody, are referred to as **anti-idiotypic antibodies** (anti-antibodies). Their specificity is determined by a particular antigenic determinant (sequence of amino acids) within the variable region of an immunoglobulin molecule that acts as the stimulating antigen (see Figure 5-8).

Antibodies in Blood Transfusion Practice (Blood Banking)

Blood banking, also known as *immunohematology,* is an area in clinical laboratory practice that involves treatment of the patient with blood or its products (clinical therapy) that must comply with specific Food and Drug Administration (FDA) regulations.

immunoglobulin classes. Two classes of immunoglobulins (IgM and IgG) play a major role in donor and recipient testing before transfusion of blood and/or its products. The pre-transfusion testing includes patient and donor blood group typing and compatibility testing (cross-match), as well as patient serum screening for presence of antibodies (immune or pre-formed) that are directed against patient red blood cell antigens.

These tests are performed to prevent adverse reactions (blood transfusion reactions) in response to incompatible blood or blood products (components) administered to the patient (see discussion of graft rejection in Chapter 6).

immunoglobulin M (IgM). IgM molecules (antibodies) are detectable as naturally occurring antibodies (hemagglutinins), produced in response to naturally occurring environmental agents.

These IgM class isohemagglutinins (anti-A and anti-B [anti-ABH] blood group antibodies) agglutinate erythrocytes of other individuals of the same species in physiologic saline (0.85%) at room temperature (Table 5-5). These antibodies are referred to as "complete antibodies" because of their structure (pentamer), consisting of ten antigen-binding sites (see Figure 5-12) in each IgM molecule that can bind to the specific antigenic determinants (epitopes) on erythrocytes, thus forming visible aggregates (agglutination) of erythrocytes.

Other examples of IgM class antibodies detected in blood banking are anti-Ii, anti-MN, anti-Lewis (Le^a, Le^b), anti-Lutheran (Lu^a), and anti-P. "Cold" antibodies (appearing at cold 4° temperature and disappearing at 37°) are also of the IgM class.

Pre-blood transfusion testing of a patient for presence of these antibodies is important for selecting (matching) appropriate donor blood (lacking the specific [complementary] antigen on the red blood cells, against which specific antibodies have been identified in the patient) to prevent transfusion reaction.

immunoglobulin G (IgG). In blood banking, IgG is sometimes referred to as an "immune" antibody or a hemagglutinin that has been produced in response to antigens on the surface of erythrocytes during incompatible blood transfusion or pregnancy (immunization).

This class of antibodies does not agglutinate erythrocytes suspended in physiologic saline. Instead, IgG molecules require potentiators (such as protein medium, enzymes, anti-human globulin reagents) to facilitate erythrocyte agglutination (bringing cells closer together) by reducing zeta potential, cross-linking, or altering IgG molecules (see Table 5-5 and Chapter 10). Thus, in blood banking, IgG molecules are known as "incomplete" antibodies and include such antibodies as anti-Ss, anti-Kell (Kk, Js^a, Js^b), Rh (CDEce), Lutheran (Lu^b), Duffy (Fy^a, Fy^b) and Kidd (JK^a, JK^b).

Detection of any one or more of these antigen-specific (blood group or type) antibodies in a patient and donor ensures that the blood selected for transfusion is compatible (lacks complementary antigen), thus preventing blood transfusion reactions. Detection of antibodies in the mother (directed against fetal erythrocytes bearing antigens not present in the mother) and administration of anti-IgG can prevent development of hemolytic disease of the newborn (destruction of fetal erythrocytes). A comprehensive discussion of these topics is within the scope of immunohematology (blood banking).

Table **5-5**	CHARACTERISTICS OF IgM AND IgG CLASSES OF ANTIBODIES RELATING TO BLOOD BANK LABORATORY PRACTICE		
	Characteristic	IgM Class	IgG Class
	Size of Ig molecule	Pentamer	Monomer
	Heavy chain type	Mu (μ)	Gamma (γ)
	Temperature	RT	37° C
	Reaction medium	Saline	High protein
	Sedimentation constant	19S	7S
	Type of antibody	Naturally occurring	"Immune" or specific
	Complement activation	Yes	Yes (except IgG$_4$)
	Passes placenta	No	Yes

Ig, immunoglobulin (antibody); *S,* sedimentation constant; *RT,* room temperature.

Suggested Readings

Abbas AK, Lichtman AH, Pober JS: Antibodies and antigens (pp 41-62). In *Cellular and molecular immunology,* ed 4, Philadelphia, 2000, WB Saunders.

Davies DR: Structural basis of antibody function, *Ann Rev Immunol* 1:87, 1994.

Hall S: Monoclonal antibodies at age 20: promise at last? *Science* 270:915, 1995.

Parker DC: T cell–dependent B cell activation, *Ann Rev Immunol* 11:331, 1993.

Roit MV: Brostoff J, Male DK: Antibodies and their receptors (pp 4.1-4.12). In *Immunology,* ed 4, St Louis, 1996, Mosby.

Snapper CM, Mond JJ: Toward a comprehensive view of immunoglobulin class switching, *Immunol Today* 14:15, 1993.

Tonewaga S: Somatic generation of antibody diversity, *Nature* 302:575, 1983.

Review Questions

HUMORAL IMMUNE RESPONSE

1-4. Associate the following cells of the immune system with their role in humoral immune response:

____ CD4+ lymphocytes
____ plasma cells
____ macrophages
____ β lymphocytes

a. MHC-restricted antigen (peptides) recognition
b. cytotoxicity
c. antigen-presenting cells
d. helper T cells
e. antigen-binding by sIg receptors
f. synthesize immunoglobulins (Ig) molecules
g. phagocytosis

5. MHC-restricted antigen (antigenic peptides) recognition is attributed to:
a. CD4+ T cells and macrophages
b. CD4+ and CD8+ T cells
c. CD8+ T cells and natural killer (NK) cells
d. all cells of the immune system

6. Cells of the immune system that are able to differentiate between self and non-self (foreign) antigens during an antigen recognition event and trigger an immune response are:
a. CD4+ and CD8+ T lymphocytes
b. CD8+ T lymphocytes and B lymphocytes
c. B lymphocytes and CD4+ T lymphocytes
d. all of the above

7. Interaction between B and T cells is necessary for inducing a humoral immune response. Select the molecules that participate in the interaction:
a. class II MHC-peptide complex
b. T cell surface receptors (TCRs)
c. CD4+ T cell-secreted cytokines
d. all of the above

8. During secondary immune response, memory B cells are stimulated by antigen to differentiate into antibody-secreting plasma cells. The most abundant class of antibodies synthesized during the secondary immune response is:
a. IgG   b. IgM
c. IgD   d. IgE

9. The encounter of B lymphocytes with a foreign antigen that produces an immune response occurs mainly in the:
a. thymus

b. bone marrow
c. lymphoid tissues
d. blood

IMMUNOGLOBULIN MOLECULES

10. Fragments, produced during proteolytic cleavage of the immunoglobulin molecule by the enzymes papain and pepsin, which retain antigen-binding function are:
    a. Fc
    b. Fab and Fc
    c. Fab
    d. Fab and $F(ab')_2$

11. Select the regions within the immunoglobulin molecule where antigen-binding occurs:
    a. constant regions
    b. hinge regions
    c. carboxyl terminals
    d. hypervariable regions

12. The regions of an immunoglobulin molecule that are associated with biologic activity during an immune response are the heavy chain:
    a. globular regions
    b. variable regions
    c. constant regions
    d. hypervariable regions

13. Within each variable heavy and light chain regions are three highly variable amino acid stretches. These hypervariable regions (protruding loops on surface of variable regions of heavy and light chain domains) are known as:
    a. antigen-binding sites
    b. complementarity-determining regions
    c. CDR1, CDR2, and CDR3
    d. all of the above

14. Immunoglobulin molecules occur in two forms. Select the form that serves as a cell surface receptor for antigens, known as:
    a. TCR/CD3+   b. CD4+
    c. BCR   d. MHC

15. Monoclonal antibodies are produced during immune response to a single antigenic stimulus (antigenic determinant or epitope) and show all the following characteristics, *except:*
    a. antigen specificity
    b. heterogeneity
    c. homogeneity
    d. preselected immunoglobulin class (isotype)

16-19. Match the following antibodies with their unique description:

    ____ heterophil
    ____ anti-idiotypic
    ____ "designer" monoclonal
    ____ polyclonal

    a. anti-immunoglobulin antibodies
    b. Igs of undefined antigen specificity, capable of reacting with cell-surface antigens on cells of other species
    c. produced in vitro by altering Ig genes and constructing new Ig genes by molecular methods
    d. diverse group of antibodies

20. In producing monoclonal antibodies, all the following methods can be used, *except:*
    a. hybridoma technology
    b. immunization of animals
    c. polymerase chain reactor (PCR)
    d. somatic cell hybridization

21. Construction of the Fab gene library involves PCR amplification of which fragments of the Ig:
    a. all variable heavy and light chain fragments
    b. constant and hinge region fragments
    c. random heavy and light chain fragments
    d. all of the above

22. The name of immunoglobulin classes (isotypes) correspond to the name of which region of the Ig molecule:
    a. heavy chain variable region
    b. light chain region
    c. variable region
    d. heavy chain constant region

23-27. Match the following Ig classes with the appropriate characteristics:

____ IgM
____ Ig G
____ Ig D
____ IgE
____ IgA

a. major Ig class expressed on surface of B cells
b. monomeric structure found in all Ig classes
c. found in trace amount in serum
d. predominant class of Ig in serum
e. major Ig class found in body secretions
f. Ig molecules lacking hinge region
g. have similar electrophoretic mobility

28. The ability of the immune system to produce an almost limitless number of Igs showing specificity for a variety of antigens is attributed to all of the following, *except:*
a. rearrangement of Ig genes
b. recombination of V, D, and J gene segments
c. diversity in amino acid sequences within the variable region
d. class-switching

29. Diversity in biologic (effector) functions associated with the various Ig classes is genetically determined and is produced by a class-switching mechanism that involves:
a. cytokines, acting as "switch factors"
b. recombination of constant region heavy chain (C_H) gene
c. B cell activator (antigen-specific CD4+ T cell)
d. all of the above

30. Genes for Ig variants (variability in constant regions of Ig) are present in all members of the same species and can be expressed as various Ig classes, also known as:
a. idiotypes
b. allotypes
c. isotypes
d. heterotypes

FUNCTIONAL CHARACTERISTICS OF IMMUNOGLOBULINS

31. An antibody showing specificity for a stimulating antigen may also bind with another antigen-containing epitope common to both antigens. This type of antibody/antigen binding is known as:
a. avidity
b. cross-reactivity
c. cross-specificity
d. affinity

32. The strength of the non-covalent bond that forms between a single epitope (antigen) and a single antibody-combining site is referred to as antibody:
a. avidity
b. affinity
c. specificity
d. all of the above

33. The segment of DNA that codes for proteins (Igs) is known as:
a. exon
b. intron
c. paratope
d. all of the above

34. The B lymphocyte has the ability to change its production of Ig class (isotype) from IgM to IgG during DNA recombination known as:
a. DNA splicing
b. heavy chain class-switching
c. variable region gene-switching
d. C to V-J-D rearrangement

35-39. Associate the following immunoglobulin (Ig) classes with their specific biologic (effector) function:

____ IgG
____ IgM
____ IgE
____ IgD
____ IgA

a. activation of complement
b. placental crossing in fetus
c. enhancement of phagocytosis
d. mucosal immunity
e. allergic reactions
f. binding to Fc receptors on certain cells
g. not identified

40. Most important immunoglobulin class associated with the body's defense against infectious agents (particularly pus forming), appearing also as a major Ig class during secondary immune response, is the:
a. IgM
b. IgG
c. IgE
d. all of the above

41. Two major classes of immunoglobulins, important in donor and recipient testing before blood transfusion to prevent adverse reactions, are:
a. IgG and IgM
b. IgG and IgE
c. IgD and IgA
d. IgM and IgA

42. All the following are important in pre-transfusion testing of patient and donor, *except:*
a. selecting donor blood for transfusion
b. preventing adverse transfusion reactions
c. detecting antigen-specific antibodies
d. identifying extracellular antigens

CHAPTER 6 _____

Immune Response to Tissue Antigens in Transplantation

Upon completion of Chapter 6, the student will be prepared to:

MAJOR HISTOCOMPATIBILITY COMPLEX/ TRANSPLANTATION (MHC)

- Define the following key terms: *allogeneic, tissue marker, histocompatibility antigens, MHC, genotype, phenotyping.*
- List names of HLA antigens that are expressed by each HLA locus on human chromosome 6.
- Differentiate between MHC I and MHC class II molecules (antigens) by stating: (1) cells on which each class of antigens is expressed, (2) functions of each class of MHC antigens, (3) cells of immune system involved in recognition of each type of MHC antigen, (4) name of antigen receptor on each cell type involved in recognition of MHC, (5) mechanism involved in recognition of each MHC class of alloantigens, (6) role of class I and class II MHC molecules in specific recognition of foreign (non-self) antigens by the immune system.
- Define the following terms used in clinical transplantation: *transplantation, graft rejection, allograft, syngeneic graft, immunosuppression, graft, cytotoxicity, autograft, xenogeneic graft, histocompatibility.*
- Name in vivo and in vitro procedures that are available for identifying each class of MHC molecules.

MAJOR HISTOCOMPATIBILITY ANTIGENS IN TRANSPLANTATION

- Describe types of host immune mechanisms responsible for rejection of donor cells expressing incompatible HLA on their surface.
- List types of immune graft rejections, classified according to the graft tissue pathology (histopathology) observed.
- State situations in which graft vs. host reaction may occur.

PREVENTION OF GRAFT REJECTION

- List two strategies used to prevent, treat, or reduce the severity of an immune graft rejection.

- Describe effect of immunosuppression of the patient on survival of the graft.

OTHER APPLICATIONS OF HISTOCOMPATIBILITY ANTIGENS IN CLINICAL IMMUNOLOGY

- Describe use of HLA genotyping (genetic profile) in disease association studies and paternity disputes.
- List laboratory tests currently available for determining genetic profiles.
- State the criteria used in direct and indirect exclusion of paternity.

Key Terms

allele - Variant of a gene located at a specific locus on a chromosome.

alloantibody - Antibody with the same specificity as the antigen (alloantigen) against which it is directed.

alloantigens - Molecules (antigens) expressed on cells of genetically dissimilar individuals (e.g., donor), which are recognized by the immune system (host) as foreign.

allogeneic - Genetically dissimilar (non-identical) members of the same species.

allograft (allogeneic graft) - Graft that is transplanted between two genetically distinct individuals of the same species. Also refers to organ transplants.

alloreactive - Refers to antigen (alloantigen)-activated antibodies or lymphocytes that show specific reactivity toward alloantigens.

autograft (autologous graft) - Graft transplanted from one area to another in the same individual.

cell lysis - Disruption of cell membrane by complement or cytotoxic T cells, resulting in cell destruction by release of cell contents. Presence of "ghost" cells (cell outlines) and stain uptake by dead cells indicate cell lysis.

cytotoxicity - Effector mechanism of cell-mediated immune response, whereby cytotoxic T cells direct their cytotoxic effect toward cells bearing foreign (e.g., incompatible HLA) antigens, causing target cell lysis.

donor - Individual who provides a graft (cells, tissue, or organs).

graft - Cells or tissues obtained from one site and transplanted to another site in the same individual. The term is also used to define a transplant taken from one individual and transplanted into another individual (usually an allograft).

graft rejection - Consequence of a host's immune response directed against donor alloantigens. Graft destruction, usually cell lysis by cytotoxicity, precedes a graft rejection.

histocompatibility antigens - Terminology used in transplantation to describe class I MHC molecules expressed on surface of all nucleated cells. Also known as *human leukocyte antigens (HLA)*.

host - Recipient of an allogeneic graft.

human leukocyte antigens (HLA) - HLA are also known as histocompatibility antigens and MHC antigens. The term is often used in transplantation and denotes identification of MHC by tissue typing procedures.

immunocompetent - Having the ability to mount an immune reaction.

immunodeficiency - Deficiency of the immune system, exhibiting reduced ability to appropriately respond to an antigenic stimulation.

immunosuppression - Deliberate or spontaneous inhibition of immune responses, resulting from immunosuppressive drug therapy (e.g., cyclosporine) or certain infections (e.g., HIV), respectively.

in vitro - Refers to studies performed in a laboratory.

in vivo - Refers to reactions observed in a live organism.

Major histocompatibility complex (MHC) - Refers to a region on human chromosome 6 that codes for MHC molecules (antigens) expressed on certain cells. MHC molecules show unique specificity in each individual and are able to discriminate between self and non-self antigens.

marker - Usually refers to tissue markers (e.g., HLA), which consist of antigens expressed on a cell surface, identifying the individual's unique genetic make-up **(genotype).** Soluble molecules may also serve as genetic markers.

target cell - Cell displaying foreign antigens, which are responsible for evoking an immune response. For example, in a cell-mediated response, cytotoxicity is directed against the target cell (causing cell lysis).

transplantation - Life-saving or life-enhancing procedure that involves replacement or enhancement of malfunctioning tissues or organs in situations that are life threatening or debilitating (wasting) to the patient.

It has been observed that tissue transplanted between **allogeneic** (genetically non-identical) individuals usually triggers an immune response causing rejection of the transplanted tissue **(allograft).** This response of the immune system to graft **alloantigens** (genetically determined dissimilar antigens), in the absence of immunosuppression (see discussion following), may occur in the form of a specific (cell-mediated or humoral) immune response and a non-specific immune response. Although antibodies (effectors of humoral immune response) may contribute to rejection of transplanted tissue, the cell-mediated immune response is the most important mechanism in graft rejection.

Graft rejection occurs when major histocompatibility antigens (class I MHC and class II MHC molecules) of the recipient do not "match" the histocompatibility antigens of the donor tissue as is typical in transplantation of **allografts.** This genetic dissimilarity is referred to as **incompatibility** between the donor and recipient MHC antigens (human lymphocyte antigens [HLA]).

The severity of the immune reaction of the graft recipient to transplanted donor tissue (graft) may be reduced in two ways: (1) by suppressing the patient's immune system with various immunosuppressive drugs or (2) by testing for histocompatibility between graft and recipient before transplantation (see discussion following).

The assumption that tissue compatibility will improve graft acceptance is based on the observation that tissue grafted between identical twins (genetically identical or **syngeneic**), does not result in graft rejection. It follows that the greater the compatibility of the graft with the recipient MHC gene products (HLA), the greater is the graft acceptance and avoidance of its rejection.

The importance of histocompatibility antigens in transplantation was first discovered in animal (mice) studies. It was observed that when histocompatibility antigens were matched, graft rejection was diminished.

Subsequently, a similar histocompatibility antigen complex (MHC), expressed on certain cells as a product of MHC genes, was discovered in humans. The basis for this discovery was an observation that antibodies in sera of transfused patients and multiparous women reacted with tissue antigens, later identified as the MHC. This observation led to the assumption that specific antibodies (leukoagglutinins) directed against tissue antigens were responsible for the reaction.

Thus MHC became particularly important in understanding graft rejection in clinical transplantation and subsequently in other procedures, where detection of the MHC molecules (HLA) assists in making such decisions as selection of HLA compatible donors in transplantation and establishing a pattern of HLA inheritance in paternity disputes.

With the advent of transplantation immunology, procedures such as histocompatibility testing and immunosuppressive therapy (discussed following) developed as essential components of pretransplantation procedures that

could predict graft survival and contribute to graft acceptance, respectively.

MAJOR HISTOCOMPATIBILITY COMPLEX/TRANSPLANTATION (MHC)

DESCRIPTION

Major histocompatibility complex (MHC) in humans is known as the *human leukocyte antigen (HLA) complex* and occupies a large region of genes located on the short arm of chromosome 6. The MHC genes (histocompatibility genes) code for protein molecules (MHC antigens) expressed on the surface of various cells.

Genetic Organization

The MHC gene region on chromosome 6 consists of separate loci designated as HLA-A, HLA-B, HLA-C, HLA-D, and HLA-DR (-DR, -DP, -DQ) (Figure 6-1). At each locus one of a number of alleles may be present (e.g., HLA-A1, HLA-A2, etc.), which codes for a MHC (HLA) antigen with specificity unique to that particular allele. MHC antigens are also known as *MHC gene products, human leukocyte antigens (HLA), histocompatibility antigens,* or *tissue compatibility antigens.*

The inheritance of MHC genes follows simple mendelian inheritance, so that each individual has two half-sets of genes (one half from each parent), which are expressed equally

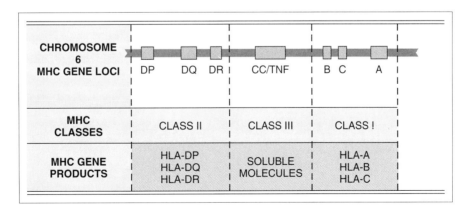

FIGURE **6-1**   **Schematic Representation of Major Histocompatibility Complex (MHC) Gene Region on Chromosome 6.**   Class I and class II MHC genes code for class I and II MHC molecules (HLA). Expressed on the surface of various cells, HLA is detectable by tissue typing techniques and serves as an unique tissue marker that reflects an individual's genetic make-up. Class III MHC genes code for soluble molecules (e.g., complement components, tissue necrosis factor). *MHC,* major histocompatibility complex; *HLA,* human leukocyte antigen; *CC,* complement component; *TNF,* tissue necrosis factor.

(maternal and paternal antigens) on the cell surface of an offspring. A combination of alleles at each locus on a chromosome is inherited from each parent as a unit (haplotype).

Three classes of MHC gene products have been identified and classified as follows:

- Class I molecules (HLA-A, HLA-B, HLA-C antigens)
- Class II molecules (HLA-D, HLA-DR, HLA-DQ, HLA-DP antigens)
- Class III molecules (PF [properdin factor]), C2, C4a and C4b [complement components], TNFα, TNFγ [tumor necrosis factor])

HLA-A, HLA-B, and HLA-C loci on chromosome 6 code for class I MHC molecules (cell surface antigens). Class II (HLA-D) region of chromosome 6 includes three subregions, (HLA-DR, HLA-DQ, HLA-DP), each with multiple loci that code for class II molecules expressed on cell membranes and the recently discovered HLA-DN and HLA-DO subregions, each containing a single genetic locus. The expression of class I and class II MHC molecules on the surface of various cells is controlled by various cytokines, such as interferon-γ (IFNγ) and tumor necrosis factor (TNF).

Genes coding for class III MHC molecules are located in the class III region on chromosome 6, between the HLA-B locus and the HLA-DR subregion (see Figure 6-1). These class III MHC molecules (gene products) are not histocompatibility antigens but are certain soluble molecules such as complement components and tissue necrosis factor, previously discussed (see Chapter 4).

Nomenclature

The official nomenclature for the HLA system is established by the HLA Nomenclature Committee of the World Health Organization (WHO) (Table 6-1). The Nomenclature Committee recognizes seven groups of antigens (HLA-A, -B, -C, -D, -DR, -DQ, -DP), with each specificity designated by a locus and a number (e.g., HLA-A2, where A is locus and 2 is the number). HLA-C antigens also have a "w" to distinguish them from complement components, while the "w" associated with HLA-D and HLA-DP antigens denotes workshop status, a provisional designation for these groups of antigens. Parenthesis by a particular antigen denotes it as original antigen from which subgroups or "splits" arise.

CLASS I MHC MOLECULES

Class I MHC molecules (antigens), also known as **human leukocyte antigens (HLA)** or **histocompatibility antigens,** are gene products that are expressed on the cell surface of all nucleated cells within the body as well as on platelets, showing highest concentration on T lymphocytes, B lymphocytes, and macrophages.

Structure

HLA antigens consist of HLA-A, HLA-B, and HLA-C molecules. These class I MHC molecules are encoded by genes of the HLA-A, -B, and -C loci of the MHC region located on chromosome 6.

Class I MHC molecules consist of a chain, containing three domains (regions) that are held together by intrachain disulfide bonds. The

Table 6-1	HLA SPECIFICITIES*						
MHC Gene	**Class I Loci**			**Class II Loci**			
Locus	A	B	C	D	DR	DQ	DP
Cell-surface antigen	HLA-A	HLA-B	HLA-C	HLA-D	HLA-DR	HLA-DQ	HLA-DP
HLA specificity	A1	B5	Cw1	Dw1	DR1	DQ1	DPw1
	A2	B7	Cw2	Dw2	DR103	DQ2	DPw2
	A203	B703	Cw3	Dw3	DR2	DQ3	DPw3

*Nomenclature devised by HLA Nomenclature Committee of the World Health Organization (1991).
"w" (e.g., HLA-Cw) distinguishes HLA antigens from "C" referring to complement components; "w" (e.g., HLA-Dw and HLA-DPw) designates workshop or provisional status; A, B, C, D, DR, DQ, DP, designate specific loci on chromosome 6.

molecules are polymorphic (many forms) glyco-proteins that are linked to a non-polymorphic beta-2 globulin. They are membrane-bound and extend through the cell membrane (trans-membrane) into the cytoplasm (see Figure 3-7).

The specificity of the HLA molecule resides within its extracellular two domains that serve as antigen-binding sites for previously pro-cessed peptides by antigen-presenting cells (APCs) to which HLA is bound. These extracel-lular domains contain the bound peptide frag-ment from the MHC–antigenic peptide complex that is presented by the APC for recognition by T cell receptors (TCR) located on the surface of a CD8+ T lymphocyte.

Function

Class I molecules are associated with three main functions (discussed following).

Specific Tissue Markers

Because class I HLA molecules are a gene product, they reflect the specific and unique genetic make-up of an individual. Serving as specific tissue markers, they may be identified by in vitro tissue typing. Reagent antibodies di-rected against a specific HLA marker are used in this tissue typing procedures (see following).

Recognition of Foreign Antigens

Class I molecules are able to bind endogenous proteins (on virally altered cells), serving both as antigen-presenting cells (APCs) and target cells. The processed endogenous proteins are bound to class I MHC molecules, forming a MHC–antigenic peptide complex, which is pre-sented to T cells (CD8+) for recognition. If the antigen is recognized as foreign, a cell-medi-ated immune response (cytotoxicity) is initi-ated. This type of antigen recognition is re-ferred to as *class I MHC–restricted antigen recognition* (see Figure 1-12).

Graft Rejection

Class I molecules, also known as *histocompati-bility antigens* or *transplantation antigens* in clinical transplantation, are the principal anti-gens recognized by a host during a clinical transplantation when MHC molecules of the transplanted donor tissue differ from those of the recipient (host). An in vivo immune re-sponse is mounted by the host against the donor cells, resulting in an immune graft rejection.

A good correlation exists between most graft rejections by the host except in graft-vs.-host reaction (One Step Further Box 6-1) and an in vitro cell-mediated cytolysis (see Histocompat-ibility Testing, described in Chapter 14).

CLASS II MHC MOLECULES

Structure

Class II antigens were first postulated to be the product of immune response (Ir) genes. Currently, genes encoding the class II anti-gens (HLA-DP, HLA-DR, and HLA-DQ), also re-ferred to as *MHC gene products*, are associated with MHC on chromosome 6. MHC consists of MHC subregions, DP, DQ, and DR, each of which contains multiple loci. Class II MHC antigens (molecules) are located on a surface of immunocompetent cells, including mono-cytes, B lymphocytes, activated T lympho-cytes, and macrophages. Although cells such as resting T cells, endothelial, and thyroid cells do not normally express class II molecules, they may be induced to do so. With the avail-ability of specific monoclonal antibodies (anti-sera), the class II antigens have been serologi-cally defined as HLA-DR, HLA-DQ, and a few HLA-DP.

All class II molecules have a similar struc-ture. They are glycoproteins, consisting of one α and one β polypeptide chains that are non-covalently linked and span the cell membrane. Each polypeptide chain has two extracellular domains (regions) held by disulfide bonds, a transmembrane segment, and an intracellular domain. The extracellular region of the chain is the binding site for attachment of processed antigenic peptide fragments (see Figure 3-7).

Function

The main function of class II MHC molecules is their participation in the following activity.

Recognition of Foreign Antigens

Recognition initiates an immune response. Briefly, antigen-presenting cells (APCs) display their cell surface–bound class II MHC molecule–processed antigen (peptide) for recognition by CD4+ helper T lymphocytes (see Figure 1-9). Whether the immune response will or will not

Box 6-1

Graft-vs.-Host Reaction

In allografts that differ from a recipient (host) at the class I and class II loci, both the CD8+ and CD4+ T lymphocytes become activated by recognizing the alloantigens (genetically dissimilar antigens within the same species) of the graft (donor tissue), thus initiating a graft rejection reaction.

A reverse situation may also occur, where T cells of the graft tissue recognize alloantigens of the host cells (incompatible MHC molecules), thus stimulating an immune reaction against the host tissue. This type of response is known as **graft-vs.-host (GVH) reaction** (Figure 6-2) and occurs when:

- There are differences in histocompatibility (transplantation antigens) between the graft (donor) tissue and the host (recipient)
- The host is immunodeficient and not able to reject foreign (incompatible) cells
- The graft cells are immunocompetent and are able to trigger an immune reaction against the host cells

A GVH reaction may result from administration or infusion of blood or various blood products containing viable (immunocompetent) lymphocytes, such as in cases of intrauterine transfusion, whole blood or packed erythrocytes transfusion, platelets, frozen cells, fresh plasma, or maternal-fetal blood transfusion. GVH reaction may also be triggered by transplantation of fetal thymus, fetal liver, or bone marrow.

The graft-vs.-host reaction (GVH) may proceed to **graft-vs.-host disease (GVHD)**, when the host becomes injured by GVH and the injury results in complete dysfunction of the affected area. This type of an immune reaction against the host is the most limiting factor in transplantation, particularly in transplantation of allogeneic bone marrow.

Classification

GVHD has been classified according to the histologic pattern observed at the site of injury:

- **Acute GVHD:** Histologic evaluation shows epithelial cell necrosis (death) in the skin, liver, and gastrointestinal (GI) tract. Clinically, GVHD is characterized by rash, jaundice, diarrhea, and pulmonary infiltrates. Enhanced susceptibility to infections may result in death from infection (sepsis).
- **Chronic GVHD:** Presence of fibrosis and atrophy of one of the target sites (skin, liver, or

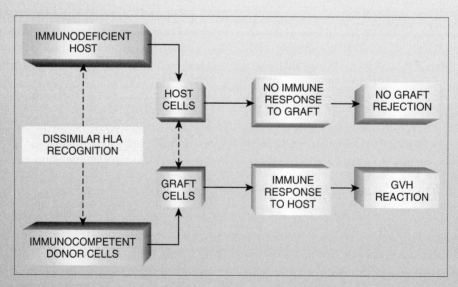

FIGURE **6-2**   **Graft-vs.-Host Reaction (GVH).**   GVH is an immune response of immunocompetent (viable) donor cells directed against a host as a result of HLA incompatibility (dissimilarity). It occurs if the host's immune system is incompetent (immunosuppressed, compromised, immunodeficient) and unable to reject the HLA incompatible graft.

Box 6-1—cont'd

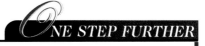

GI tract) is observed. This may lead to dysfunction of the affected site and may be fatal when complete dysfunction occurs. Chronic GVHD is associated with severe cellular immunodeficiency and may be seen in patients who have received transfusion of potentially immunocompetent cells within 5 to 30 days. GVHD may also be the result of maternal-fetal transfusion or immunotherapy with bone marrow transplantation. Secondary infection is a frequent complication in GVHD.

Mechanism

Although the mechanism involved in this type of immune reaction and the production of cell necrosis is not fully understood, natural killer (NK) cells are implicated as effector cells of an immune response at the graft-vs.-host reaction site. These NK cells (effector cells) are seen attached to the dying epithelial cells at the site of the reaction. It is believed that the NK cells, when activated by IL-2, become lymphokine-

activated killer cells (LAK). Because LAK cells are not MHC-restricted, they are able to lyse normal cells without specific recognition of their alloantigens.

Treatment

Acute and chronic GVHD are treated by immunosuppression. Although there is no adequate treatment available once the GVHD is established, cyclosporine may be useful.

Prevention

Prevention of GVHD is essential. Therefore any patient who has immunodeficiency and requires administration of blood products should receive cells (whole blood, packed erythrocytes, platelets) that have been previously (1) typed for HLA antigens, (2) tested for compatibility (histocompatibility test or cross-match), and (3) irradiated (3000 to 6000 R of radiation) to destroy viable (immunocompetent) lymphocytes.

---

occur depends on recognition of the MHC-antigen complex by the CD4+ cells as non-self or self. This mechanism for recognition of a particular antigenic stimulus is in the context of "MHC restriction" (see One Step Further Box 3-3).

MAJOR HISTOCOMPATIBILITY ANTIGENS IN TRANSPLANTATION

Transplantation of an allogeneic (genetically dissimilar) graft is the best understood and most practiced procedure in transplantation immunology, used to correct an existing functional deficit (organ or tissue) in a patient. However, the genetic dissimilarity that exists between the donor major histocompatibility antigens (MHC class I and class II) on donor cells and the recipient MHC (class I and class II MHC antigens) is the major reason for an immune reaction that causes graft rejection.

The severity of the immune reaction (graft rejection) by the host to transplanted donor tissue (graft) may be reduced mainly by suppressing the patient's immune system with various immunosuppressive drugs and by testing for histocompatibility between the graft

and the recipient before transplantation (see discussion following).

The assumption that tissue compatibility will improve graft acceptance is based on the observation that tissue grafted between identical twins (genetically identical or syngeneic), does not result in graft rejection. It follows that, the greater the compatibility of the graft with the recipient MHC gene products (HLA antigens), the greater the graft acceptance and avoidance of its rejection.

TYPES OF GRAFTS

Clinical transplantation (transfer) of graft (organ or tissue transplant) from one individual to another individual of the same species is referred to as an **allogeneic graft (allograft).** However, other sources of grafts are also available for research studies (e.g., xenografts).

Nomenclature

The following terms describe various grafts that have been used in research and clinical practice:

- *Allogeneic graft (allograft):* Graft transplanted between two genetically different

Table 6-2   CLINICAL TRANSPLANTATION

Graft	Preventive Measures*	Indications
Kidney	ABO and HLA testing/HLA matching (patient/ donor)	End-stage renal failure
Liver	Immunosuppressive and ALG therapy, ABO blood group match	Progressive liver disease (cirrhosis, tumors)
Bone marrow	HLA and ABO match, antibiotic/chemotherapy/ radiotherapy	Immunodeficiency, leukemia, and lymphomas
Skin	Not required (autografts), immunosuppression (allografts)	Burns
Cornea	Not required (no blood vessels)	Keratitis, ulcerations
Heart	HLA typing and HLA antibody screening, immunosuppressive and ALG therapy	End-stage cardiac dysfunction
Pancreas, islet (IL) cells	Immunosuppression	Complications of diabetes (uremia)

*Required pretransplantation testing and treatment of graft recipient to prevent or minimize immune reaction against a graft (graft rejection).
ABO, blood group antigens located on erythrocytes; *HLA*, human leukocyte antigens; *ALG*, anti-leukocyte globulin; *IL*, islets of Langerhans (insulin-producing tissue).

individuals of the same species, containing alloantigens (molecules recognized by the recipient immune system as foreign). Immune response is initiated against the graft, resulting in graft rejection (see discussion of prevention of graft rejection following).

- *Autologous graft (autograft):* Describes a graft (tissue) transplanted from one body site of an individual to another site (donor tissue and recipient site are on same individual and therefore genetically identical). No graft rejection is anticipated.
- *Syngeneic graft (syngraft):* Graft transplanted between two genetically identical individuals. Graft rejection does not occur (complete compatibility between MHC molecules of donor [source of graft] and MHC molecules of the recipient [host]).
- *Xenogeneic graft (xenograft or heterograft):* Graft from one species transplanted into another species. This type of transplantation is not well understood although it is believed that the main obstacle to xenogeneic transplantation is the presence of naturally occurring antibodies.

Clinical Transplants

Advances in transplantation procedures and testing such as immunosuppressive drug therapy (e.g., cyclosporin), histocompatibility testing, and monoclonal antibody therapy have improved the success rate of various grafts, such as renal (kidney) transplants. These advances have opened new possibilities for using other organs and tissues in clinical transplantation. A limiting factor in transplantation continues to be the unavailability of donor organs.

Starting with the first successful kidney transplantation (1954), which is the current protocol used to treat end-stage renal disease, other organs and tissue grafts have subsequently been successfully transplanted (Table 6-2). With the increasing success (reduced graft rejection), transplantation procedures are now no longer used only as life-saving emergency procedures. Most common and successful transplantation procedures involve the following grafts, briefly described.

Corneal Transplants

Replacement of a cornea is a common and highly successful form of therapy in non-healing corneal ulcerations, which does not require immunosuppression of the recipient before the transplantation. Graft rejections are infrequent because of a technique that involves placement of small corneal grafts in a central location to avoid contact with the highly vascular surrounding area (containing lymphocytes). Corneal tissues do not contain blood vessels.

Bone Marrow Graft

This graft consists of intravenous infusion of allogeneic or autogeneic (autologous) hematopoietic stem cells to correct reduced bone marrow function. In autologous bone marrow transplantation, stem (progenitor) cells are obtained from the patient before treatment (e.g., chemotherapy) and infused back after treatment to restore the normal bone marrow function reduced by chemotherapy.

Reduced bone marrow function may also be associated with an existing defect or reduction in hematopoietic stem cells, such as is seen in various blood dyscrasias or abnormalities (e.g., acute leukemia), in immunodeficiency states, and in certain metabolic diseases.

Complications associated with bone marrow transplantation include acute or chronic GVHD and microbial infections. However, pretreatment of the patient with immunoglobulins (intravenous administration) and antithymocyte or antilymphocyte globulin reduces the possibility of complications, particularly GVHD. Histocompatibility testing (particularly HLA-D related), before transplantation, increases success of the allograft.

Kidney Transplants

First successful organ transplantation (1954) consisted of a transfer of a syngraft (kidney from a monozygous twin). Subsequently, improvement in administration of immunosuppressive drugs and advances in histocompatibility testing increased the success rate of transplantation. The availability of allogeneic (genetically dissimilar living or cadaveric donor) kidney (renal) transplants has also increased the availability of kidney transplants and their rate of success.

pretransfusion laboratory testing in renal transplants. Specific donor and recipient (host) testing before renal transplantation is essential and includes:

- Erythrocyte ABO blood group testing (ABO antigens are present on erythrocytes and vascular endothelium).
- ABO compatibility cross-match between donor and recipient. Transplantation of an

incompatible graft results in very rapid graft rejection (hyperacute rejection) because of preexisting natural antibodies (isohemagglutinins) that injure the graft endothelium.

- Tissue typing (HLA -A, -B, -C, -DR, and DQ antigens) to match donor with HLA-compatible recipient.
- Histocompatibility procedure (e.g., mixed leukocyte reaction [MLR]) evaluates an in vitro immune response between the donor and host MHC molecules (HLA antigens). The stronger the MLR (incompatibility), the greater the possibility of graft rejection (decreased graft survival).

posttransplantation immunosuppression. Immunosuppression (e.g., immunosuppressive drugs, anti-lymphocyte monoclonal antibodies) is indicated in patients (graft recipients) to prevent or treat graft rejection.

Contraindication to Transplantation

An existence of infection or debilitating disease (e.g., cancer) is a contraindication to transplantation.

IMMUNE RESPONSE TO GRAFTS

As previously discussed (see Clonal Selection, Chapter 3), T cells are normally selected during a "clonal selection" process to recognize only foreign peptides (antigens) within the self major histocompatibility complex (MHC) context. This MHC-restricted antigen recognition by T cell antigen receptors (TCRs) plays an important role in preventing the immune system from reacting against its self-antigens.

In tissue transplantation, the recipient's T cells recognize donor MHC molecules (antigens) on the cells of a graft as self or non-self. An immune response (graft rejection) is triggered when donor MHC molecules differ from the MHC molecules of the recipient.

Molecular Basis for Recognition of Alloantigens

Role of T Cell Receptors in Alloantigen Recognition

Research findings indicate that recognition of donor alloantigens (genetically dissimilar antigens) by the immune system and subsequent

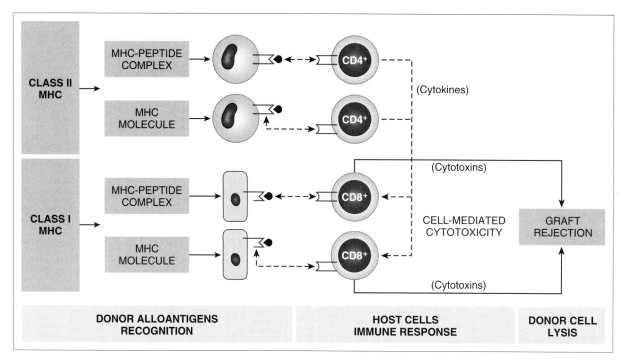

FIGURE **6-3**   **Recognition of Alloantigens.**   Recognition of class I and class II MHC molecules (HLA) occurs in two ways. T cell receptors (TCRs) on the surface of host CD4+ or CD8+ T lymphocytes recognize donor MHC antigens on antigen-presenting cells and endothelial cells. Alternately, the recognition proceeds by a MHC-restricted recognition (recognition of MHC-peptide complex). Graft rejection is a consequence of cell-mediated cytotoxicity (mediated by CD8+ cells). Involvement of CD4+ T cells in the process is through secreting of cytokines that induce differentiation of CD8+ cells to cytotoxic T cells. *MHC,* major histocompatibility complex.

rejection of cells bearing these incompatible antigens is accomplished through the recipient's T cell receptors (TCRs).

The molecular basis for the recipient's TCR recognition of alloantigens, expressed on donor cells (graft), occurs in two ways (Figure 6-3).

recognition of donor major histocompatibility antigens (MHC molecules). In this process, host TCRs recognize donor MHC molecules that have been complexed with donor peptides and expressed on cells of the graft. It is believed that **recognition of donor MHC molecules** (not donor MHC-bound peptides) is the major mechanism in graft rejection and that it is a cross-reaction of host TCRs (previously selected in the thymus to recognize only self MHC).

recognition of donor MHC-bound peptides. Non-self antigens (donor-derived peptides) that are bound to donor MHC molecules

and expressed on cells of the graft are recognized by the host's TCRs. In this type of recognition (MHC restricted), the host TCRs **recognize donor MHC-peptide complex** (rather than donor MHC molecules).

Alloantigen Recognition by Helper and Cytotoxic T Cells

In allografts that differ from the host at both class I MHC and class II MHC, two subpopulations of host T lymphocytes (T cells [CD4+] and CD8+ T cells) are activated during recognition of alloantigens in two ways (see Figure 6-3).

allograft recognition by CD4+ T lymphocytes. The host CD4+ T cells are activated by allogeneic class II molecules located on the surface of antigen-presenting cells (donor APCs).

Once activated, the helper (CD4+) T cells produce cytokines (co-simulators), which activate other cells (i.e., cytotoxic CD8+ T lym-

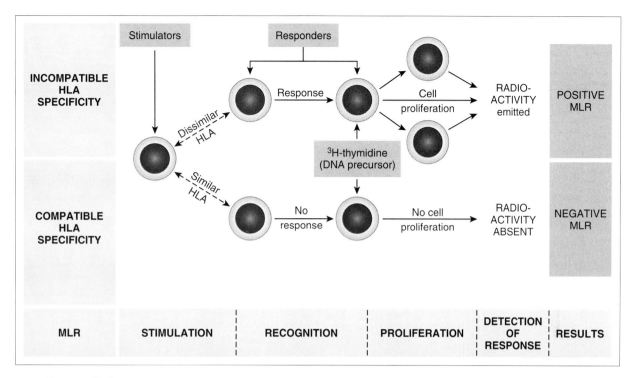

FIGURE **6-4** **Lymphocyte Matching Technique Using Mixed Leukocyte Reaction (MLR).** MLR is an example of an in vitro technique that is used to determine the degree of histocompatibility (compatibility or incompatibility) between recipient (responder) mononuclear cells (T cells, B cells, NK cells) and donor (stimulator) mononuclear cells. Dissimilarity (incompatibility) in HLA specificities between the two cell populations results in recipient immune response against donor cells. (See also text.) *MLR,* mixed leukocyte reaction; *HLA,* human leukocyte antigen; *³H,* tritiated (radiolabeled).

phocytes, B lymphocytes [antibody-secreting plasma cells], and macrophages) as follows:

- IL-2 and IFNγ activate CD8+ cytotoxic T cells
- IL-2, IL-4, and IL-5 activate B cells
- TNFβ (lymphotoxin) and IFNγ act as macrophage-activating factor (MAF)

These newly cytokine-activated and proliferating cells are capable of rejecting the MHC incompatible graft by the mechanisms of specific (cell mediated and humoral) and non-specific (inflammatory reaction) immune responses, discussed later in the chapter.

allograft recognition by CD8+ lymphocytes. Alternatively, CD8+ T cells may be directly stimulated (activated) by allogeneic class I MHC molecules expressed on the surface of all cells of a graft, with required helper T cell participation (see Figure 6-3).

It is also possible to stimulate CD8+ T cells in vitro by alloantigens (HLA) and T cell mito-gens, such as phytohemagglutinin (PHA) and concanavalin A (Con A). An example of al-loantigen (HLA) stimulation is a mixed leuko-cyte reaction (MLR), described following.

In Vitro Recognition and Response to Alloantigens (Mixed Leukocyte Reaction)

The most powerful immune response to geneti-cally incompatible allografts (graft rejection) results when the host's CD8+ and CD4+ T lymphocytes recognize dissimilar donor MHC class I and MHC class II antigens, respectively.

The response of the immune system to in-compatible tissue HLA antigens can be evalu-ated by an in vitro study (Figure 6-4), known as **mixed leukocyte reaction (MLR).** MLR can be used to predict the success of a graft or cell-mediated rejection of graft by the host's immune system.

MLR is induced by culturing together (by cell culture technique) two cell populations (e.g., donor and recipient) of HLA-incompatible blood–derived mononuclear cells (T cells, B cells, natural killer [NK] cells, mononuclear phagocytes). When differences in MHC antigens exist in the two cell populations cultured, many mononuclear cells of one cell population are stimulated and proliferate on recognition of alloantigens present on the other cell population.

When both cell populations are immunocompetent (able to proliferate) and either of the two populations serves as an inducer of response and a responder to the non-self HLA stimulus, the reaction is known as a **two-way MLR**. In a **one-way MLR** (see Figure 6-4), one cell population is inactivated (not able to proliferate or differentiate into effector cells), while the other remains immunocompetent, serving as a responder. The quantity of immune response or cell proliferation that occurs during an MLR may be measured by the amount of radioactivity emitted by ^{3}H-thymidine (radiolabeled DNA precursor), which becomes incorporated into the newly synthesized DNA as the cells respond and proliferate (multiply) in the culture medium.

The greater the incompatibility in the MHC antigens between the donor and recipient (quantitated by MLR), the greater is the potential for a graft rejection.

GRAFT REJECTION

Graft rejection (destruction and elimination) is an outcome of a non-specific and specific immune reaction of the host (recipient) to a graft that displays allogeneic MHC antigens (genetically dissimilar HLA) not present in the recipient.

Exceptions are seen in (1) certain "privileged" anatomic sites (e.g., in utero location of fetus containing antigens incompatible with the mother) and (2) graft-vs.-host reaction, where the graft reacts to host alloantigens (see Box 6-1).

Mechanisms in Graft Rejection

In a rejection of an incompatible graft, patient CD4+ cells play a central role during induction of an immune response to donor cells, expressing MHC antigens with specificity that differs from the patient MHC antigens. There are several mechanisms responsible for a graft rejection, which include (Figure 6-5):

- **Cell-mediated immune response (cell-mediated cytotoxicity)**
- **Humoral immune response (antibody-dependent cell-mediated cytotoxicity and antibody-dependent complement-mediated cytotoxicity)**
- **Non-specific immune response (inflammation)**

Class I and class II MHC molecules, bound with self-peptides and expressed on cells of the graft, are the main targets of the host's immune response, which may occur as follows.

Cell-Mediated Cytotoxicity

During cell-mediated immune response directed by a host against donor alloantigens (genetically dissimilar antigens), activation of cytotoxic (CD8+) T lymphocytes (CTLs) occurs in two ways (Figure 6-6).

- Host CD4+ lymphocytes recognize alloantigens, presented as a class II MHC–peptide complex by donor-derived antigen-presenting cells (APC). As CD4+ cells are activated, they secrete cytokines, which in turn activate effector cells (i.e., B cells, CD4+ cells, CD8+ cells, and macrophages [MQ]) that are involved in rejection of an HLA-incompatible graft.
- Host CD8+ T lymphocytes recognize class I MHC–antigen complex on graft cells through their T cell receptors (TCR) and are activated. Activated CD8+ cells proliferate and differentiate into cytotoxic (CD8+) T lymphocytes (CTLs), which are capable of rejecting a graft by direct lysis of the target cells (graft endothelial and parenchymal cells expressing an MHC-antigen complex of different specificity). Cytokines secreted by antigen-activated CD4+ cells provide the necessary "help" in the form of cytokines (IL-2, IFNγ).

Antibody-Dependent Cytotoxicity (Complement Mediated)

Host B lymphocytes, activated by IL-2, IL-4 and IL-5 cytokines (produced by antigen activation of host CD4+ T lymphocytes), differentiate into antibody-secreting plasma cells, which produce specific anti-graft (donor anti-HLA) antibodies. These alloantibodies bind to

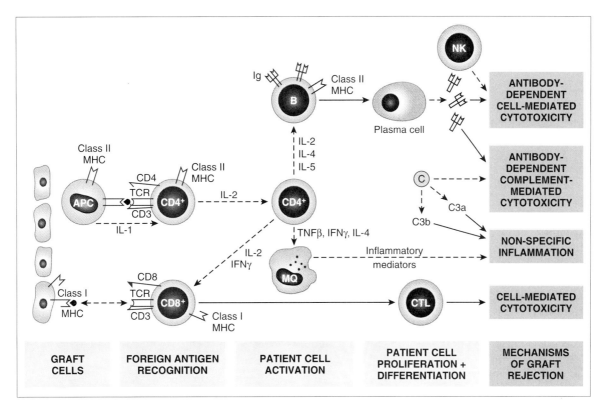

FIGURE **6-5** **Diagrammatic Presentation of Major Mechanisms and Components Involved in Graft Rejection.** (See Mechanisms in Graft Rejection in text.) *MHC,* major histocompatibility complex; *Ig,* immunoglobulin; *IL,* interleukin; *TCR,* T cell receptor; *IFN,* interferon; *TNF,* tissue necrosis factor; *MQ,* macrophage; *CTL,* cytotoxic T cells (CD8+); *C,* complement.

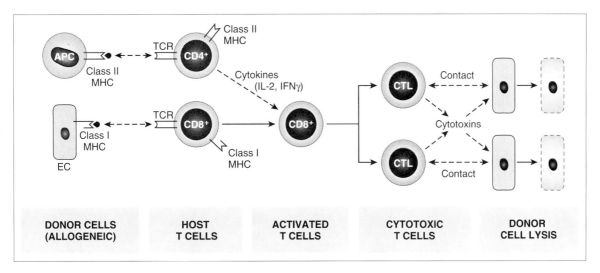

FIGURE **6-6** **Cell-Mediated Cytotoxicity in Graft Rejection.** Incompatible donor MHC (class I and class II alloantigens), carrying self-components (donor antigens) as a MHC-peptide complex, activate T host lymphocytes. CD8+ and CD4+ T cell activation occurs by host TCR recognition of donor class I MHC and class II MHC, respectively. CD8+ cells proliferate and differentiate into CTLs under the influence of CD4+ signals (cytokines). Lysis (cytotoxicity) of donor cells (allogeneic cells) occurs by CTL cell-to-cell contact (CTL-to-donor cell) and by action of cytotoxins elaborated by the CTLs. *APC,* antigen-presenting cell; *EC,* endothelial cell; *TCR,* T cell receptor; *MHC,* major histocompatibility complex; *IL,* interleukin; *IFN,* interferon; *CTL,* cytotoxic T cell.

HLA molecules of the same specificity and activate complement (which attaches to their Fc portion of the molecule). Antibody-activated complement is responsible for lysing donor endothelial cells expressing class I alloantigens (Figure 6-7). Inflammatory mediators (C3a and C5a complement components), released during complement activation, participate in an inflammatory reaction in the graft rejection.

Antibody-Dependent Cytotoxicity (Cell Mediated)

This effector mechanism in graft rejection proceeds as follows: alloantibody (produced as described previously) binds to a specific antigen located on a target cell (graft). Natural killer (NK) cells bind to the antibody (antigen/antibody complex on the target cell) through its Fc receptor for the antigen-bound antibody (IgG class), causing target cell lysis (see Figure 6-7).

Inflammation

Inflammation is a non-specific immune response in graft rejection, mediated by host T cells, inflammatory cells, and soluble mediators (see Chapter 1).

Cytokines in Graft Rejection

Experimental data illustrates that CD4+ helper T lymphocytes play a central role in induction of graft rejection (immune response to foreign HLA). Other cells and soluble molecules (i.e., **cytokines**) also participate in this process (see Figure 6-5).

Cytokines in Cell-Mediated Graft Rejection

In a *cell-mediated immune response* to an incompatible HLA-bearing graft (see Figure 6-5), the most important cytokines involved are:

- **IL-2** and **IFNγ**, which activate cytotoxic T lymphocytes.

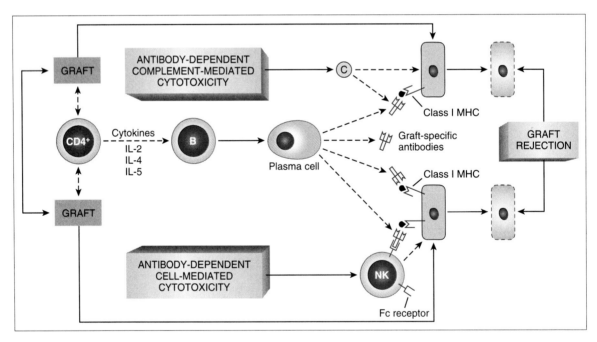

FIGURE **6-7** **Antibody-Dependent Cytotoxicity (Complement Mediated and Cell Mediated).** In this effector mechanism of graft rejection, the initiation of graft rejection occurs with activation of host CD4+ lymphocytes by donor alloantigens (graft). Activated CD4+ cells produce cytokines that stimulate B cells to differentiate into antibody-secreting plasma cells. Antibodies are graft-specific (anti-graft). Cytotoxicity is mediated by either complement or NK cells. In **complement-mediated antibody-dependent cytotoxicity,** donor cell lysis is caused by complement activated by specific antibodies that have bound to target class I MHC alloantigens. In **cell-mediated antibody-dependent cytotoxicity,** NK cells bind by Fc receptors to antibody/antigen (class I MHC) on the target cell, causing cell lysis. *IL,* interleukin; *C,* complement; *NK,* natural killer cell; *MHC,* major histocompatibility complex; *Ig,* immunoglobulin (antibody).

- **IFNγ,** which is responsible for (1) inducing the expression of MHC molecules (antigens), (2) increasing activity of antigen-presenting cells (APC), and (3) increasing the expression of adhesion molecules, is needed for adhesion of blood-derived leukocytes before their migration into tissues.
- **IFNγ, TNFβ,** and **IL-4,** which are gamma interferon (IFNγ), tumor necrosis factor (TNFβ) (previously known as macrophage-activating factor [**MAF**]), and lymphotoxin (IL4), are involved in activating the macrophages.

Cytokines in Antibody-Mediated Graft Rejection

In *humoral immune response,* graft-specific antibodies participate in graft rejection by causing damage to the graft endothelium. The cytokines that participate in humoral immune response are:

- **IL-2, IL-4,** and **IL-5,** which activate B lymphocytes to differentiate into plasma cells that secrete graft-specific antibodies.

Types of Graft Rejection

Immune graft rejection is typically classified according to graft tissue pathology (histopathology) rather than immune mechanisms responsible for graft rejection (see previously). The classification is as follows.

Hyperacute Graft Rejection

This rejection is characterized by rapid (within minutes) thrombosis (blood clots) within the graft blood vessels (intravascular thrombosis) in recipients who already have antibodies against the graft.

mechanism. Graft rejection is induced by pre-existing antibodies that bind to endothelium and activate complement. Complement activation contributes to the thrombosis and occlusion (blockage) of vessels within the graft, thus causing irreversible obstruction of blood flow (ischemic damage) before inflammation and subsequent graft cell lysis (*antibody-dependent complement-mediated cytotoxicity,* see Figure 6-7).

The preformed antibodies are believed to be natural antibodies (e.g., antibodies against ABO blood group antigens [anti-ABO] expressed on red blood cells). However, anti-ABO antibodies are not a major clinical problem because all graft donors and recipients are tested and selected according to the same ABO blood type.

Currently, it is believed that hyperacute rejection is caused by host antibodies directed against alloantigens on donor endothelial cells. These antibodies are pre-formed during blood transfusion, previous transplantation, or multiple pregnancies.

Acute Graft Rejection

There are two types of acute graft rejections, which occur within days or weeks of the transplantation:

acute vascular graft rejection. This rejection is characterized by necrosis (death) of individual cells of the graft blood vessels.

mechanism. Rejection is mediated (1) by IgG class of antibodies directed against endothelial cell alloantigens (MHC molecules) and involves activation of complement (*antibody-dependent complement-activated cytotoxicity,* see Figure 6-7) and (2) response of (CD8+) T cells to alloantigens on endothelial cells, causing cell lysis, or cell necrosis by elaborating cytokines, which activate inflammatory cells (see Figure 6-5 and Chapter 1).

acute cellular graft rejection. This rejection is characterized by lymphocyte and macrophage infiltration (invasion) of graft parenchymal cells.

mechanism. Recognition and lysis of foreign cells in this type of graft rejection is thought to be mainly mediated by CD8+ cytotoxic T cells responding to alloantigens (see Figure 6-6). Other possible effector mechanisms in acute cellular rejection of a graft are delayed-type hypersensitivity (see Chapter 7) and natural killer (NK) cell–mediated lysis (antibody-dependent cell-mediated cytotoxicity, see Figure 6-7).

Chronic Graft Rejection

Chronic type graft rejection is a slow process and takes months or even years to occur. It is characterized by fibrosis (formation of fibrous tissue), resulting in loss of normal organ structure.

mechanism. Although the mechanism of chronic rejection is less well understood, it is believed that it may occur as a slow cell-mediated rejection or as a result of deposition of antigen-antibody (immune) complexes or antibodies within the tissue (graft), particularly when the patient has received immunosuppressive treatment.

PREVENTION OF GRAFT REJECTION

As previously described, transplantation of foreign (donor) tissue that is not compatible (genetically not identical) with the recipient (host) will induce a cell-mediated and humoral im-

mune response in the host, causing immune rejection of the incompatible donor tissue (graft).

The immune graft rejection may be prevented, treated, or its severity reduced by performing the following **pretransplantation procedures and testing** (see Chapter 14, Histocompatibility Testing):

- **Immunosuppression:** Suppressing the immune system of the graft recipient (see following).
- **Pretransplantation laboratory testing:** Assessing compatibility between the donor tissue and the host (Figure 6-8), thus predicting success of the graft.

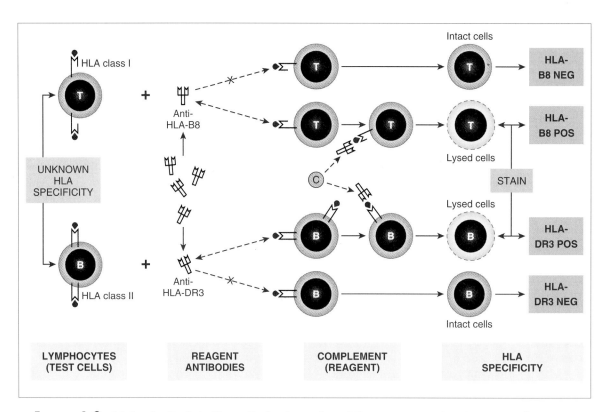

FIGURE **6-8** **Molecular Basis in Tissue Typing Procedure (Microcytotoxicity).** Commercially prepared antisera (monoclonal antibodies) of known HLA specificity are reacted with mononuclear cells (T and B cells) of unknown specificity. Antigen/antibody complex will form on the cell surface when the antigen and reagent antibody are of the same specificity. The antigen specificity is determined by the presence of test cell lysis (cytotoxicity), visible as a stain uptake by cells reacted with antibody of known HLA specificity. Cell lysis is caused by reagent complement (rabbit), which is activated by attaching to an antigen-bound antibody on the cell surface. In this diagrammatic presentation of a microcytotoxicity procedure (an example of **complement-mediated antibody-dependent cytotoxicity** [see also Figure 6-7 and text]), T cells have HLA-B8 specificity, while B cells show HLA-DR3 specificity. *HLA,* human leukocyte antigen; *anti,* against (refers to antibody against a specific antigen); *C,* complement.

IMMUNOSUPPRESSION IN TRANSPLANTATION

The need for a safe and effective immunosuppressive therapy, which could suppress or inhibit an unwanted immune response, became increasingly important as transplantation of various tissues and organs increased.

Consequently, research efforts in clinical transplantation to increase the success rate of transplants through immunosuppression produced gratifying results with the identification of new drugs and the expanding use of already existing immunosuppressive drugs.

Immunosuppression with Drugs

Three types of immunosuppressive drugs were identified and adopted as an acceptable means of non-specifically inhibiting immune responses to grafts.

Steroids (Prednisone, Methylprednisone)

Steroids suppress inflammatory and immune reactions. Among the various mechanisms that contribute to these effects of corticosteroid therapy are:

- *Alteration of leukocyte circulation,* as evidenced by an increase in neutrophils and a striking reduction in lymphocytes (mostly CD4+ helper T cells), consequently reducing the production of CD8+ cytotoxic T cells (thus minimizing cytotoxic effect on the graft)
- *Impairment in macrophage activity* or reduction in the number of monocytes (macrophages), causing an impairment in macrophage antigen-presenting activity and phagocytic activity (thereby reducing immunity to infections)
- *Reduction in monocytes,* responsible for the apparent reduction in an inflammatory reaction (anti-inflammatory function of corticosteroids)

Cytotoxic Drugs (Cyclophosphamide, Azathioprine, Methotrexate, Chlorambucil)

This group of drugs has a cytotoxic effect on the proliferating (replicating) lymphocytes and other cells. The use of cytotoxic drugs has been expanded from its use in cancer therapy to treatment of autoimmune disorders, such as rheumatoid arthritis and systemic lupus erythematosus (SLE). Currently, azathioprine is the cytotoxic drug of choice for inhibiting immune response to grafts (graft rejection).

Cyclosporine (Cyclosporin A)

This drug is the most important immunosuppressive agent used in clinical practice. It has opened the field of modern transplantation by reducing rejection of such transplants as heart and liver.

Cyclosporin A differs from other immunosuppressive compounds in that it selectively impairs helper (CD4+) T lymphocyte activities (inhibits production of IL-2 cytokine), thus inhibiting generation of antigen-specific cytotoxic T lymphocytes. Cyclosporine is not cytotoxic.

Other Immunosuppressive Methods

Use of other means (such as polyclonal and monoclonal antibodies directed against lymphocytes) of inducing immunosuppression in clinical transplantation and in experimental or standard procedure for treatment of disease states (e.g., autoimmune diseases) has also shown promising results.

Anti-Lymphocyte Antibodies (Polyclonal)

These non-specific polyclonal antibodies, capable of reacting with multiple T cell membrane antigens, are produced by animal immunization with human lymphocytes (thymocytes, splenic cells, thoracic duct lymphocytes, or blood lymphocytes).

It has been observed in animal studies that polyclonal antibodies impair cell-mediated immune responses by decreasing the number of lymphocytes. During treatment of organ rejection and significant graft-vs.-host reactions (GVH, see One Step Further Box 6-1) with polyclonal antibodies, several difficulties have been observed because of (1) lack of standardization (e.g., dose), (2) cross-reactivity between other cell types, and (3) recognition of these heterologous (from different species) antibodies by the host as foreign, thus triggering an immune response (cause of serum sickness).

Anti-Lymphocyte Antibodies (Monoclonal)

Monoclonal antibodies (from a single cell line) are produced by hybridoma technology (see One Step Further Box 14-1), are selective in their reactivity, and show *specificity for lymphocytes* (e.g., anti-CD3, a monoclonal antibody targeting CD3 receptor on mature T cells). Monoclonal antibodies show no cross-reactivity with other cells. They may be used in a predetermined quantity to treat graft rejections and GVH reactions in bone marrow transplants.

OTHER APPLICATIONS OF HISTOCOMPATIBILITY ANTIGENS IN CLINICAL IMMUNOLOGY

POPULATION STUDIES

In investigating genetic differences between various populations (population genetics of the HLA system), a quantitation/comparison of the distribution (frequencies) of HLA alleles among different populations is performed. Genetic differences observed may be a reflection of population migration or evolutionary factors impacting on the genome (complete set of inherited factors) and the possible association with diseases (see discussion following).

The HLA gene frequencies are estimated by typing HLA (tissue-typing procedure, Figure 6-8) expressed in a racially or ethnically homogenous (uniform) population. The gene or allele frequencies occurring within the study population are then calculated using a mathematical equation.

Comparison of HLA distribution (frequencies) shows a significant difference in unlike racial and ethnic populations. Therefore HLA testing may also be used to place an individual in a certain origin and ancestry.

DISEASE ASSOCIATION STUDIES

Numerous factors have been associated with an individual's susceptibility to disease. Among these, many have an immune basis. A statistically significant association has been established between an HLA type and the occurrence of certain diseases, such as the well-documented HLA-B27 antigen and ankylosing spondylitis (inflammation of the vertebrae). It has been proposed that both the class I MHC and class II MHC molecules (HLA) may be directly involved in susceptibility to disease (Table 6-3).

More than 3000 diseases are now associated with the HLA system, and additional HLA (and HLA-associated) markers are continually being

Table 6-3	SELECTED HLA-DISEASE ASSOCIATION (CAUCASIANS)	
Antigen	Associated Disease	Approximate RR*
HLA-B27	Ankylosing spondylitis	82
HLA-DR4	Rheumatoid arthritis	61
HLA-DR3/4,	Insulin-	
HLA-DR3,	dependent	3
HLA-DR4,	diabetes	6
HLA-DQw8	mellitus	32
HLA-DR3	Sjögren's syndrome,	6
	Graves' disease	4

*RR (relative risk): calculated value that predicts the probability an individual has for developing a disease associated with a particular HLA antigen (marker) as compared to negative controls (individuals without the HLA marker). The higher the RR number, the stronger is the disease association.

detected with the availability of advanced technology (e.g., molecular techniques). These HLA markers can be used to assist in diagnosis of a particular disease and to increase our understanding of the HLA type and disease association, such as:

- *Linkage of diseases with HLA region on chromosome 6 (e.g., linkage disequilibrium)*
- *The genetics of the diseases (pattern of inheritance of a disease and position of a disease gene on known genetic marker regions, such as the HLA region)*
- *The etiology (cause) of HLA-associated diseases*

Family Studies

Family studies (two- or three-generation families) may be conducted to determine a positive disease association (genetic link) between HLA and a particular disease. Parents and offspring are HLA-typed in these studies and **relative risk (RR)** calculated to establish the probability of a genetic marker (HLA) association with a particular disease. The higher the number obtained, the stronger the association and, therefore, the risk or chance that an individual with a particular HLA marker has of developing a particular disease in comparison to one that lacks the same marker (e.g., HLA-B27).

Mechanisms in HLA-Associated Diseases

Several mechanisms have been proposed in HLA association with certain diseases but may differ according to the particular disease:

- *HLA may be similar to viral antigens in production of an altered immune response*
- *HLA may serve as a receptor for etiologic agents (i.e., bacterial and viral antigens)*
- *HLA genes may be linked to other genes that control certain immune responses*

PATERNITY TESTING

The most reliable way of identifying an individual is to establish the individual's genotype (genetic profile) through laboratory testing (i.e., typing for gene products [HLA, MNS, and Rh markers] expressed on various cells). Because each individual has a unique set of genes, it is possible to distinguish one individual from another and to evaluate relationships (genetic similarity) by tissue typing with HLA antisera of known specificities (see Figure 6-8).

Procedures

Genetic profiles (genotypes) may be established by detecting genetic markers (cell-surface antigens and soluble molecules) using such laboratory tests as:

- *Serologic procedures for blood group antigens (ABO, MNSs, Rh, Kell, Duffy, Kidd systems)*
- *Lymphocyte cytotoxicity (tissue typing) for histocompatibility antigens (HLA)*
- *Molecular HLA typing techniques (DNA)*
- *Electrophoretic procedures (transferrin, serum protein molecules)*

Genotypes are currently used in courts to assist with establishing true parentage in disputed paternity (i.e., genotypes of the alleged father, biologic mother, and child, whose antigens are well developed at birth). Because procedures are not available in all laboratories, genotype may be established even by limited testing as long as HLA determinations are included.

Exclusion of Paternity

There are several assumptions that are important in paternity testing:

- *The mother is truly the mother*
- *RBC and HLA are expressions of genes (co-dominant)*
- *Test results are valid*

When these assumptions are met, exclusion of the alleged father can be established according to the following criteria:

- *Direct exclusion:* Direct exclusion occurs when a genetic marker is present in the child but not in the father. The presence of a genetic marker in a child but not in the father or mother indicates that these are not the child's biologic parents (*obligatory genes* must be transmitted to the offspring by mother or father or both).
- *Indirect exclusion:* Indirect exclusion can be established when the genetic markers (obligatory gene products) that must be transmitted by the alleged father are not present in the child. This type of exclusion is not as convincing as the direct exclusion because certain antigens cannot currently be identified.

Non-Exclusion of Paternity

In cases where exclusion of the alleged father is not possible, the probability of paternity may be calculated using gene frequencies of the antigens tested.

These statistical analyses are based on probability theory and the Hardy-Weinberg equilibrium. Basically, the probability that the alleged father is the biologic father is compared with the probability that a random man could contribute the same obligatory gene(s).

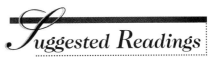

Suggested Readings

Abbas AK, Lichtman AH, Pober JS: Transplantation immunology (pp 363-383). In *Cellular and molecular immunology*, Philadelphia, 2000, WB Saunders.

Bias WB, Zachary AA, Rosner GL: Genetic and statistical principles of paternity determination: histocompatibility and transplantation immunology. In Rose NR, et al, editors: *Man-*

ual of clinical laboratory immunology, Washington, DC, 1997, American Society for Microbiology.

Bodmer JG, Marsh SE, Albert ED, et al: Nomenclature for factors of the HLA system, *Tiss Antigens* 44:1-18, 1994.

Jackson AL: Summary of the Fifth International Workshop on Human Leukocyte Differentiation Antigens, *Clin Immunol Newsletter* 24(4):1191-1197, 1995.

Review Questions

MAJOR HISTOCOMPATIBILITY COMPLEX/TRANSPLANTATION (MHC)

1. Major histocompatibility complex (MHC) antigens in humans are also known as:
   a. human leukocyte antigens (HLA)
   b. MHC gene products
   c. histocompatibility antigens
   d. all of the above

2. All of the following statements refer to the genetics of the HLA (MHC) system, *except:*
   a. MHC is located on human chromosome 6
   b. loci of the HLA system have a linear arrangement on the chromosome (i.e., HLA-A, HLA-B, HLA-C, HLA-D)
   c. MHC genes code for cell surface HLA molecules
   d. MHC genes code for complement components

3. Variants of a gene that occupies a specific locus on the chromosome are known as:
   a. specificities
   b. alleles
   c. antigens
   d. none of the above

4. A genotype (genetic profile) of an individual is the most reliable way of identifying the individual and establishing kinship (genetic similarity). An individual's unique set of genes may be detected by:
   a. microcytotoxicity (tissue typing)
   b. antibody-dependent complement-mediated cytotoxicity
   c. molecular (DNA) typing technique
   d. all of the above

5-7. Match the following classes of MHC antigens with the following descriptive terms:

   ____ class I MHC
   ____ class II MHC
   ____ class III MHC

   a. genes of this class code for complement components
   b. coded by genes of HLA-A, -B, -C loci
   c. involved in MHC-restricted antigen recognition
   d. HLA-D/DR

8-13. The following cell surface markers may be defined by descriptive phrases (listed a through h). Match each phrase with the appropriate marker:

____ class II MHC molecule   ____ sIg
____ class I MHC molecule   ____ TCR
                                ____ CD4+
                                ____ CD8+

a. B cell surface immunoglobulin
b. T cell antigen receptor
c. recognizes self vs. non-self antigens
d. found on immunocompetent cells
e. found on all nucleated cells
f. helper T cell
g. cytotoxic T cell
h. B cell antigen receptor

14. In a cell-mediated immune response to HLA alloantigens, CD8+ T cells differentiate into CD8+ cytotoxic T cells by stimulation with the following cytokines:
a. interleukin-2 (IL-2) and interferon (IFNγ)
b. IL-2, IL-4, and IL-5
c. IL-4, IFNγ, and tumor necrosis factor (TNFβ)
d. all of the above

15. Serologic tissue typing technique used for detection of MHC gene products (histocompatibility antigens) is:
a. mixed leukocyte reaction (MLR)
b. microcytotoxicity
c. RFLP tissue-typing procedure
d. oligonucleotide probe

16. HLA typing is used primarily in all the following situations, *except:*
a. establishing HLA disease association
b. genetic counseling
c. establishing HLA compatibility
d. paternity dispute

MAJOR HISTOCOMPATIBILITY ANTIGENS IN TRANSPLATATION

17. The most common and highly successful allograft (i.e., infrequently rejected) is the:
a. kidney
b. heart
c. cornea
d. bone marrow

18. In transplanting solid organs (e.g., kidney), success is observed when the following pretransplantation procedure(s) is/are performed:
a. immunotherapy with cyclosporine A
b. detection of donor-specific alloantigens
c. HLA/ABO antigen matching and immunosuppression
d. HLA typing and immunosuppression

19. The term *allogeneic* refers to a relationship between:
a. different sites on same individual
b. different species
c. genetically dissimilar members within the same species
d. genetically identical members of the same species

20. Select the good predictor(s) of a possible allogeneic graft (allograft) rejection:
a. incompatible HLA antigens
b. HLA-specific antibodies
c. positive mixed lymphocyte reaction
d. all of the above

21. Graft rejection by a recipient may be triggered by:
a. host immunodeficiency
b. inappropriate host immunosuppression
c. MHC gene coding for class I HLA
d. recognition of incompatible donor class I HLA

22. Select the mechanism(s) involved in graft rejection:
    a. cell-mediated cytotoxicity
    b. antibody-dependent cytotoxicity
    c. antibody-dependent complement-mediated cytolysis
    d. all of the above

23. Hyperacute graft rejection may occur as an outcome of:
    a. cell destruction by cytotoxic T cells
    b. presence of pre-existing antibodies
    c. cell-mediated cytotoxicity
    d. complement-dependent cytotoxicity

24. A graft-vs.-host (GVH) reaction occurs in situations when:
    a. graft cells are immunocompetent
    b. the host is immunodeficient
    c. HLA specificities differ between the host and donor
    d. all of the above

25. GVH may be triggered by transfusion or transplantation of:
    a. whole blood
    b. platelets
    c. bone marrow
    d. all of the above

PREVENTION OF GRAFT REJECTION

26. Increased graft survival is predicted when donor and recipient HLA show compatibility in their lymphocyte cross-match. Increased graft survival is the result of:
    a. inhibition of cytotoxic T cell response
    b. inhibition of antibody production
    c. reduced cytokine production
    d. reduction in alloantigens

27. The ability (immunocompetence) of T cells to proliferate in response to an alloantigenic stimulus may be evaluated by:
    a. microcytotoxicity
    b. mixed lymphocyte reaction
    c. flow cytometry
    d. all of the above

OTHER APPLICATIONS OF HISTOCOMPATIBILITY ANTIGENS IN CLINICAL IMMUNOLOGY

28. Ankylosing spondylitis is the most prevalent disease associated with a specific HLA genotype. Select the HLA antigen associated with this abnormality:
    a. HLA-B5
    b. HLA-A2
    c. HLA-DR1
    d. HLA-B27

29. In paternity testing, when a genetic marker that should be transmitted from the alleged father is absent in a child, the type of exclusion is known as:
    a. direct exclusion of paternity
    b. indirect exclusion of paternity
    c. probability of paternity
    d. all of the above

30. Genetic profile (genotype) of an individual may be established by detecting genetic markers by the listed procedures. When not all procedures are available, one procedure that is absolutely required to establish the genotype is:
    a. molecular (DNA) typing techniques
    b. tissue typing (HLA)
    c. blood group typing (ABO, MNSs, Rh, Kell, Duffy, Kidd)
    d. electrophoresis (serum protein molecules [allotypes])

31. Select one statement that describes criteria for direct exclusion of paternity:
    a. statistical analysis based on probability theory
    b. absence of obligatory gene (must be transmitted) in child but present in the alleged father
    c. genetic marker is present in the child but not in the alleged father
    d. none of the above

CHAPTER 7

Abnormal Immune Responses

Learning Objectives

Upon completion of Chapter 7, the student will be prepared to:

- In general terms, define the following inappropriate responses of the immune system: hypersensitivity, autoimmunity, immunodeficiency, and hypergammaglobulinemia.
- Name three malfunctions in immunoregulation that may lead to an inappropriate immune response.

HYPERSENSITIVITY

- Describe the mechanism of tissue injury in the four types of hypersensitivity reactions, giving an example of an abnormality associated with each reaction.
- Name two categories of inappropriate immune response that are the result of an exaggerated immune response to an antigen.
- Compare the mechanisms of tissue injury in localized and generalized allergic reactions to an allergen.

AUTOIMMUNITY

- Define the following terms: *self-tolerance, homeostasis, regulatory mechanisms, tissue injury, autoantibodies.*
- State three local and systemic changes causing loss of tolerance to self-antigens (autoantigens) and development of an autoimmune response.
- Describe the following conditions, which may give rise to the development of autoimmune disorders: alterations in lymphocytes, tissue alterations, genetic factors, environmental factors.
- Name three mechanisms by which tissue injury occurs in autoimmune disease.
- List four examples of autoantibodies directed against organ-specific self-antigens.
- Describe the main function of T lymphocytes in maintaining self-tolerance.

IMMUNODEFICIENCY

- List components of the immune system that cause an abnormally low immune response when present in a lowered or defective state.

- Describe the origin of the defect or deficiency in the following primary (hereditary) and secondary immunodeficiency disorders: B cell immunodeficiency, T cell immunodeficiency (primary and secondary), combined B cell and T cell immunodeficiency.
- List major complement components that have been associated with immunodeficiency disorders.

HYPERGAMMAGLOBULINEMIA

- Define *monoclonal* and *polyclonal gammopathies,* including their origin, and give two examples for each type of abnormality.
- State the main difference between monoclonal and polyclonal antibodies.
- Name two laboratory procedures that may be used to detect specificity of an elevated class of antibodies.

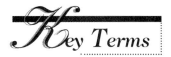

Key Terms

agammaglobulinemia - Immunodeficiency that is characterized by absence of gamma globulins, giving rise to recurrent infections.

allergen - Any foreign antigen or agent (e.g., house-dust mite, pollen) that is able to induce antibody (IgE)-mediated hypersensitivity reaction (allergy).

anaphylaxis - Generalized and severe hypersensitivity reaction that is characterized by vasodilation (dilatation of blood vessels) and constriction of smooth muscles, with clinical symptoms such as bronchospasm (constriction of bronchus). May lead to death.

anergy - Failure of the immune system to respond to an antigenic stimulus (tolerance).

autoantibodies - Immunoglobulins produced in response to specific self-antigens (autoantigens). Because of antigen specificity, they may be used as "markers" in laboratory detection of the stimulating antigen, thus facilitating identification of a particular autoimmune response.

autoimmune disease - Characterized by tissue injury caused by an autoimmune response (response to self-antigens).

autoimmunity - Abnormality in the induction or maintenance of self-tolerance, leading to immune response to self-antigens.

cytotoxicity - Cell-mediated immune response that results in tissue injury through destruction of target cells (cells expressing specific antigens).

edema - Accumulation of excessive amounts of fluids in tissues.

effector cells or molecules - Components of the immune system that participate in the last stage of an immune response (effector phase) by producing the end effect (resolution of the immune response).

hypersensitivity - Exaggerated or inappropriate form of immune response, occurring on subsequent contact with the same antigen, causing inflammation and tissue injury.

immune complexes - Antigen/antibody complexes produced in vivo (within any living organism) by binding of antibody with the specific antigen that induced its production.

immunodeficiency (immunocompromised) - State of deficiency in an immune response, resulting from absence or failure of normal function of one or more of the components of the immune system.

immunosuppression - Restraint of an immune response by deliberate use of chemicals or radiation or by deficiency in any component of the immune system.

monoclonal - Single clone of cells.

polyclonal - Refers to two or more types of cell clones.

self-reactive (autoreactive) - Response of the immune system against autoantigens (self-antigens), such as cell-surface receptors, basement membrane antigens of kidney glomeruli, or hormone receptors.

self-tolerance - State of unresponsiveness of the immune system to self-antigens. It is an acquired characteristic of lymphocytes in each individual resulting from a selective process, by which self-reactive lymphocyte clones are eliminated before their functional maturity.

sensitivity - Quick and acute cell-mediated immune response to an antigen that has been previously encountered by the individual.

sensitization (priming) - Process by which an antibody molecule is bound to an antigen, either as a first step in an in vitro antigen/antibody reaction or as an in vivo sensitization (coating) of a cell with antibodies that bind with the specific cell membrane antigens (e.g., blood group antigens on erythrocytes).

target cell or organ - Specific cells, expressing epitopes (antigenic determinants) on their cell surface, which are targeted by mediators (e.g., cells, antibodies) of an immune response.

tolerance - State of immune unresponsiveness to a particular antigenic determinant (epitope).

The immune system in all healthy individuals has the ability to respond to a multitude of foreign antigenic stimulators. As discussed in previous chapters, the immune response consists of a variety of components and mechanisms that collaborate to protect an individual from infection by bacteria, viruses, and other infectious agents.

Among the mechanisms involved in immune response, there are regulatory mechanisms (controls) that ensure that the immune response is appropriate, does not become uncontrollable, and does not react against its own tissue antigens.

The regulatory mechanisms (controls) originate during the developmental stage of the immune system (i.e., during cell maturation) as well as during the course of the immune response (i.e., as the mature lymphocytes respond to an antigen).

Malfunction of any one of the regulatory mechanisms results in a variety of inappropriate immune responses with a potential to cause tissue damage, such as is seen in **hypersensitivity** and **autoimmunity.** The abnormal responses may be caused by such factors as:

- Failure to control immune responses
- Inability to maintain tolerance to self-antigens
- Failure to distinguish between self and non-self antigens

Other inappropriate or abnormal responses of the immune system that are of concern in clinical immunology are **hypergammaglobu-linemia** and **immunodeficiency.**

Thus the principal abnormalities associated with an inappropriate or abnormal immune response are:

- **Hypersensitivity:** Exaggerated responses causing tissue damage.
- **Autoimmunity:** Elevated immune response to self-antigens causing tissue injury.
- **Immunodeficiency:** Deficient or compromised immune response against infectious agents because of deficiency in any one of the components of the immune system, resulting in secondary (opportunistic) infections.
- **Hypergammaglobulinemia:** Immunoproliferative disorder characterized by increased or unregulated production of immunoglobulins.

Presence of any of the listed abnormalities may be confirmed through clinical laboratory testing, discussed in Section II of this text.

ℋYPERSENSITIVITY

Hypersensitivity has been defined as a normal but exaggerated or uncontrolled immune response to a persistent antigen, which results in inflammation and possible tissue injury (see Figure 1-5).

The original classification of hypersensitivity was first proposed by Coombs and Gall as type I, type II, type III, and type IV hypersensitivity. Although this classification continues to be used, a more recent classification defines the principal mechanism responsible for a particular cell or tissue injury occurring during an immune response (Table 7-1).

The first three types of hypersensitivity are antibody-dependent, while the fourth type is cell mediated, although some overlapping between the various types does occur (see discussion following).

IMMEDIATE HYPERSENSITIVITY OR ALLERGY (TYPE I)

Immediate hypersensitivity reaction (type I) is mediated by an antibody (IgE) and occurs immediately after a second or subsequent contact with the same antigen, commonly referred to as an *allergen* (e.g., pollen, certain food). The immune response that follows the contact with a particular allergen is commonly referred to as an *allergic reaction* or *allergy.*

Table 7-1 FOUR TYPES OF HYPERSENSITIVITY

Type	Immune Reaction (Cells/Molecules)	Mediators	Mechanism of Tissue Injury	Clinical Disorders
Type I	Antibody-mediated (immediate) hypersensitivity	IgE, mast cell granules (histamine, cytokines)	Allergic and anaphylactic reactions	Hay fever, asthma
Type II	Antibody-dependent complement- or cell-mediated hypersensitivity	Complement, effector cells (MQs, PMNs)	Target cell lysis, cell-mediated cytotoxicity	HDN, Goodpasture's syndrome
Type III	Immune complex–mediated hypersensitivity (immune complex disease)	Antigen/antibody complexes, complement, MQs, cytokines, mast cells	Immune complex deposition, inflammation	SLE, serum sickness
Type IV	T cell–mediated hypersensitivity (DTH)	Antigen-specific T cells, T cell cytokines	Inflammation, cellular infiltration	Contact sensitivity, tuberculin skin test

Ig, immunoglobulin; *MQs*, macrophages; *PMNs*, polymorphonuclear leukocytes; *HDN*, hemolytic disease of the newborn; *SLE*, systemic lupus erythematosus; *DTH*, delayed-type hypersensitivity.

Mechanism of Tissue Injury

Although the role of IgE was initially described as a protective mechanism against parasitic infections (mainly worms), it has a well-defined role in host tissue injury during an allergic response.

During the first contact, the stimulating antigen triggers a series of events (responses of the immune system) at the site of antigen entry, resulting in the production of IgE. On subsequent contact with the *same* antigen, the newly synthesized IgE binds to the Fc receptors on mast cells and basophils, thus coating the cells. This process of coating a cell by an antibody is known as "sensitization" and the cells are thus "sensitized."

Subsequent binding and cross-linking of the stimulating antigen with the antigen-specific IgE on the surface of sensitized cells causes calcium ions (Ca^{2+}) to enter into these cells, resulting in release of cellular granules (Figure 7-1). Other molecules (anaphylatoxins), mainly products of complement activation (C3a and C5a), may also induce release of granules containing various mediators (see discussion of inflammation, Chapter 1).

The unbound or free IgE produced in response to the stimulating antigen (antigen specific) can be detected in blood by such a laboratory procedure as radioallergosorbent test (RAST, discussed in Chapter 13). RAST test results show a good correlation with an in vivo skin test for the same allergen.

Clinical Manifestations

The released mediators (e.g., prostaglandins, eosinophils, chemotactic factors [ECF], and histamines) trigger the clinical symptoms observed in an allergic reaction (allergy) although environmental and genetic factors also contribute to these symptoms.

The allergic reaction may be either a local inflammation (see Chapter 1, Figure 1-5) or a generalized anaphylaxis (IgE-mediated immune response) with symptoms such as those found in hay fever, asthma, or eczema.

Localized Reaction

A localized reaction occurs as an *immediate response* to mediators released from mast cell degranulation. It is characterized by a cutaneous

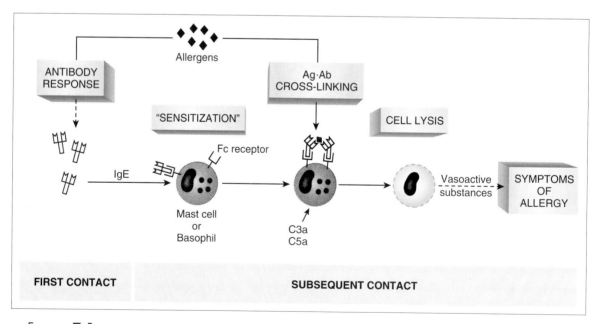

FIGURE **7-1**   **Mechanism of Tissue Injury in Type I Hypersensitivity.**   The reaction, also known as *immediate hypersensitivity,* is antibody mediated. IgE molecules are produced and bound to Fc receptors on mast cells and basophils (sensitization) in response to first contact with the allergen (antigen). On second contact, the same allergen cross-links IgE molecules on the sensitized cells and triggers cell degranulation. Released granules (e.g., histamines) within minutes produce symptoms of allergy and anaphylaxis. (See also text.) *Ig,* immunoglobulin; *C,* complement; *Ag,* antigen; *Ab,* antibody; *Fc,* antibody receptor.

reaction that appears as a "wheal and flair reaction," local edema, and itching at the site of introduction of the particular allergen (e.g., skin test, bee sting).

This simple immediate reaction to an allergen may be used as a skin test to diagnose an allergy or confirm sensitivity to a specific antigen.

Generalized Reaction

This type of antigen-specific immune reaction, also known as *anaphylaxis,* is produced by such mediators as cytokines and vasoactive amines (e.g., histamine released from mast cells). The reaction is characterized by distention of blood vessels (vasodilation), smooth muscle constriction, bronchospasm (constriction of bronchioles), and edema (accumulation of excessive fluid) that may lead to death.

ANTIBODY-DEPENDENT CYTOTOXIC HYPERSENSITIVITY (TYPE II)

In type II hypersensitivity, destruction of target or tissue cells, which express certain antigens on their surface, occurs by a process of antibody-dependent cytotoxicity (cell lysis). Cytotoxic cell destruction may be either **complement mediated** or **cell mediated.**

Mechanism of Tissue Injury
Antibody-Dependent, Complement-Mediated Cytotoxicity

In antibody-dependent, complement-mediated cytotoxicity, cytolysis or tissue damage (target cell membrane damage) occurs through a series of immunologic events (Figure 7-2) that take place when antibody (IgM and some classes of IgG) bind with cell surface antigen

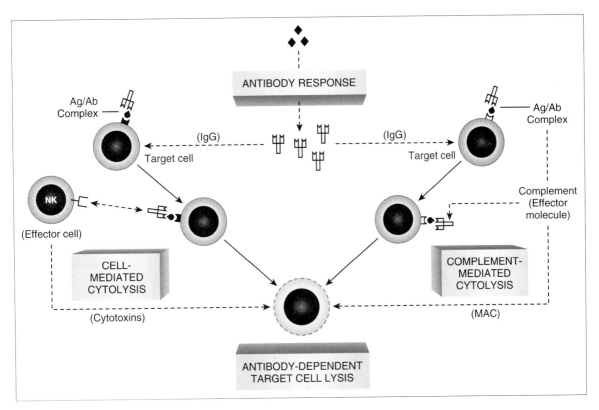

FIGURE **7-2** **Tissue Damage in Type II Hypersensitivity.** This antibody-dependent cytotoxic response may occur in two ways: (1) Cell-mediated cytotoxic destruction of target cells. Specific antibodies (IgG), bound to surface antigens on target cells, bind to Fc receptors on effector cells, releasing cytotoxic substances that destroy the target cells. (2) Complement-mediated target cell lysis. Antigen/antibody complex, formed on target cells, activates complement through the classical pathway. The activation (cascade) culminates in formation of a membrane attack complex (MAC) and disruption of the target cell membrane, causing cell lysis. *Ag,* antigen; *Ab,* antibody; *Ig,* immunoglobulin, *NK,* natural killer cell; *MAC,* membrane attack complex.

and activate complement. Complement fragments (C3b and C3d) thus generated participate in the reaction by binding to the target cell membrane and assemble there to form a membrane attack complex (MAC). MAC (C5b through C9) is inserted into a target cell membrane, causing cell lysis (see Figure 4-3).

Other complement fragments produced (i.e., C3a and C5a) attract macrophages and neutrophils to the reaction site and stimulate mast cells and basophils to produce additional chemotactic molecules (see Chapter 1, Figure 1-5).

Antibody-Dependent, Cell-Mediated Cytotoxicity

This type of cytotoxicity depends on initial binding of specific antibodies to target cell surface antigens. The antibody-coated cells are destroyed (lysed) by effector cells (NK cells and other leukocytes expressing Fc receptors), which attach by their Fc receptors to the Fc portion of the antibody coating the target cell. Target cell destruction (lysis) occurs when cytotoxic substances are released by the effector cells (see Figure 7-2).

Clinical Manifestations

The following are examples of type II hypersensitivity.

Blood Transfusion Reaction

The reaction occurs when the patient's immune system reacts against incompatible antigens expressed on transfused donor blood erythrocytes (red blood cells), to which antigen-specific antibodies have been *formed during previous exposure.*

The previously produced antibodies form antigen/antibody complexes on donor erythrocytes, thus activating complement (classical pathway). The C5b through C9 fragments are assembled to form a membrane attack complex (MAC) that causes intravascular hemolysis (incompatible donor cell lysis within patient blood vessels).

Hemolytic Disease of the Newborn (HDN)

The disease is characterized by destruction (hemolysis) of the fetal erythrocytes because of the presence of maternal antibodies (IgG) against incompatible fetal erythrocyte antigens (mainly RhD antigens) inherited from the father.

The maternal antibodies to specific antigens on fetal erythrocytes are produced during a *previous pregnancy* or *through a blood transfusion* that contains antigens not expressed on the mother's erythrocytes. The previously formed antigen-specific antibodies pass into fetal blood circulation during subsequent pregnancies, causing destruction of fetal red blood cells that results in HDN.

Goodpasture's Syndrome (Glomerulonephritis)

This tissue injury, which is responsible for severe glomerulonephritis, occurs as follows: (1) antigen/antibody complexes form along the basement membrane of glomeruli (smallest structural units of the kidney), (2) complement (classical pathway) is activated by antigen/antibody complexes, (3) resulting membrane damage is complement mediated (C5 through C9), (4) subsequent accumulation of neutrophils and release of their enzymes at the site of antibody deposition (usually IgG) causes cell-mediated cytotoxicity.

Specific autoantibodies, forming antigen/antibody complexes with antigens expressed on the glomerular basement membrane, may be visualized by fluorescent microscopy as an evenly distributed fluorescent layer of antibodies. The pattern is characteristic for type II hypersensitivity and is observed in bullous skin disease (Figure 7-3, *A*) and differs in appearance from the granular pattern, observed in type III hypersensitivity (discussed following).

IMMUNE COMPLEX–MEDIATED HYPERSENSITIVITY (TYPE III)

Type III hypersensitivity, also known as *immune complex disease,* occurs when immune complexes (antigen/antibody complexes that are produced as the antigen comes in contact with a specific antibody in vivo) are not effectively removed by phagocytes and are deposited in various tissues and organs (e.g., kidney, joint, skin, lung) (Figure 7-3, *B*). Tissue damage occurs at the site of the immune complex deposition (e.g., glomerular basement membrane) (Figure 7-4).

Immune complex formation may occur as a result of (1) autoimmune disease (e.g., rheumatoid arthritis), (2) persistent infection (e.g.,

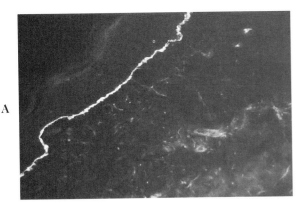

A

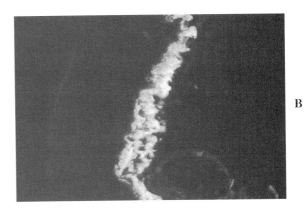

B

FIGURE **7-3**   **Autoantibodies in Bullous Skin Disease.**   **A,** Direct immunofluorescence staining of a skin biopsy from a patient with bullous (blistering) pemphigoid, depicting a linear reaction of IgG autoantibodies with the epithelial basement membrane. **B,** Indirect immunofluorescence reaction of glomerular basement membrane antibodies on primate kidney sections. (Courtesy Dr. V. Kumar, IMMCO, Buffalo, NY.)

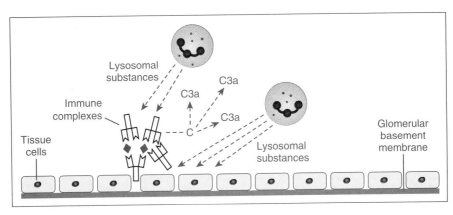

FIGURE **7-4**   **Schematic Representation of Tissue Damage (Type III Hypersensitivity).**   Tissue damage is triggered by deposition of immune complexes along the glomerular basement membrane. The mechanism of tissue damage involves (1) immune complex activation of complement (C) by deposited immune complexes, (2) attraction of polymorphonuclear leukocytes through chemotactic property of C3a fragment to the site of immune complex deposition, and (3) release of lysosomal substances that produce the tissue injury.

viral hepatitis), and (3) repeated inhalation of antigenic material (e.g., moldy hay [farmer's lung]).

Deposition of immune complexes is promoted by such factors as (1) increased vascular permeability in the presence of vasoactive amines (e.g., histamine), (2) high blood pressure and turbulence (e.g., glomerular capillaries), and (3) the size, antigen affinity for tissue, and class of antibody of the immune complex (e.g., IgG and anti-IgG rheumatoid factor, both produced in joint synovium, combine to form immune complexes that cause inflammation).

The characteristic pattern of antigen/antibody complex deposits at various sites may be visualized by fluorescent microscopy as granular deposits (see Figure 7-3, B).

Mechanism of Tissue Injury

Normally, immune complexes that occur in vivo (IgM or IgG molecules binding to specific antigens) are cleared by phagocytes (macrophages) within the liver and spleen. However, any defect in phagocytosis or other factors (e.g., large size of circulating complexes) allow formed immune complexes to remain within the blood and to deposit in various tissues (e.g., kidney, joints).

At these sites, the deposited antigen/antibody complexes activate the complement system, which generates anaphylotoxins (e.g., C3a). Mast cells and basophils are stimulated by anaphylotoxins to release chemotactic factors and various amines (e.g., histamine). These factors increase vascular permeability, thus allowing effector cells (neutrophils) to enter the site of immune complex deposition. A local inflammatory reaction develops. Tissue injury occurs as lysosomal enzymes are released by the effector cells, which accumulate at the site of immune complex deposition (see Figure 7-4).

As complement is used in the previously described reaction, serum complement levels are lowered, and immune complexes are detectable in blood by immunologic procedures (see Complement Assays in Chapter 14). Thus lowered serum complement levels and presence of immune complexes are laboratory findings that support the diagnosis of immune complex disease.

Clinical Manifestations

Persistence of immune complexes in blood circulation is not in itself harmful to the body. However, **immune complex disease** may occur when these circulating complexes are not cleared by phagocytosis and are then deposited in certain tissues.

Serum Sickness

Serum sickness is a self-limiting systemic immune complex disease (affecting lymph nodes and joints). It is caused by passive immunization (now less frequently used), such as administration of pre-formed antibodies or gamma globulins (usually horse serum, see Chapter 1) to prevent infectious or toxic diseases (e.g., tetanus).

Systemic Lupus Erythematosus (SLE)

SLE is characterized by presence of autoantibodies, which form immune complexes with autoantigens and are deposited within the kidney glomeruli. The resulting type III hypersensitivity is responsible for the glomerulonephritis (inflammation of blood capillary vessels in

the glomeruli) that is associated with SLE (see Chapter 13, One Step Further Box 13-2).

Microscopic evaluation (immunofluorescent technique) of glomeruli and other renal tissue from patients with SLE shows a characteristic pattern of immune complex deposits (uneven or granular pattern, see Figure 7-3). This and other diagnostic procedures for SLE are discussed in Section II of this text.

T Cell–Mediated Hypersensitivity (Type IV)

T cell–mediated hypersensitivity is also known as **delayed-type hypersensitivity (DTH)**. It occurs when an antigen (e.g., TB) that remains within a macrophage after phagocytosis is encountered by previously activated T cells for a second (or subsequent) time.

DTH reaction does not require participation of complement or antibody.

Mechanism of Tissue Injury

DTH is mediated by T lymphocytes, which had previous exposure (primary contact) with a particular stimulating antigen. These antigen-specific T lymphocytes release cytokines following a secondary or subsequent contact with the same non-self antigen (see Secondary Immune Response, Chapter 1). The released cytokines induce an inflammatory reaction and activate and attract macrophages, causing cellular infiltration and a resulting edema at the tissue site (Figure 7-5).

Clinical Manifestations

DTH reaction may be used for an in vivo evaluation of cell-mediated immune response to a particular antigen (see Figure 7-5), thus establishing the existence of sensitivity to that antigen.

Contact Sensitivity

This skin disease, also known as *allergic contact dermatitis*, is an inflammatory response characterized by skin eruptions, lesions, blistering, scaling, and edema at the area of contact with various natural or synthetic allergens, such as poison ivy or certain metals.

Diagnosis of contact sensitivity is confirmed by patch testing (immunologic skin

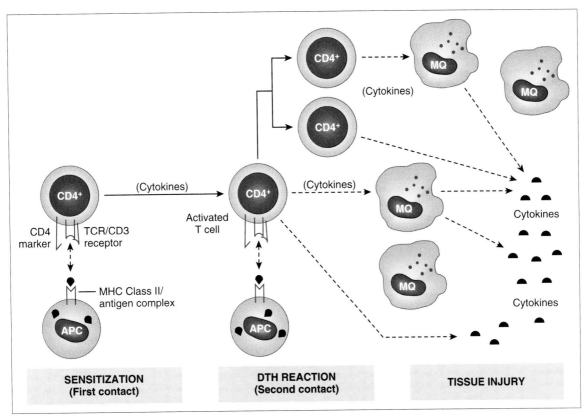

FIGURE **7-5** **Delayed-Type Hypersensitivity (DTH).** This type IV hypersensitivity may be used to evaluate in vivo a cell-mediated immune response. First exposure to an antigen or "sensitizing agent" (e.g., PPD-tuberculin) activates helper T lymphocytes. On second contact with the same antigen, activated T cells proliferate and secrete cytokines that attract and activate macrophages (MQ). Cytokines secreted by activated CD4+ cells and macrophages are responsible for tissue injury in DTH. *MHC,* major histocompatibility complex; *TCR/CD3,* T cell receptor complex; *CD4,* helper T cell marker; *APC,* antigen-presenting cell; *MQ,* macrophage.

test), a well-established procedure that uses common sensitizing agents (stimulating antigens) to induce the reaction. Contact sensitivity may persist for many years and even for a lifetime.

Tuberculin and Other Skin Tests
These intradermal tests (injection of test antigen or allergen) measure in vivo cell-mediated immune response by evaluating delayed immune response (after 12 hours or more) at the injection site. They are performed mainly for the detection of immunity to certain infections and the effectiveness of the cell-mediated immune response.

The more common sensitizing agents used in DTH procedure are PPD (purified protein derivative) in the tuberculin skin test and

Candida (C. albicans) in the skin test for detection of specific immune response against this infective organism.

AUTOIMMUNITY

Regulation of a normal immune response is through such control mechanisms as "feedback" by soluble products (e.g., antibodies, cytokines) and cell-to-cell interactions (e.g., B cell–T cell). These regulatory mechanisms are required to either heighten or reduce an immune response, so that it is only as intense as is necessary to contain the invading microorganism. Also, the regulatory mechanisms allow the immune response to "shut-down" and return to its normal state of equilibrium *(homeostasis).*

In the presence of certain genetic defects or overwhelming infections, the regulatory mechanisms may become ineffective, giving rise to an uncontrolled and exaggerated immune response, such as is seen in *hypersensitivity* (discussed previously) or *autoimmunity* (see discussion following).

TOLERANCE TO SELF-ANTIGENS

Self-tolerance is a state of unresponsiveness to "self"-antigens (autoantigens) that are located on various cells and tissues of the body.

Tolerance to self-antigens can be attributed to a certain population of lymphocytes, the T lymphocytes, that are able to distinguish between self and non-self (foreign) antigens and to respond only to non-self antigens (see antigen-recognition, Chapter 1). This ability of the T cells is an evolutionary process (not inherited) that serves as the main regulatory mechanism in an immune response and is vital

for the normal development and survival of an individual.

Normally, precursor T lymphocytes (T cell clones) with a potential to react against self-molecules are eliminated or inactivated, mainly in the thymus (see Immunologic Tolerance in Chapter 1 and Figure 1-16). This ability to delete or inactivate self-reactive T cell clones prevents the immune system from responding to "self"-antigens (Figure 7-6).

AUTOIMMUNE RESPONSE (LOSS OF SELF-TOLERANCE)

Malfunction of the mechanisms that maintain self-tolerance allows the immune system to inappropriately respond to "self-antigens," a condition that is referred to as **autoimmune response.**

Autoimmune response is an antigen-specific response of the immune system that may be either cell mediated or humoral. It is catego-

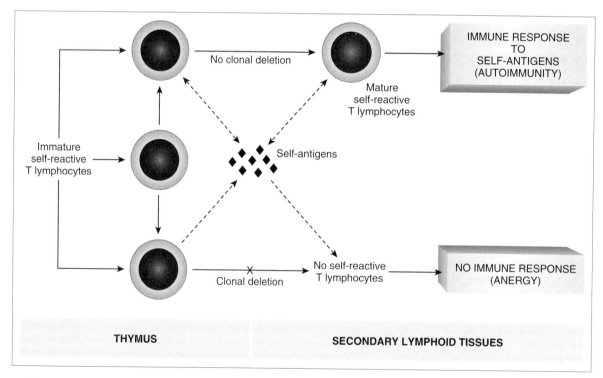

FIGURE **7-6**   **Immune Response to Self-Antigens.**   Deletion of self-reactive (autoreactive) clones of T cells occurs in the thymus, thus preventing immune response against self-antigens. In situations where autoreactive cells are not deleted and are permitted to mature, their contact with self-antigens results in an autoimmune response, with a possibility of tissue injury (autoimmune disease). (See also text.)

rized as an abnormal response in that it is directed against self-antigens (epitopes), such as:

- Cell-surface receptors
- Erythrocyte surface proteins
- Basement membrane antigens of kidney glomeruli
- Hormone receptors
- Nucleoproteins

The autoimmune response occurs only in the presence of self-reactive (autoreactive) T cells (see Figure 7-6 and discussion following) and shows loss of tolerance to self-antigens, as a result of such factors as:

- Inadequate control of immune responses (regulatory failure)
- Failure to maintain tolerance to self-antigens
- Inability to distinguish between self and non-self antigens

Factors Affecting Development of Autoimmunity

The following local and systemic conditions have been linked to the development of an autoimmune response.

Alterations in Lymphocytes

Alterations or changes may occur in B lymphocytes, T lymphocytes, or both populations, as follows:

- *Abnormal selection of lymphocytes:* Failure in deletion or inactivation of clones of self-reactive (autoreactive) T lymphocytes during cell maturation in the thymus or B lymphocyte clones in the bone marrow.
- *Cross-reactions ("shared antigens"):* Microorganisms that bear antigens that cross-react with self-antigens (epitopes) are able to activate self-reactive (autoreactive) T cells. The activated autoreactive T cells are now able to recognize and react against self-antigens, thus producing an autoimmune response. For example, rheumatic fever (myocarditis), which occurs after a streptococcal throat infection, is caused by cross-reaction of anti-streptococcal antibodies with proteins of patient myocardium.
- *Increased production of cytokines:* Increased production of cytokines (cell-to-cell signals) by T cells (CD4+ and CD8+

subsets) is responsible for DTH (delayed-type hypersensitivity) reaction with tissue injury.
- *Polyclonal stimulation of lymphocytes:* This type of stimulation of lymphocytes will induce non-specific (antigen-independent) response of self-reactive lymphocytes (not deleted during development) and the production of multiple autoantibodies, which have been associated with non-organ specific autoimmune disease.

Local (Tissue) Alterations

Autoimmunity may also develop as a consequence of certain alterations that occur locally during inflammation or tissue injury, such as:

- Release of previously removed (sequestered) self-antigens
- Alterations in the structure of self-antigens

Genetic Factors

Studies of autoimmune diseases in animal models (mice) have implicated certain genes in the development of autoimmunity, thus showing heredity as a possible factor.

In humans, for example, individuals who have inherited a particular major histocompatibility complex (MHC) of genes, such as HLA-DR4, have a higher probability of developing an autoimmune skin disease known as pemphigus vulgaris (blistering skin disease).

Environmental Factors

Such factors as drugs and ultraviolet radiation may produce alterations in certain self-antigens. The immune system will then recognize the altered self-antigens as non-self and will generate an autoimmune response.

SCOPE OF AUTOIMMUNE DISEASES

Autoimmune diseases have been categorized as *organ-specific* and *organ–non-specific*.

Organ-Specific Autoimmune Diseases

In **organ-specific autoimmune diseases** (Table 7-2), the immune response is directed primarily against antigens located in a particular organ. Organs most commonly targeted are the

Table **7-2**	**EXAMPLE OF ORGAN-SPECIFIC AUTOIMMUNE DISORDERS**		
Disease	Organ Involved	Autoantibody Specificity*	Clinical Manifestations
Addison's disease	Adrenal gland	Cells of adrenal cortex	Hypoadrenalism
Thyrotoxicosis	Thyroid	TSH receptors	Thyroid hyperactivity
Myasthenia gravis	Skeletal or heart muscle	Acetylcholine receptors (at neuromuscular junction)	Muscle weakness
Goodpasture's syndrome	Kidney	Glomerular basement membrane	Glomerulonephritis (inflammation)
Diabetes mellitus (type I)	Pancreas	Islets of Langerhans	Insulin-dependent hyperglycemia

*Diagnostic "markers."
TSH, thyroid-stimulating hormone.

thyroid, adrenals, pancreas, and stomach. For example, in Hashimoto's thyroiditis, the autoantibodies are specific for the thyroid.

Organ–Non-Specific Autoimmune Diseases

In **organ–non-specific autoimmune disease** the response may be directed against antigens of many tissues of the body, such as the kidney, skin, joints, and muscle. For example, in systemic lupus erythematosus (SLE), although the main organ targeted is the kidney (see Figure 7-4), predominant antibodies present in patient serum are directed against cell nuclei (see Chapter 13, One Step Further Box 13-2).

TISSUE INJURY IN AUTOIMMUNE DISEASES

In certain situations, a particular autoimmune response may be pathogenic (i.e., may cause local, organ-specific, or systemic tissue injury). The condition is known as **autoimmune disease.**

Tissue injury may occur through any of the following mechanisms:
- Antibody-mediated cytotoxicity (type II hypersensitivity) or antigen-specific antibodies (autoantibodies)
- Immune complex deposition (type III hypersensitivity) or antigen/antibody complexes
- Cell-mediated immune responses or antigen-specific T lymphocytes (as mediators)

Antibody-Mediated Cytotoxicity
Antigen-specific antibodies produced during an autoimmune response are known as *autoanti-*

bodies. These autoantibodies (IgG and IgM class) are directed against specific tissue or cells (Table 7-3), thus causing tissue damage (cytolysis) through a *cytotoxic hypersensitivity reaction (type II),* previously discussed and illustrated (see Figure 7-2).

Autoantibodies are designated according to the specific antigen (self-antigen) that induced their production and are classified as *organ-specific* and *organ–non-specific autoantibodies.*

Organ-Specific Autoantibodies
These antibodies are directed against antigens that are specific for a particular organ (see Table 7-2), such as the following:
- *Cell surface receptors:* For example, antibodies against cells of the adrenal cortex (Addison's disease)
- *Biologically active molecules (hormones):* For example, anti-intrinsic factor (IF) antibody detectable in the majority of pernicious anemias
- *Specific tissue/organ antigens:* For example, anti-glomerular basement membrane antibodies (anti-GBM) suggestive of the presence of Goodpasture's syndrome (glomerulonephritis)

Organ–Non-Specific Autoantibodies
These antibodies do not show specificity for any one organ but may be directed against multiple organs.

For example, antibodies to nuclear antigens, known as *anti-nuclear antibodies (ANA)* (see Table 7-3), are associated with untreated systemic lupus erythematosus (SLE) and multiple organ involvement and are detectable in most cases of SLE (99%).

Table 7-3	EXAMPLE OF AUTOANTIBODIES ASSOCIATED WITH SPECIFIC AUTOIMMUNE DISORDERS		
Antigen-Specific Autoantibodies	Disorder	Effector Mechanism	Clinical Manifestations
ANA, anti-dsDNA, anti-Sm	Systemic lupus erythematosus (SLE)	Immune complex–mediated tissue injury (type II hypersensitivity)	Multiple organ involvement
Anti-IF Abs	Pernicious anemia (B$_{12}$ malabsorption)	IF-blocking Abs	Abnormal erythropoiesis
Anti-TSH receptor Abs	Hyperthyroidism (Graves' disease)	Blocking of TSH receptor	Increase in thyroid hormones
Anti-RBC surface Abs	Autoimmune hemolytic anemia	Complement-dependent cell lysis	Erythrocyte lysis (hemolysis)
Anti-basement membrane Abs	Glomerulonephritis (Goodpasture's syndrome)	Complement, neutrophils	Renal failure

TSH, thyroid-stimulating hormone; *Abs,* antibodies; *RBC,* red blood cell (erythrocyte), *IF,* intrinsic factor; *ANA,* anti-nuclear antibody; *dsDNA,* double-stranded DNA; *Sm,* Smith.

Immune Complex Deposition

Immune complexes (antigen/antibody complexes) are formed when antigen-specific antibodies combine with the corresponding antigen. They are normally removed from circulation by phagocytes. In autoimmune disease, the immune complexes are not effectively removed and are deposited at various sites (tissue and organs), where they cause tissue injury by mechanisms previously described (see Figure 7-4).

Cell-Mediated Immune Response

T cells are essential for maintaining tolerance to self-antigens because of their ability to discriminate between self and non-self antigens. However, in the presence of autoreactive (self-reacting) T cells, the ability to recognize and tolerate self-antigens is lost, and an autoimmune response with tissue injury may occur.

Autoimmune response with tissue injury may also occur in the presence of T cells showing specificity to foreign protein antigens located within or on the surface of the individual's own cells.

Tissue injury in both situations occurs through T lymphocytes, which function as mediators in the cell-mediated immune response responsible for the injury (see type IV hypersensitivity). The mechanisms include delayed-type hypersensitivity reaction (DTH, see Figure 7-5) by T cell–secreted cytokines and cytotoxicity (cytolysis of target cells by cytotoxic T lymphocytes, see Figure 7-2).

It is also possible for an individual to have more than one autoimmune disease because of an overlapping that exists between the various diseases. For example, clinical manifestations observed in rheumatoid arthritis are also present in SLE.

LABORATORY EVALUATION

Autoantibodies are used extensively in clinical immunology as diagnostic "markers" for a particular autoimmune disease. This is possible because of their antigen specificity and their ability to bind with only the particular antigen that evoked their production (i.e., corresponding self-antigen). Thus laboratory detection of specific autoantibodies in patient serum or within specific tissue (see Immunofluorescence Assays, Chapter 13) is a powerful tool for confirming diagnosis, differentiation, and prognosis of certain autoimmune diseases (see Table 7-3 and One Step Further Boxes 13-2 and 13-3).

For example, the presence of anti-mitochondrial antibodies (AMA) (antibodies against cellular structures [mitochondria]) is associated with many cases of primary biliary

Table 7-4 SELECTED EXAMPLES OF PRIMARY AND SECONDARY IMMUNODEFICIENCY DISORDERS

Type of Disorder	Primary Abnormality	Origin of Defect	Specific Defect
PRIMARY (CONGENITAL) IMMUNODEFICIENCY			
X-linked (Bruton's) agammaglobulinemia	Reduced B cells and all Ig classes	Mutated gene on X chromosome	Blocked B cell maturation
IgG subclass deficiency	Decrease in one or more IgG subclasses	Defect in Ig isotype switching	Blocked B cell differentiation
Common variable immunodeficiency	Normal or decreased B cells; variable decrease in Ig isotypes	B cell defect (intrinsic)	Defective B cell differentiation to plasma cells
DiGeorge syndrome (thymic hypoplasia)	Normal B cells and Ig levels, reduced or absent T cells	Abnormal development of thymus	Defect in T cell maturation
SCID (autosomal recessive)	Decreased T and B cells, reduced Ig levels	Enzyme deficiency (PNP), toxic effect mainly on T cells	Abnormal T and B cell development
SCID (X-linked)	Decreased T cells, normal or increased B cells, lowered Ig level	IL-2 receptor chain gene mutation	Defective T cell development and growth
CGD	Granulomas (nodules of phagocytes)	Intracellular H_2O_2 not produced	Defective phagocytosis
SECONDARY (ACQUIRED) IMMUNODEFICIENCY (TO INFECTION)			
AIDS (HIV infection)	Reduced helper (CD4+) T lymphocytes	HIV-induced loss of CD4+	Lysis of CD4+ cells by viral budding
SECONDARY (ACQUIRED) IMMUNODEFICIENCY (TO MALIGNANCY OR THERAPY)			
Malignant lymphoma (Hodgkin's disease)	Deficiency in DTH responses (anergy)	T cell abnormality (cause not known)	Impaired T cell function
Drug therapy (immunosuppression)	Reduction in lymphocytes	Destruction of lymphocytes, PMN and MQ precursors	Cytotoxic effect

Ig, immunoglobulin; *SCID,* severe combined immunodeficiency disorder; *PNP,* purine nucleoside phosphorylase; *IL,* interleukin; *CGD,* chronic granulomatous disease, H_2O_2, hydrogen peroxide; *AIDS,* acquired immunodeficiency syndrome; *HIV,* human immunodeficiency virus; *DTH,* delayed-type hypersensitivity, *PMN,* polymorphonuclear neutrophils; *MQ,* macrophage.

cirrhosis (liver disease). Detection of AMA facilitates differential diagnosis of this form of cirrhosis from other forms of cirrhosis and hepatitis.

IMMUNODEFICIENCY

The effectiveness of defense against any infectious organism and its toxic products depends mainly on the normal function of the immune system. Therefore a defect or deficiency in any one or more of the main components of the immune system (e.g., B lymphocytes, T lymphocytes, phagocytic cells, or complement components) may result in an abnormally low immune response, referred to as **immunodeficiency.**

The deficiency may affect natural immune responses (e.g., defect in phagocytosis or complement system) or specific immune responses (e.g., abnormality in function, development, or activation of cells of the immune system [T and/ or B lymphocytes]) although both natural and specific immune responses may be involved. For example, as previously discussed in Chapter 3, macrophages function as phagocytic cells in natural immune responses and as antigen-presenting cells (APCs) in specific immune responses. Therefore deficiency in macrophages will impair both types of immune responses.

Patients with immunodeficiencies, generally, are more susceptible to infections and certain cancers.

Most immunodeficiencies may be diagnosed by clinical evaluation and various *laboratory screening tests* such as immunoglobulin quantitation, and leukocyte count and differential, among others (see Section II of this text). Additional *immunologic studies* (e.g., evaluation of T cells and T cell subsets) may be necessary to diagnose certain immunodeficiencies (see Flow Cytometry, Chapter 14).

Immunodeficiency disorders have been classified into two general categories (Table 7-4):

- **Primary immunodeficiencies:** Known as *congenital* or *hereditary,* these immunodeficiencies are caused by a genetic defect that is inherited and becomes evident as an increased susceptibility to infections in infancy and early childhood (e.g., DiGeorge's syndrome). Treatment of these disorders is currently limited to managing the infection and replacing abnormal components through transplantation (e.g., bone marrow in SCID and administration of gamma globulins in X-linked agammaglobulinemia, see discussion following.)
- **Secondary immunodeficiencies:** Also known as *acquired immunodeficiencies* (e.g., acquired immunodeficiency syndrome [AIDS]), these disorders develop later in life, secondary or subsequent to infection and cancers as well as to treatment with immunosuppressive drugs, or to diabetes, burns, or malnutrition.

Immunodeficiency disorders may also be defined according to the component of the immune system that shows the defect:

- *B cell deficiencies*
- *T cell deficiencies*
- *Combined B cell and T cell deficiencies*
- *Defect in phagocytic function*
- *Complement deficiencies*

B CELL IMMUNODEFICIENCY DISORDERS

The main deficiency observed in hereditary (primary) B cell immunodeficiency is in the production of antibodies (immunoglobulins). The deficiency may be the result of an abnormal development and function of B lymphocytes and leads to various recurrent infections with *pyogenic (pus-forming) microorganisms,* such as streptococci and pneumococci, as well as an increased susceptibility to certain viruses (e.g., polio).

As presented in Chapter 5, immune responses to many infectious microorganisms are normally antibody mediated. Thus any deficiency in antibody production, which may be detected as lowered serum immunoglobulin levels, will adversely affect the individual's ability to protect against infections.

Origin of Defect
The origin of these hereditary defects may be either at the B lymphocyte maturation stage (pre-B cell to B cell) or in the B lymphocyte response to an antigen, such as is seen in heavy chain class-switching defect (deficiency in IgG and IgA, with increased IgM levels).

Abnormality in helper (CD4+) T lymphocytes may also adversely affect antibody production. As previously discussed (see Chapter 5), T cell recognition of foreign antigens and T cell–secreted cytokines is essential for a normal antibody response.

Clinical Manifestations
The extent of B cell immunodeficiency (see Table 7-4) may be limited to a single class deficiency (e.g., IgA or IgG subclass deficiency) or it may involve a complete absence of B lymphocytes and serum immunoglobulins (e.g., *X-linked agammaglobulinemia* in male infants, also known as *Bruton's agammaglobulinemia*).

Bruton's Agammaglobulinemia
In this relatively rare X chromosome–linked agammaglobulinemia, the pre-B cells are present. However, because of a defective (mutated) gene located on the X chromosome, the pre-B cells cannot mature. Thus B cells and lymphoid tissue (e.g., tonsils) are absent, resulting in severe depression or absence of all classes of immunoglobulins (i.e., IgA, IgM, IgD, IgE or IgG).

The defective gene in this disease is carried by a female (XX) who shows no abnormality because of the presence of another normal X chromosome. However, males (XY) that inherit the abnormal X chromosome show absence of antibodies in their serum (agammaglobulinemia).

During infancy (first 6 to 12 months), protection from recurrent bacterial infection is provided by maternal IgG (maternal IgG crosses the placenta to infant). After depletion of maternal IgG, administered gamma globulin maintains the protection.

T CELL IMMUNODEFICIENCY DISORDERS

Deficiencies that affect T lymphocytes mainly impair cell-mediated immune response although humoral immune response may also be affected because of reduced help from CD4+ T cells. These deficiencies may be diagnosed by a decreased number of total blood T lymphocytes and a lowered proliferation of T cells in response to antigens or to T cell activators (e.g., phytohemagglutinin [PHA] mitogen) introduced into an in vitro tissue culture. A deficiency in vivo (delayed-type hypersensitivity [DTH], see previously) is also observed in T cell immunodeficiency.

T cell immunodeficiency disorders have been classified as:

- *Primary or congenital T cell immunodeficiency*
- *Secondary or acquired T cell immunodeficiency*

Primary (Congenital) T Cell Immunodeficiency

In congenital immunodeficiency, the primary defect is in maturation and function of the T lymphocytes, which leads to impaired cell-mediated immune responses with an increased susceptibility to infections caused by viruses, fungi, protozoa, and intracellular bacteria.

Origin of Defect

T cell immunodeficiency may be an outcome of defective maturation of T lymphocytes caused by an abnormal development (hypoplasia) of the thymus. It is characterized by a reduction or absence of blood T cells.

Defects in T cell activation and function in response to various antigenic stimuli have also been linked with T cell immunodeficiencies (e.g., Nezelof's syndrome).

Although the molecular basis and clinical significance of abnormal T cell responses have not been fully defined, it has been suggested that the deficiency may be caused by (1) defective surface receptors, (2) defective cytokine production, or (3) impaired cell-to-cell communication (signals).

Clinical Manifestations

For example (see Table 7-4), in *congenital T cell deficiency (DiGeorge syndrome)*, an abnormal (not hereditary) embryonic development of the thymus is responsible for the defective T cell maturation and other associated abnormalities (e.g., congenital heart disorder) that are associated with this disorder.

DiGeorge syndrome is characterized by a reduction or absence of T lymphocytes in the blood, which results in an impaired cell-mediated immune response. Individuals with DiGeorge syndrome also show abnormal humoral immune response (particularly IgG antibody response) because of the absence of helper (CD4+) T lymphocytes that are required for humoral immune response.

The severity of the immunodeficiency depends on the degree of impairment in the development of the thymus.

Secondary (Acquired) T Cell Immunodeficiency

T cell immunodeficiency may also be acquired as a secondary condition to an infection. This type of deficiency is associated with an increased susceptibility to malignant tumors and infections that are caused by a variety of opportunistic microorganisms.

Origin of Defect

Acquired T cell deficiencies may be caused by a loss of CD4+ T cell functions, such as is observed in infection with human immunodeficiency virus (HIV).

Clinical Manifestations

For example, *acquired immunodeficiency syndrome (AIDS)* (see Chapter 15, One Step Further Box 15-3) is a secondary immunodeficiency condition induced by HIV infection of CD4+ T cells, macrophages, and dendritic cells within the lymph nodes.

The condition is characterized by a decrease in the number of CD4+ T cells and by an impairment of antigen-specific CD4+ function (see Table 7-4). As discussed in previous chapters, CD4+ cells are required for normal humoral and cell-mediated immune responses. Thus, the impairment of helper (CD4+) T cell function is accompanied by lowered production of IL-2 (CD4-secreted interleukin), affecting the activation of T cell subsets and cytotoxic T cells.

Additional manifestations associated with the infection of CD4+ cells with HIV are (1) increased susceptibility to secondary infections with various opportunistic microorganisms, (2) ineffective destruction of target cells (virally infected cells) by cytotoxic T cells (CD8+), and (3) incidence of a certain rare skin cancer (Kaposi's sarcoma).

COMBINED B CELL AND T CELL IMMUNODEFICIENCY DISORDERS

These disorders affect both B and T lymphocytes. The immunodeficiency may be caused by primary lymphoid deficiencies or may be associated with other hereditary disorders.

Origin of Defect
Several conditions that are responsible for T and B cell combined immunodeficiencies have been identified:

- Defect in maturation of T and B lymphocytes, causing reduction in T and B cells and serum immunoglobulins
- Enzyme deficiency, leading to accumulation of toxic substances
- Abnormal maturation of bone marrow stem cells, resulting in reduction of T and B cells, other cells, and serum immunoglobulin levels

Clinical Manifestations
For example, in *severe combined immunodeficiency disease (SCID)*, there is a defect in B and T cell development from bone marrow stem cells, decrease in lymphocytes (lymphopenia), and a deficient humoral and cell-mediated immune response (see Table 7-4). Individuals with this inheritable disease are susceptible to microbial infections, such as *Candida*, cytomegalovirus, and *Pneumocystis carinii*. Survival beyond the first year without treatment is rare. Bone marrow transplantation cures these infants.

OTHER IMMUNODEFICIENCY DISORDERS

Other immunodeficiency disorders may occur following certain therapeutic procedures or because of an abnormality in phagocytic cells (i.e., macrophages and polymorphonuclear leukocytes) and complement components.

These components of the immune system (i.e., phagocytes and complement) serve as the principal mediators of natural immunity ("first line of defense" against infectious organisms) although their participation in the specific immune responses is also well defined. Thus any disorder associated with these components will result in an immunodeficiency that is characterized by recurrent bacterial and fungal infections.

Deficiency Secondary to Chemotherapy/Radiation
The most commonly occurring immunodeficiency disorder (secondary) is caused by therapy in cancer patients. This is because many therapeutic agents and radiation are capable of destroying bone marrow cells and lymphocytes in treated patients, thus producing manifestations associated with immunodeficiency.

Deficiency Caused by Deliberate Immunosuppression
Immunosuppressive agents, such as cytotoxic agents and corticosteroids, are administered during a transplantation procedure to a recipient (patient) to prevent immunologic rejection of a particular graft. This treatment suppresses immune responses, mainly by inhibiting activation of T lymphocytes, thus producing symptoms of immunodeficiency.

Deficiency Resulting from Defect in Phagocytic Function
Immunodeficiency produced by defective phagocytosis may be an outcome of either (1) an *inherited defect* in the metabolic pathways of phagocytic cells or (2) a *deficiency in other factors*, such as antibodies, complement components, adhesion molecules (integrins), or lymphokines (IL-2).

Inherited (genetic) defects in phagocytosis may lead to immunodeficiency with increased susceptibility to various infections because of an ineffective destruction of infectious microorganisms.

For example, *chronic granulomatous disease (CGD)* is an inherited disorder that is characterized by recurrent bacterial and fungal infections (usually at an early age) because of a defect in phagocytosis.

In patients with CGD, the normal intracellular "respiratory burst" in antigen-activated phagocytes is defective; i.e., hydrogen peroxide (and superoxide radicals) are not produced. Because of the absence of hydrogen peroxide, destruction of phagocytosed organisms does not occur, resulting in formation of granulomas (nodules of activated phagocytes).

Deficiency Caused by Congenital Defects in Complement Components

Genetic (congenital) defects in practically all the complement components of the classical and alternative pathways have been associated with certain immunodeficiencies.

Immunodeficiencies resulting from deficiency in complement components are characterized by an increased susceptibility to infection with pyogenic and certain intracellular bacteria and a tendency to develop immune complex disease.

For example, *C3 deficiency* and *factor H or factor I deficiency* are responsible for frequent infections with pyogenic bacteria, which may be fatal. As discussed in previous chapters, C3 opsonization of bacteria to enhance phagocytosis plays a significant role in the destruction of infectious organisms.

Also *deficiencies in terminal complement components (C5b through C9)* limit formation of the membrane attack complex (MAC), thus restricting complement-mediated lysis of infected cells. Certain intracellular bacteria, such as *Neisseria* species (*N. gonorrhea* and *N. meningitides*) are then allowed to persist within the infected cells and to disseminate throughout the body.

Finally *deficiencies in C1, C4, or C2 components* of the classical pathway are associated with an impaired clearance of immune complexes from the blood circulation. This promotes immune complex deposition in blood vessel walls and tissues, where they activate complement pathway and produce inflammation at the site of deposition (see type III hypersensitivity). Resulting tissue injury is associated with immune complex or autoimmune disease, such as systemic lupus erythematosus (SLE) (see Box 13-3).

HYPERGAMMAGLOBULINEMIA (IMMUNOPROLIFERATIVE DISORDERS)

Hypergammaglobulinemia is an abnormality that is associated with certain immunoproliferative disorders, also known as *gammopathies*. It is characterized by an increased proliferation of antibody-producing plasma cells (B lymphocyte lineage) that leads to increase in production of antibodies (immunoglobulins).

Antibodies produced by a single clone of antibody-producing plasma cells are known as **monoclonal antibodies.** Antibodies secreted by two or more classes (idiotypes) of immunoglobulins (Igs) are known as **polyclonal antibodies.**

Thus, abnormalities associated with increased production of monoclonal and polyclonal antibodies are designated as **monoclonal** and **polyclonal gammopathies,** respectively, and differ by certain characteristics presented in Table 7-5.

MONOCLONAL GAMMOPATHIES

Monoclonal gammopathies, also referred to as *plasma cell dyscrasias,* are characterized by an uncontrolled proliferation of a single clone or line of antibody-producing cells (plasma cells of the B cell lineage) at the expense of other clones.

The *excessive antigen-independent proliferation of plasma cells* originates from a malignant change within a single clone of the B cell line, referred to as a *plasma cell tumor.* Malignant transformation usually leads to an increased production of one class or subclass of immunoglobulins that is associated with a particular monoclonal gammopathy.

For example, in most multiple myeloma patients (52%), the monoclonal antibodies produced are of the IgG class. Other well-defined excessive plasma cell proliferation (monoclonal gammopathies) includes Waldenstrom's macroglobulinemia and heavy-chain disease, among others.

Table 7-5	SELECTED DIFFERENTIAL CHARACTERISTICS OF MONOCLONAL AND POLYCLONAL GAMMOPATHIES	
Characteristic	Monoclonal Gammopathy	Polyclonal Gammopathy
Antigenic stimulation	Antigen-independent (malignant transformation, plasma cell tumor)	Antigen-dependent (complex antigens)
Immune response (uncontrolled plasma cell proliferation)	Single clone of B lymphocytes involved	Two or more B lymphocyte clones respond
Class of antibodies produced	Single Ig class (mainly monoclonal IgG)	More than one Ig class involved (polyclonal IgG, IgA, IgM)
IEP pattern (gamma region)	Single peak (spike), sharply defined and narrowly based	Broad-based diffuse peak

Ig, immunoglobulin; *IEP,* immunoelectrophoresis.

POLYCLONAL GAMMOPATHIES

Polyclonal gammopathy is defined as a protein abnormality that is manifested as a *secondary condition* to such primary abnormalities as acute and chronic infections, autoimmune connective tissue disorders (rheumatoid), and liver disease.

The disorder is characterized by *increased production of more than one immunoglobulin (Ig) class* that involves several clones of plasma cells. Each of these Ig classes shows a different antigen specificity that corresponds to the epitope on the complex antigen that stimulated its production.

LABORATORY EVALUATION

In order to detect the presence of increased serum immunoglobulin levels, it is necessary to identify the abnormal class of immunoglobulin and its antigen specificity and to differentiate monoclonal from polyclonal immunoglobulins (Table 7-5), it is necessary to perform the following selected laboratory procedures (see Section II of this text):

- *Serum protein electrophoresis:* This procedure separates serum proteins into several regions. Increased levels of a particular monoclonal immunoglobulin class (gene product) appear as a single, narrow-based, sharply defined peak or spike in the gamma region of electrophoretically separated serum proteins (Figure 7-7).

Serum protein electrophoresis may also be used to detect a broad-based increase in the gamma region that indicates presence of polyclonal immunoglobulins (polyclonal gammopathy) (see Figure 7-7 and Chapter 11).

- *Immunoelectrophoresis (IEF) and immunofixation:* These procedures detect specificity of a particular class of antibodies (in the gamma fraction of serum proteins), which have been produced in excess. IEP also allows semi-quantitation of the immunoglobulins (see Chapter 11).
- *Radial immunodiffusion or nephelometry:* Methods of quantitation of immunoglobulins in serum are discussed in Chapter 11.
- *DNA hybridization, immunoblotting, and DNA probing:* Newer biotechniques for detection of abnormal genes responsible for the excessive production of a particular class of monoclonal antibodies are discussed in Chapter 15.

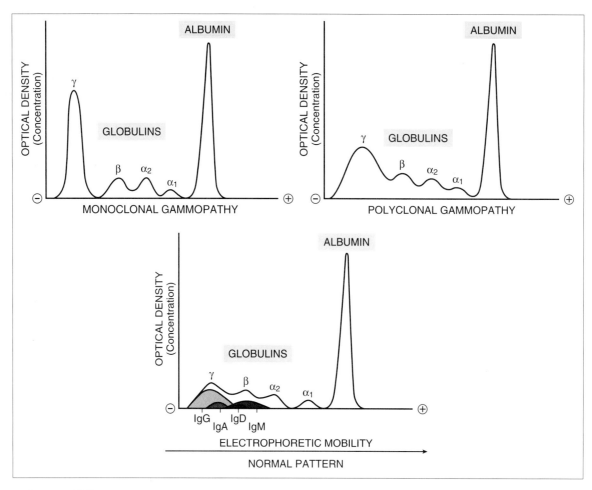

FIGURE **7-7**   **Serum Protein Electrophoretic (SPE) Patterns.**   SPE patterns seen in monoclonal and polyclonal gammopathy compared with normal electrophoretic pattern. Note presence of a discrete spike in gamma (γ) region of serum globulins in monoclonal gammopathy. A broad-based elevation in the serum globulin region is seen in polyclonal gammopathy.

𝒮uggested Readings

Gaspari AA: Advances in the understanding of contact hypersensitivity, *Am J Con Derm* 4:138, 1993.

Kotzin BL: Systemic lupus erythematosus, *Cell* 85:303-306, 1996.

McMichael AJ, Phillips RE: Escape of human immunodeficiency virus from immune control, *Annu Rev Immunol* 15:271-296, 1997.

Rose NR, Bona C: Defining criteria for autoimmune disease, *Immunol Today* 14:426, 1993.

Sideras P, Smith ECI: Molecular and cellular aspects of x-linked agammaglobulinemia, *Advan Immunol* 59:135, 223, 1995.

Theofilopoulos AN: The basis of autoimmunity, *Immunol Today* 16:90, 150, 1995.

Review Questions

HYPERSENSITIVITY

1. An exaggerated response of the immune system to an antigenic stimulus may be a result of all of the following mechanisms, *except:*
   a. failure to regulate an immune response
   b. clonal deletion
   c. failure to maintain self-tolerance
   d. inability to discriminate between self and non-self antigens

2. An excessive or uncontrolled immune response to an allergen, which may lead to tissue damage and may be more harmful to the host than the actual stimulating antigen, is known as:
   a. autoimmunity
   b. hypersensitivity
   c. infection
   d. all of the above

3. Which of the following events is involved in an allergic reaction:
   a. mast cell degranulation
   b. binding of IgE molecules to mast cells
   c. specific antigen binding to Fc receptors on mast cells and cross-linking the previously bound IgE molecule cell
   d. all of the above

4. In type II hypersensitivity, destruction of target cells is antibody dependent and occurs through:
   a. complement-mediated cytotoxicity
   b. complement-mediated cell lysis
   c. cell-mediated cytotoxicity
   d. all of the above

5-8. Match following types of hypersensitivity with associated mechanism of tissue injury:

   ____ type I   a. immune complex
   ____ type II   deposition
   ____ type III   b. target cell lysis
   ____ type IV   c. allergic reaction
                   d. contact sensitivity
                   e. inflammation

9. All of the following statements describe immediate hypersensitivity (allergic reactions), *except:*
   a. mast cells bind IgE via their Fc receptors
   b. the response occurs on a second or subsequent encounter with the same antigen
   c. complement is required for antigen binding with antibody
   d. IgE is the antibody molecule that mediates the reaction

10. Immune complex formation is promoted by:
    a. persistent infection
    b. autoimmune disease
    c. viral hepatitis
    d. all of the above

AUTOIMMUNITY

11. Breakdown in self-tolerance may be attributed to all the following conditions, *except:*
    a. abnormal selection of T lymphocytes
    b. genetic predisposition
    c. cross-reaction between foreign and self-antigen
    d. deficiency in T lymphocytes

12. Tolerance or unresponsiveness to self-antigens is attributed to cells that have the ability to recognize self and non-self antigens. These cells are:
    a. B lymphocytes
    b. T lymphocytes
    c. macrophages
    d. all of the above

13. Autoimmune response is a loss of self-tolerance that results in an antigen-specific response against which of the following antigens:
    a. erythrocyte surface antigens
    b. cell surface receptors
    c. hormone receptors
    d. all of the above

14. Indicate which of the following autoimmune diseases is *not* organ-specific:
    a. systemic lupus erythematosus
    b. Goodpasture's syndrome
    c. diabetes mellitus (type 1)
    d. Addison's disease

15. Detection of antigen-specific autoantibodies in serum or tissue is of diagnostic value in establishing the type of autoimmune disease because autoantibodies:
    a. bind only with a specific self-antigen
    b. may cause autoimmune disease
    c. are specific reagents for laboratory tests
    d. all of the above

IMMUNODEFICIENCY

16. Select an immunodeficiency disorder that is limited to an abnormality of the humoral immune response:
    a. multiple myeloma
    b. Bruton's X-linked agammaglobulinemia
    c. DiGeorge syndrome
    d. severe combined immunodeficiency disease (SCID)

17. Immunodeficiency may be the result of:
    a. a defect in phagocytosis
    b. a defect in complement function
    c. a defect in development of T lymphocytes
    d. all of the above

18. Individuals that are immunosuppressed are more susceptible to:
    a. certain cancers
    b. recurrent bacterial and fungal infections
    c. opportunistic organisms
    d. all of the above

19. Secondary or acquired immunodeficiency may occur after all of the following conditions, *except:*
    a. organ and tissue transplantation
    b. treatment with immunosuppressive drugs
    c. diabetes
    d. infections

20. In B cell (hereditary) immunodeficiency, the main manifestations observed include all of the following, *except:*
    a. defective phagocytosis
    b. abnormal antibody-mediated immune response
    c. abnormal humoral response
    d. reduced serum immunoglobulins

21. In primary (congenital) T cell immunodeficiency, the following conditions may be observed:
    a. a defect in T cell activation
    b. defective maturation of T cells
    c. impaired cell-mediated immune response
    d. all of the above

22. Severe combined immunodeficiency (SCID) is characterized by:
    a. a defect in T cell and B cell development
    b. susceptibility to microbial infections
    c. a deficient humoral and cell-mediated immune response
    d. all of the above

23. Which conditions may give rise to immunodeficiency disorders:
    a. defective phagocytosis
    b. chemotherapy in cancer patient
    c. a defect in certain complement components
    d. all of the above

HYPERGAMMAGLOBULINEMIA

24. Excessive antigen-independent proliferation of plasma cells in monoclonal gammopathy may be caused by:
    a. malignant changes within a single clone of B cells
    b. increased production of a single clone of antibodies
    c. increased production of multiple clones of antibodies
    d. all of the above

25. Differentiation between monoclonal and polyclonal gammopathy is possible by per-

forming serum protein electrophoresis. The separated proteins show a characteristic broad band (peak) within the gamma region of an electrophoretogram, indicating presence of:

a. monoclonal and polyclonal immunoglobulins
b. polyclonal immunoglobulins
c. monoclonal immunoglobulins
d. all of the above

SECTION II

DIAGNOSTIC LABORATORY IMMUNOLOGY

Section II begins with an overview of the scope of laboratory testing that includes various test panels and state-of-the-art immunologic and molecular techniques that provide information in support of clinical diagnosis of existing immunologic disease states, infections, and malignancies.

Included in the introductory chapters is a description of test quality management (i.e., quality assurance and control, proficiency testing, and test reliability features [sensitivity and specificity]) adopted by laboratories to ensure reliable test results. Important laboratory safety procedures, infection control, hazardous materials and waste management, and preparation for laboratory testing that includes method evaluation, method comparison, and specimen preparation and processing complete this introductory information.

Discussions in subsequent chapters cover basic principles of antigen-antibody reactions and immunologic laboratory procedures that use these reactions as their foundation. These procedures are categorized and discussed according to the major similarities in their protocol, such as the principle of the test (e.g., precipitation reaction), labels (e.g., fluorochrome-labeled immunoassays), separation of molecules (e.g., electrophoresis), and evaluation of the end-product of these reactions (e.g., nephelometry).

Among advanced immunologic and molecular techniques included are flow cytometry (e.g., cell sorting, immunophenotyping, HLA and tumor phonotyping, DNA analysis), functional tests (e.g., cell cultures and microcytotoxicity tests), monoclonal antibody production, DNA synthesis and isolation, nucleic acid amplification (e.g., polymerase chain reaction [PCR]), and nucleic acid hybridization (e.g., Southern blotting and in situ hybridization). One Step Further Boxes provide examples of specific infections and disease states associated with the immune system, which may be diagnosed using the discussed techniques.

Inclusion of molecular methods in this book reflects recent technologic advances, expanded diagnostic possibilities, and the sophistication of clinical immunology laboratory practice.

CHAPTER 8

Scope of Laboratory Testing

Upon completion of Chapter 8, the student will be prepared to:

INDICATIONS FOR IMMUNOLOGIC TESTING

- List the major indications for immunologic testing.
- Explain the reason for use of immunologic procedures in preference to viral cultures in the diagnosis of viral infections.
- State two conditions associated with bacterial infections in which immunologic testing is preferred.
- State three circumstances in which laboratory evaluation of a patient's immune competence is indicated.
- List laboratory procedures that constitute the test panel for evaluation of immune competence.
- Explain the effect of B cell immunodeficiency on the immune response to infectious agents.
- Define tumor-specific markers, tumor-associated (non-specific) markers, tissue-specific tumor markers, phenotypic markers, and malignant tumor.
- List an example of each of the following: tumor-specific marker, tumor-associated marker, B cell phenotypic marker, T cell phenotypic marker, and marker present in most lymphoblastic leukemias and lymphomas.
- List the major pre-transplantation tests performed on the donor and the potential graft recipient.
- Explain the reason for performing HLA antibody screening on the serum of a potential recipient.
- List two examples of organ-specific autoantibodies and organ–non-specific autoantibodies and the autoimmune disorder associated with each type of autoantibody.
- Explain which of the laboratory tests used to identify immunoglobulin disorders can differentiate monoclonal from polyclonal gammopathy.
- Name one immunoassay that is able to detect specific allergic reaction by quantifying allergen-specific IgE.

allergic reaction - Type I hypersensitivity reaction (e.g., hay fever and asthma) characterized by increased serum levels of immunoglobulin E (IgE).

antigen-specific antibodies - Molecules produced in response to an antigenic stimulus, showing the same specificity as the antigen and the ability to specifically bind with the antigen that induced their production.

autoantibodies - Immunoglobulins (antibodies) that are directed against self-antigens such as cell surface molecules, cytoplasmic components, or the cell nucleus. These antigen-specific antibodies are used in the diagnosis of autoimmune disorders.

crossmatch - Procedure used to detect the presence of antibodies in a patient's serum that are specific for the donor's HLA antigens. An incompatible crossmatch indicates a probable graft rejection.

diagnosis - Determination of the nature of a disease or abnormality or differentiating one disease from another (differential diagnosis).

dyscrasia - Abnormal condition or a clinical disorder (e.g., blood dyscrasia).

hyperactivity (of the immune system) - Inappropriate or exaggerated immune response.

immune competence - Ability of the immune system, through its mechanisms of normal response, to effectively eliminate or minimize any foreign (non-self) antigenic substance or configuration.

immunodeficiency - Hereditary or acquired defect or deficiency in any one or more components of the immune system, characterized by increased susceptibility to infections and malignant tumors.

leukemia - Hematologic malignancy (neoplasm) that is characterized by proliferation of malignant cells in the bone marrow or blood.

lymphoma - Solid tissue mass formed by localized proliferation of lymphoid cells.

monitor - On-going check on the status or progress of a condition or a particular situation.

monoclonal - Originating from a single genetically identical clone (line) of cells.

polyclonal - Originating from more than one clone of cells.

screening tests - Tests performed as an initial evaluation of suspected abnormality.

specific tests - Tests that have the ability to detect only those antigens or antibodies for which they have been designed and to show negative results in specimens in which the specific antigens or antibodies are absent.

tissue typing - Antisera with specificity for each of the human leukocyte antigens (HLA), used to identify these antigens on the surface of leukocytes.

tumor marker - Antigenic molecule or biochemical substance that is expressed by a tumor cell as a surface molecule or shed into body fluids (e.g., blood), used in screening for malignancies (neoplasm, cancer, carcinoma) or in clinical diagnosis of tumors (abnormal cell clones).

———•—•—●—•—•———

Use of laboratory testing in the earlier stages of immunology practice consisted primarily of detecting the presence of antibodies as an indicator of a particular infection as well as serologic identification of microorganisms responsible for the particular infection (causative or etiologic agents).

More recently, however, with the introduction of new technology and instrumentation into the clinical laboratory (e.g., molecular techniques and flow cytometry) and improvement in immunodiagnostic techniques (i.e., sensitivity, specificity, efficiency, and effectiveness), laboratory practitioners now have better tools for immunologic testing.

In addition, production of almost an unlimited number of predetermined antigen-specific monoclonal antibodies (mAb), readily available from commercial sources as reagent antibodies, have greatly expanded methods of detection and quantitation of antigens and antibodies. This has opened new possibilities for identifying specific markers on the cell surface of various cells.

With these improvements in immunologic techniques and the introduction of new tech-

nology, evaluation of various components and responses of the immune system to specific antigens has become more comprehensive.

INDICATIONS FOR IMMUNOLOGIC TESTING

Immunologic testing is an important source of information for establishing clinical diagnoses and for monitoring treatment of disease. The following are major **indications for testing:**

- *Detection of immune response to infectious agents:* Bacterial, viral, and parasitic
- *Evaluation of immune competence:* Post-immunization, post-immune reconstitution, post-immunosuppression
- *Detection of deficiencies of the immune system:* Hereditary and acquired immunodeficiency, deficiency in complement components
- *Evaluation of hyperactivity of the immune system:* Hypersensitivity or allergy, immunoproliferative disorders, autoimmunity
- *Diagnosis of malignancies:* Tumors, leukemias, and lymphomas
- *Pre-transplantation testing:* Histocompatibility in organ and tissue transplantations
- *Monitoring:* Treatment and progress of immune disorders

TESTING FOR IMMUNE RESPONSE TO INFECTIOUS AGENTS

In the past, detection of an infection consisted mainly of culturing, isolation, and identification of the causative infectious microorganism through standard microbiology procedures, such as direct identification of the microorganism, culturing techniques, and testing for microbial use of various biochemical components.

These time-consuming methods depended on the availability of a specimen (e.g., collected during the acute phase of an infection) and the time required for growth of the organism in a growth-supporting culture medium.

However, currently, with the availability of vast numbers and specificities of immunologic procedures, commercially prepared reagents, readily obtainable serum specimens, and the convenience of specimen transport and storage

Table 8-1	DETECTION OF ANTIGEN-SPECIFIC ANTIBODIES IN SELECTED INFECTIOUS DISEASES		
Infection	Antigen	Antibody Detected	Methods of Detection
Diphtheria (*Corynebacterium diphtheriae*)	Diphtheria toxin	Specific antitoxin	EIA, PHA
Legionella (*L. pneumophilia*)	Polyvalent Ag (4 strains)	Anti-*Legionella*	IFA, ELISA
Lyme disease (*Borrelia burgdorferi*)	Borrellia Ag	Antigen-specific antibody	ELISA, IFA
Gonorrhea (*Neisseria gonorrhoeae*)	Gonococcal Ag (e.g., LPS)	Anti-LPS	EIA, Immunoblot
Rheumatic fever (Post-streptococcal infection)	Streptolysin O DNase (B) isozyme (Streptococcal exotoxins)	Anti-ASO Anti-DNase (B)	ASO assay ELISA

EIA, enzyme immunoassay; *PHA*, passive hemagglutination; *IFA*, indirect immunofluorescence assay; *Ag*, antigen; *Ab*, antibody; *LPS*, lipopolysaccharide; *ASO*, anti-streptolysin O; *DNase*, deoxyribonuclease; *ELISA*, enzyme-linked immunosorbent assay.

(see Chapter 9), use of immunologic tests has become a highly desirable tool for the diagnosis of various infections.

The following discussion focuses on the more commonly encountered infections.

Detection of Infections

Immune response to a specific microorganism may be evaluated by a variety of immunologic tests that measure the various components of the immune system as well as their functional competence. *However, the most widely used tests are those that detect antibody response to a specific organism (Table 8-1).*

Detection of antigen-specific antibodies (humoral immune response) when an infectious disease is suspected has two major clinical applications:

- *Diagnosis of primary infection (recent infection)*
- *Detection of immunity (past infection)*

Primary Infection

Existence of initial (acute) infection requires demonstration of antigen-specific IgM in a patient's serum, which has been collected during the first week of the infection. The IgM is the first immunoglobulin class to appear when the immune system responds to an antigen. As IgGs are subsequently produced (see Ig class-switching, Chapter 6), the IgM level falls.

A recent infection may be demonstrated by a four-fold or higher increase in antigen-

Table 8-2	RECOMMENDED POST-IMMUNIZATION TESTING		
Effectiveness of Immunization			
Vaccine	Specific IgG	Methods of Detection	
Hepatitis B Ag (HBsAg)	HBV Ab	EIA (quantitative)	
Varicella Ag (chickenpox)	VAR ZOS Ab	Latex agglutination	
HAV	HAV Ab	EIA	
Measles	Rubella Ab	ELISA	

Ag, antigen; *Ab*, antibody; *HBs*, hepatitis B surface Ag; *HAV*, hepatitis A virus; *VAR ZOS*, varicella zoster; *EIA*, enzyme immunoassay; *ELISA*, enzyme-linked immunosorbent assay.

specific IgG titer between the acute and the convalescent (recovering from infection) serum specimens (see concept of titer, Chapter 9).

Past Infection

IgG is detectable within 1 to 2 weeks after initial or *primary infection*. It peaks at 4 to 8 weeks and declines, remaining detectable throughout life, thus showing immunity to the particular infectious agent (Table 8-2). Immunity is a function of immunologic memory and can be conferred through immunization (see Chapter 1). It is detectable in the same way as is the previous infection.

Re-infection, a secondary immune response to the same infectious agent, produces low titer of IgM and a higher titer of antigen-specific IgG at onset of the infection, with a rapid increase in IgG titer that peaks at a higher level than during primary infection (primary immune response). The concept of **primary** and **secondary immune responses** is discussed in Chapter 1.

In *congenital infection,* IgM or IgA detected in fetal, cord, or newborn blood represents a fetal response to an infection, whereas detectable IgG is of maternal origin (passed through placenta to fetus).

Laboratory Testing for Viral Infections

In testing for viral infections, detection of antigen-specific antibodies is the diagnostic tool of choice (Table 8-3). This is particularly true in situations that require specialized isolation conditions, for organisms such as Epstein-Barr virus (EBV) and human herpes virus. Immunologic testing is also preferred when propagation (growth in cultures) of such highly dangerous viruses as human immunodeficiency virus (HIV) is to be avoided.

Screening Profiles (Test Panels)

Test panels presented in Table 8-4 are commonly used screening profiles for the diagnosis of specific *viral infections.*

Laboratory Testing for Bacterial Infections

Diagnosis of most acute bacterial infections, such as group A streptococcal infection, is based on positive cultures of the organisms obtained from an infected site, blood, or cerebrospinal fluid (CSF). Positive results from commercially prepared "rapid test" kits may also be used to detect group A streptococcal antigen, but cultures of the organism may be required when negative results are obtained.

However, immunologic procedures are the methods of choice when testing for past infection or for conditions following an acute infection, such as post-streptococcal rheumatic fever or post-streptococcal glomerulonephritis, in which the streptococcal organisms may no longer be present. In these cases, detection of exotoxin-specific antibodies (e.g., anti-streptolysin O) demonstrates the presence of the post-streptococcal condition (see Table 8-1).

Table 8-3 DETECTION OF ANTIGEN-SPECIFIC IMMUNOGLOBULINS IN SELECTED VIRAL INFECTIONS

Immunoglobulin Class	Indication for Testing
IgG	Detection of immunity (HAV, HBV, VZV, measles, mumps)
IgM	Preferred method of diagnosis (EBV, HAV, HBV, HCV, measles, mumps, rubella)
IgG	(HCV, HIV-1, 2)
IgM and IgG	Differentiation between primary and recurrent infection (maternal) (CMV, HSV)
IgG	Evaluation of blood/blood products (HBV, CMV, HCV, HIV-1, 2)

HAV, hepatitis A virus; *HBV,* hepatitis B virus; *VZV,* varicella-zoster virus; *EBV,* Epstein-Barr virus; *HCV,* hepatitis C virus; *HIV,* human immunodeficiency virus, types 1 and 2; *CMV,* cytomegalovirus; *HSV,* herpes simplex virus.

TESTING FOR IMMUNE COMPETENCE

Immune competence is the ability of an individual's immune system to produce a normal humoral and cell-mediated immune response to a specific antigen. Immunologic tests currently used to evaluate the individual's immune competence (Box 8-1) may be categorized as follows:

- *Tests that evaluate various components of the immune system:* Enumeration of particulate and soluble components, such as cells and antibodies, respectively is discussed in subsequent chapters.
- *Tests that evaluate functional competence of the immune system:* Evaluation of immune response to antigen or mitogen, as evidenced by in vitro cell proliferation in cell cultures is discussed in Chapter 14.

Results of *non-specific tests* may also provide general information regarding the patient's immune competence (Table 8-5). In fact, when these test results are normal and the clinical history is negative, there is a high probability that the cellular and soluble components of the

Table 8-4   TEST PANELS FOR SELECTED VIRAL INFECTIONS

Antibodies Detected	Infectious Agent	Methods of Detection
HEPATITIS A, B, AND C PANEL		
Anti-HCV	HCV	EIA
Anti-HAV (IgM)	HAV	EIA
Anti-HAV (total)	HAV	EIA
Anti-HBsAg	HBV	EIA
Anti-HBcAg	HBV	EIA
TORCH (IgG, IgM) PANEL		
Toxoplasma antibodies	*Toxoplasma gondii*	ELISA
Rubella antibodies	Rubella virus (German measles)	EIA, latex agglutination
CMV antibodies	Cytomegalovirus	EIA
HSV antibodies	Herpes simplex virus (HV)	EIA
MMR/VZV (IgG) PANEL		
Rubeola antibodies	Rubeola virus (measles)	ELISA
Mumps antibodies	Mumps virus	EIA
Rubella antibodies	Rubella virus (German measles)	Latex agglutination
Varicella-zoster antibodies	Varicella-zoster virus (chickenpox)	Latex agglutination
EBV PANEL		
EBV-VCA (IgG/IgM) antibodies	EBV—viral capsid Ag	ELISA
EBV-EA antibodies	EBV—early Ag	ELISA
EBV-NA antibodies	EBV (EBNA)—nuclear Ag	ELISA

Ig, immunoglobulin; *anti*, antibodies directed against a specific antigen; *HCV*, hepatitis C virus; *EIA*, enzyme immunoassay; *Ag*, antigen; *HBs*, hepatitis B surface (antigen); *HBc*, hepatitis B core (antigen). *TORCH*, toxoplasma-rubella-cytomegalovirus-herpes; *MMR/VZV*, measles-mumps-rubella/varicella-zoster virus; *HAV*, hepatitis A virus; *HBV*, hepatitis B virus; *EBV*, Epstein-Barr virus; EBNA, Epstein-Barr nuclear antigen; *EIA*, enzyme immunoassay; *ELISA*, enzyme-linked immunosorbent assay.

Box 8-1   SCREENING TESTS FOR EVALUATION OF IMMUNE COMPETENCE

- Complete blood count (CBC) with differential and platelet count
- Total T lymphocytes (CD3)
- Helper T lymphocytes (CD3, CD4)
- Suppressor cytotoxic T lymphocytes (CD3, CD8)
- Helper/suppressor T cell ratio
- Total B lymphocytes (CD19)
- Natural killer cells (CD16, CD56)

Indications for Laboratory Evaluation

Laboratory testing for a patient's immune competence is performed in various circumstances, particularly to determine the effectiveness of a therapeutic procedure, such as:

- *Immunosuppression* (induced by drugs or radiation)
- *Immune reconstitution* (following bone marrow grafting or cancer therapy)
- *Immunization effectiveness* (presence of antigen-specific antibodies, see Table 8-2)

Testing for immune competence may also be performed when *autoimmune* or *immunodeficiency disorders* are suspected.

Test Panels

Tests that evaluate the individual's immune status (i.e., the competence of the immune system) include initial screening tests (Box 8-1), tests that evaluate humoral and cell-mediated immune responses (see Table 8-5), and more

immune system are also normal (see Chapters 3 and 4). However, by performing the immunologic tests presented in Table 8-6, it is possible to obtain more reliable information regarding the functional status (immune competence) of the immune system.

Table 8-5	NON-SPECIFIC TESTS FOR CELL-MEDIATED AND HUMORAL IMMUNE RESPONSES		
Type of Immune Response	Methods of Detection	Parameters Measured
Cell mediated	White blood cell count (WBC) and differential	Number and type of leukocytes
	Skin test (DTH)	Lymphocyte function
Antibody mediated (humoral)	Rate nephelometry, RID	Serum Ig (IgG, IgA, IgM) concentration

DTH, delayed type hypersensitivity; *RID,* radial immunodiffusion; *Ig,* immunoglobulin(s).

Table 8-6	SELECTED SPECIFIC TESTS FOR EVALUATION OF IMMUNE COMPETENCE		
	Methods of Detection	
Parameters Measured	Quantitation	Functional Assays
Total T cells	Flow cytometry (mAbs to CD2, CD3, CD5, CD7)	Activation of all T cells with mitogens (cell proliferation)
T cell subsets (helper/cytotoxic or suppressor)	Flow cytometry (mAbs to CD3, CD4, CD8)	CD8+ T cell function (cytotoxicity)
Total B cells	Flow cytometry (mAbs to CD19, CD20, CD22)	Serum Ig levels (RID or rate nephelometry for IgG, IgA, IgM); activation of B cells with mitogen
Immunoglobulins	Antibody titer to specific antigen or microorganism by ELISA, RIA, Ag-Ab reactions	Not routinely performed
NK cells	Flow cytometry (mAbs to CD56, CD16a)	Antibody dependent, cell-mediated cytotoxicity (ADCC) or cell lysis
Monocytes/MQs	Flow cytometry (mAbs to CD13, CD14, CD33)	Not routinely performed
Complement (C)	Hemolytic complement activity (CH50)	Not routinely performed
C components	ELISA, rate nephelometry, electroimmunodiffusion	Antibody-mediated cell lysis

mAbs, monoclonal antibodies; *CD,* cluster of differentiation; *Ig,* immunoglobulin; *RID,* radial immunodiffusion; *ELISA,* enzyme-linked immunosorbent assay; *RIA,* radioimmunoassay; *Ag,* antigen; *NK,* natural killer cells; *MQs,* macrophages.

specific tests (see Table 8-6) that evaluate the cellular and soluble components of the immune system.

TESTING FOR IMMUNODEFICIENCY

Normal function of the immune system depends on the integrity of all of its components, both cellular and soluble (see Chapter 1). Because immune responses to various antigens (epitopes) depend on the interaction between these various components of the immune system, a defect or deficiency in any one com-

ponent can affect the other components, thus producing an adverse effect on the normal immune response (see Chapter 7).

Immunodeficiency Disorders
Deficiencies of the immune system can be classified as follows (see Chapter 7 and Table 7-4):
- *Primary immunodeficiencies*
- *Secondary immunodeficiencies*

Primary Immunodeficiencies
These immunodeficiencies are also known as *hereditary* or *congenital immunodeficiencies*

Table 8-7   SELECTED SCREENING TESTS FOR IMMUNODEFICIENCIES

Testing	Suspected Deficiency	Methods of Detection
Number and type of lymphocytes	Any deficiency	CBC and differential
Number of neutrophils	Phagocytosis	CBC and differential
Neutrophil function	Phagocyte defect	NBT test, chemiluminescence
ANCA	Wegener's Disease, rheumatoid arthritis (vasculitis)	IFA, EIA
B cell function, antibody production (IgG, IgA, IgM levels)	Humoral immune response	RID, ELISA, nephelometry
T cell function, number of T cells and T cell subsets (CD3, CD4, CD8)	Cell-mediated immune response	DTH skin tests (*Candida* or PPD antigens), flow cytometry
Complement	Complement deficiency	CH_{50}, serum C3 level

CBC, complete blood count; *Ig*, immunoglobulin; *NBT*, nitroblue tetrazolium; *ANCA*, antineutrophil cytoplasmic autoantibodies; *IFA*, immunofluorescence antibodies; *EIA*, enzyme immunoassay; *DTH*, delayed type hypersensitivity; *PPD*, purified protein derivative; CH_{50}, complement hemolytic activity; *RID*, radial immunoassay; *ELISA*, enzyme-linked immunosorbent assay.

Table 8-8   TESTS FOR SELECTED DISEASES ASSOCIATED WITH COMPLEMENT COMPONENT DEFICIENCIES

Disease	Component	Methods of Detection
LE-like syndrome	C1q, C4,	RID, nephelometry, latex agglutination
Severe recurrent infections	C3	Same as above
Neisserial infections	C5	Same as above
Recurrent bacterial infections	Factor H or I	Same as above

LE, lupus erythematosus; *C*, complement; *RID*, radial immunodiffusion.

and include deficiency of B cell (humoral) immune responses, T cell (cell-mediated) immune responses, combined B cell and T cell responses, and defects in complement and neutrophil function.

The particular defect is inherited, becoming evident in infancy and early childhood as an increased susceptibility to infections. This is the characteristic finding in DiGeorge's syndrome (T cell deficiency) and severe combined immunodeficiency (SCID, T and B cell defect).

Secondary Immunodeficiencies

These deficiencies are also known as *acquired immunodeficiencies* and develop later in life as a secondary condition to infection, cancers, treatment with immunosuppressive drugs, diabetes, burns, or malnutrition. They are charac-

terized by increased susceptibility to malignant tumors and to infections with opportunistic microorganisms as seen in acquired immunodeficiency syndrome (AIDS).

Deficiency in Components of the Immune System

Immunodeficiency disorders have been also defined according to the component of the immune system that shows the defect. Defects in the following components are known and may be identified through various immunologic procedures (presented in Tables 8-7, 8-8, 8-9, and 8-10):

- *B cell deficiency*
- *T cell deficiency*
- *Combined B cell and T cell deficiency*
- *Defect in phagocytic function*
- *Complement deficiencies*

Table 8-9	TESTS FOR EVALUATION OF B CELL IMMUNODEFICIENCY DISORDERS*	
Parameters Measured	**Methods of Detection**	
Total serum proteins	Serum electrophoresis	
Ig class quantity (IgG, IgM, IgA)	Nephelometry, RID	
B cell count	Flow cytometry (mAbs to CD19, CD20, CD22)	
IgG subclass quantity (IgG1, IgG2, IgG3, IgG4)	RID, ELISA, nephelometry	

*Evaluation of humoral (antibody) response.
Ig, immunoglobulin; *RID*, radial immunodiffusion; *CD*, cluster of differentiation; *ELISA*, enzyme-linked immunosorbent assay; *mAb*, monoclonal antibody.

Table 8-10	TESTS FOR EVALUATION OF T CELL IMMUNODEFICIENCY DISORDERS*	
Parameters Measured	**Methods of Detection**	
Total lymphocyte count	WBC and differential	
Total T cell count	Flow cytometry (mAbs to CD2, CD3, CD5, CD7)	
T cell subsets	Flow cytometry (mAbs to CD3, CD4, CD8)	
T cell function	Delayed type hypersensitivity reaction (DTH), mixed lymphocyte reaction (MLR)	

*Evaluation of cell-mediated immune response.
WBC, white blood cell (leukocyte) count; *mAb*, monoclonal antibody; *CD*, cluster of differentiation.

Laboratory Evaluation of Immunodeficiency

Two types of laboratory tests are available for evaluation of immunodeficiency disorders. These are:

- *Screening tests as an initial evaluation of suspected immunodeficiency (see Table 8-7)*
- *Specific tests for suspected immunodeficiency disorders (see Tables 8-8, 8-9, and 8-10)*

For example, laboratory testing for suspected *acquired immunodeficiency syndrome (AIDS)*, induced by the human immunodeficiency virus (HIV), includes antibody detection, antigen detection, testing for viral nucleic acid, and cultures for HIV (see One Step Further Box 15-3). Screening tests for AIDS are presented in Table 8-11.

TESTING FOR MALIGNANCY

Transformation from a normal cell into a malignant cell may result from a variety of events, such as mutations in tumor suppressor genes, regulatory genes, or oncogenes, or it may be induced by various physical, chemical, or viral carcinogens (cancer-producing substances).

Thus, a **malignant tumor,** also known as a **neoplasm, carcinoma,** or **cancer,** is a clone or a mass of transformed cells derived from normal (self) tissue. These abnormal cell clones (tumor cells) show loss of their specific function and biochemical characteristics and normal morphologic characteristics (appearance).

Tumor Markers

Tumor markers are certain gene products or molecules expressed by various transformed (malignant) cells. The following gene products represent tumor markers that are most widely used in screening for malignancies, in clinical diagnosis, and in monitoring of malignancies (Table 8-12):

- **Antigenic molecules:** Referred to as *tumor antigens,* expressed on the surface of specific tumor cells
- **Certain biochemical substances:** Expressed by tumor cells and shed into body fluids, such as blood and urine

Classification of Tumor Markers

The most common classification of tumor markers is according to the site of origin, although some classifications are based on the markers' biochemical characteristics or their tumor specificity. The following classification is based on tumor markers' site of origination:

- **Tumor-associated markers:** Expressed as surface molecules by certain normal or malignant cells from the same cell line
- **Tumor-specific markers:** Expressed as surface molecules on tumor cells

Table 8-11	TEST PANEL FOR ACQUIRED IMMUNODEFICIENCY SYNDROME (AIDS)	
Type of Test	Parameter Detected	Methods of Detection
Screening tests	Antibodies to HIV-1 and HIV-2	EIA
Confirmatory tests	Antibodies to HIV antigens (p24, gp41, gp120/160)	Western blot test
Monitoring disease	T cell subset ratio (helper/ suppressor)	Flow cytometry (mAbs to CD3, CD4, CD8)
	HIV RNA—viral load	PCR or bDNA

HIV, human immunodeficiency virus, types 1 and 2; *mAb,* monoclonal antibody; *RNA,* ribonucleic acid; *EIA,* enzyme immunoassay; *PCR,* polymerase chain reaction; *p,* core antigen (protein product of HIV gag gene); *gp,* envelope proteins (HIV env gene product); *bDNA,* branch deoxyribonucleic acid.

- **Tissue-specific tumor markers:** Expressed by a tumor that develops from a particular tissue type and bears the same self-antigen (marker) as the normal tissue, thus not inducing an immune response

Detection of Tumor Markers

The basic principle in detecting a particular antigen (marker) is to react the suspected antigen with an antigen-specific antibody (tracer or labeled antibody) that has been labeled with a detectable "signal," such as fluorescein (fluorescent), luminol (chemiluminescent), ^{125}I (radioisotope), or peroxidase (enzyme), depending on the selected procedure. When the particular antigen is present, the formed antigen/antibody complex is detected by the selected "signal."

Currently, tumor markers may be detected by such techniques as:

- **Immunoassay procedures:** Enzyme immunoassays (EIA), radioimmunoassays (RIA), chemiluminescence assays (CIA)
- **Immunocytochemical characteristics:** Immunofluorescence (IFA), immunocytochemical assay (ICA)
- **Molecular techniques**
- **Commercial kits**

Evaluation of Leukemias and Lymphomas

Leukemia is a hematologic neoplasm (malignancy). It is characterized by proliferation of malignant cells that are detected in bone marrow and blood, whereas *lymphoma* is characterized by a localized proliferation of lymphoid cells that form a solid tissue mass.

In both conditions, the type of neoplasm present must be characterized for proper clinical diagnosis and prognosis of malignancy. The

Table 8-12	DETECTION OF SELECTED TUMOR MARKERS IN SERUM
Marker*	Malignancy Identified
TUMOR-ASSOCIATED (NON-SPECIFIC) MARKERS	
CEA	Primary colorectal cancer, GI, breast, lung, ovarian, prostatic, liver, and pancreatic malignancies
AFP	Non-seminomatous testicular cancer, primary hepatocellular carcinoma
HCG	Hydatidiform mole, choriocarcinoma, testicular neoplasm
TUMOR-SPECIFIC MARKERS	
CA 27.29 (CA 15-3)	Breast carcinoma
CA 125	Ovarian carcinoma
CA 19-9	GI cancer
PSA	Prostatic cancer
Calcitonin	Thyroid (medullary) malignancy

*Antigens detected by EIA or chemiluminescence.
EIA, enzyme immunoassay; *CEA,* carcinoembryonic antigen; *AFP,* alpha-fetoprotein; *HCG,* human chorionic gonadotropin; *CA,* cancer antigen; *PSA,* prostate-specific antigen.

following analysis for evaluation of hematologic malignancy is currently available:

- *Morphologic evaluation:* Stained blood or bone marrow smear
- *Immunophenotyping:* Detection of cell membrane, cytoplasmic, or nuclear antigens (flow cytometry, mAbs) (Table 8-13) (see Chapter 14)
- *DNA analysis (cell-cycle analysis):* Detection of total DNA at various phases of cell

Table 8-13	IMMUNOPHENOTYPING IN ANALYSIS OF SELECTED LYMPHOCYTIC LEUKEMIAS AND LYMPHOMAS
Antigen	**Cell Association**
B CELL–ASSOCIATED ANTIGENS (PHENOTYPIC MARKERS)	
sIg	Surface immunoglobulin (sIg) on mature B cells, absent on plasma cells
CD10 (CALLA)	Marker for common acute lymphoblastic leukemia, CD10 antigen is present on normal and acute lymphoblastic leukemia (ALL) B cells, absent on mature (circulating) B cells
T AND NK CELL–ASSOCIATED ANTIGENS (PHENOTYPIC MARKERS)	
CD3	Cell surface marker on T cells and most T cell neoplasms
CD4	Cell surface marker, present on helper T cell subset, monocytes and macrophages, and on many T cell lineage neoplasms
CD8	Cytotoxic/suppressor T cell subset marker, present also on many subpopulation sets of NK cells
CD9	Marker for acute leukemia
MISCELLANEOUS MARKERS	
TdT	Terminal deoxyribonucleotidyl transferase, a marker present in most lymphoblastic leukemias and lymphomas, not present in B and T cell lineage neoplasms

growth cycle (cell proliferation) (see Chapter 14)

TESTING FOR HISTOCOMPATIBILITY IN TRANSPLANTATION

Since complete tissue compatibility and successful retention of grafts is only possible between identical twins who have the same histocompatibility antigens (HLA), grafts obtained from all other donors are eventually rejected by the recipient, unless the recipient undertakes an immunosuppressive therapy before transplantation.

The graft rejection occurs because of some degree of antigen mismatching that exists between the donor and the recipient as a result of the extensive polymorphism (variability) of the HLA antigen system.

However, the greater the compatibility between the donor and recipient HLA, the greater is the graft survival. Thus pre-transplantation testing for histocompatibility between a graft donor and graft recipient is important to ensure the best survival of the graft (see Chapter 6).

Indications for Laboratory Testing

The following are the major *pre-transplantation tests* that are performed on the donor and the potential recipient (Table 8-14):

- *Tissue typing (HLA class I and class II)*
- *Crossmatching*
- *HLA antibody screening/identification*

Tissue Typing

Identification of human leukocyte antigens (HLA) on the surface of various leukocytes is performed by flow cytometry using antisera (monoclonal antibodies [mAbs]) with specificity for each antigen (see Chapter 14).

Tissue typing can also be performed by a *serologic procedure (lymphocytotoxicity)* and a *cellular method,* known as *mixed lymphocyte culture (MLC)* (discussed in Chapter 14), or by *molecular methods (DNA analysis)* that are based on amplification of DNA sequences by polymerase chain reaction (PCR) (discussed in Chapter 15).

Crossmatching

This pre-transplantation procedure is highly sensitive and specific for HLA antigens. It is performed to detect the presence of antibodies (anti-HLA) in the patient's serum that are specific for the potential donor's HLA antigens. A positive or incompatible crossmatch indicates the presence of antibodies directed against the donor's HLA antigens and the possibility of a powerful immune response against these antigens on the donor's graft (organ, tissue, or cells), causing graft rejection.

Table 8-14 PRE-TRANSPLANTATION EVALUATION

Test	Patient Specimen	Donor Specimen	Method
HLA type (class I and II antigens)	T/B cells	T/B cells	Lymphocytotoxicity (HLA-specific antisera), flow cytometry (HLA-specific mAb), DNA analysis
ABO/Rh (D) type	RBCs	RBCs	Anti-A, anti-B, and anti-D antisera
HLA Ab screen			
Class I (HLA Ab)	Serum	N/A	T cell panel (HLA-A, -B, and -C)
Class II (HLA Ab)	Serum	N/A	B cell panel (HLA-DR, -DQ)
Crossmatch			
Blood lymphocytes or T/B lymphocytes	Serum	Lymphocytes	Cytotoxicity, flow cytometry
MLC	Lymphocytes	Lymphocytes	Cellular assay

MLC, mixed lymphocyte culture; *HLA,* human leukocyte antigen; *Ab,* antibody; *mAb,* monoclonal antibody; *DNA,* deoxyribonucleic acid; *RBC,* red blood cell (erythrocyte); *ABO/Rh,* antigens (markers) on RBCs; *N/A,* not applicable.

The simplest procedure for a crossmatch is the standard *lymphocytotoxicity method.* In this procedure, an incompatible or positive crossmatch (visible T cell or B cell cytotoxicity) indicates presence of antibodies to class I HLA or class II HLA antigens, respectively.

Flow cytometry crossmatch is another procedure used in pre-transplantation. It is more sensitive than visual serologic crossmatch and has the capability to detect patient serum-derived HLA-specific antibodies on donor lymphocytes. Other crossmatch techniques are listed under pre-transplantation procedures (see Table 8-14 and discussion in Chapter 6).

HLA Antibody Screening

Screening for HLA antibodies that may be present in a patient's serum is performed to identify those antibodies (class I and class II) that are directed against the potential donor's HLA antigens. Presence of donor-specific antibodies indicates that the recipient has been "sensitized" to those antigens and is capable of mounting a strong immune response against the transplant (see discussion of graft rejection in Chapter 6).

Antibody screening uses serologic procedures with commercially prepared panels of T and B cells with known HLA specificities (see Table 8-14).

TESTING FOR HYPERACTIVITY OF THE IMMUNE SYSTEM

Hyperactivity of the immune system is manifested by various clinical disorders that result from an inappropriate or exaggerated immune response, such as:

- **Inappropriate immune response** to self-antigens as a result of loss of self-tolerance as seen in *autoimmune disorders*
- **Heightened immune response** to harmless antigens or allergens (with possible tissue injury) as seen in *hypersensitivity reactions* or *allergic reactions*
- **Abnormality of antibody-producing cells** as seen in *B cell malignancy* or *monoclonal gammopathy,* showing increased production of a single type of immunoglobulin (monoclonal) by the abnormal B cell lineage

Autoimmune Diseases

Autoimmune diseases occur when there is loss of self-tolerance and the immune system responds to self-antigens by producing *autoantibodies* that are capable of causing tissue damage. Thus autoimmune diseases have been classified according to the site of the autoimmune response (i.e., **organ-specific** [localized] or **systemic** [affecting multiple organs]).

Organ-Specific Diseases

In this type of autoimmune disease, the autoantibodies show specificity for antigens ex-

Table 8-15 AUTOANTIBODIES* IN SELECTED AUTOIMMUNE DISORDERS

Autoantibody Specificity	Autoimmune Disorder
ORGAN-SPECIFIC AUTOIMMUNE DISORDERS	
Cells of adrenal cortex (adrenal gland)	Addison's disease (hypoadrenalism)
TSH receptors (thyroid)	Graves' disease (hyperthyroidism)
Islets of Langerhans (pancreas)	Insulin-dependent diabetes (hyperglycemia)
Glomerular basement membrane (kidney)	Goodpasture's syndrome (glomerulonephritis)
SYSTEMIC AUTOIMMUNE DISORDERS (ORGAN NON-SPECIFIC)	
ds-DNA, Sm, nRNP	Systemic lupus erythematosus (SLE) (rheumatic disease)
Intrinsic factor (IF)	Pernicious anemia (B_{12} malabsorption)
RBC surface	Autoimmune hemolytic anemia (cell lysis)
Scl-70, centromere	Scleroderma (connective tissue disorder)

*Diagnostic markers
TSH, thyroid-stimulating hormone; *ds-DNA,* double-stranded deoxyribonucleic acid molecule; *Sm,* Smith antigen; *nRNP,* nuclear ribonucleoprotein antigen, *Scl-70,* scleroderma antigen; *RBC,* red blood cell (erythrocyte).

pressed within a particular organ, indicating the presence of organ-specific autoimmune disease. For example, detection of autoantibodies with specificity for cells of the adrenal cortex confirms the presence of Addison's disease (Table 8-15).

Systemic Diseases

Systemic autoimmune diseases (organ–non-specific) are characterized by the presence of one or more autoantibodies directed against surface antigens, cytoplasmic components, or the nucleus of the cell. These autoantibodies are not specific for any one organ but show association with multiple organs.

For example, antibodies to nuclear antigens, known as *anti-nuclear antibodies (ANA),* are associated with untreated systemic lupus erythematosus (SLE) and involve multiple organs (see Chapter 13, One Step Further Box 13-2). Laboratory testing (Table 8-16) for SLE, rheumatoid arthritis, and other rheumatic diseases is performed in conjunction with clinical diagnosis to establish, differentiate, and/or confirm the existence of a specific rheumatic disease.

Detection of Antigen-Specific Autoantibodies

Autoantibodies are antigen-specific (i.e., show specificity for the particular self-antigen that induced their production). Their specificity makes them excellent "diagnostic markers" for certain autoimmune diseases.

Table 8-16 TEST PROFILE FOR RHEUMATIC DISEASES*

Parameter Tested	Methods
ESR	Micro-ESR, or Westergren method
CRP	Latex agglutination test or nephelometry
C3, C4	Nephelometry
ANA	EIA or IFA
Anti-DNA	IFA
ENA	ELISA, immunodiffusion, IFA
CIC	Raji cell technique, ELISA
RF	Latex agglutination or nephelometry

*Systemic autoimmune disorder.
ESR, erythrocyte sedimentation rate; *CRP,* C-reactive protein; *C3, C4,* complement components; *ANA,* anti-nuclear antibody; *anti-DNA,* deoxyribonucleic acid; *ENA,* extractable nuclear antigen; *CIC,* circulating immune complexes; *RF,* rheumatoid factor (anti-Fc of IgG); *ELISA,* enzyme-linked immunosorbent assay; *IFA,* immunofluorescence antibody; *EIA,* enzyme immunoassay.

Thus diagnosis of suspected autoimmune disease can be established by detection and identification of autoantibodies in *serum* or *within a specific tissue or organ* that is associated with a particular autoimmune disease (see Table 8-15).

The following are examples of diseases in which specific autoimmune responses have been identified:

- *Multiple sclerosis:* Antibodies against myelin protein cause destruction of the myelin sheath of axons. These autoantibodies are identified by radioimmunoassay (RIA).

- *Myasthenia gravis:* Antibodies to acetylcholine receptors block binding of acetylcholine and are destroyed because of activation of complement. Detection of these autoantibodies is by RIA.
- *Goodpasture's syndrome:* Antibodies directed against the glomerular basement membrane cause glomerulonephritis and renal failure. Antibodies are detected by RIA and immunofluorescence (IF).
- *Graves' disease (hyperthyroidism):* Antibodies directed against thyroid-stimulating hormone (TSH) receptor stimulate the receptor, causing continuous release of thyroid hormone. Elevated levels of thyroid hormone provide the diagnosis.
- *Hashimoto's thyroiditis:* Anti-thyroglobin antibodies cause a gradual destruction of the thyroid gland, resulting in hypothyroidism. RIA, indirect immunofluorescence, and agglutination techniques can detect anti-thyroglobulin and anti-peroxidase antibodies.
- *Insulin-dependent diabetes mellitus:* Antibodies to islet cells cause progressive destruction of beta cells in the pancreas, resulting in decreased production of insulin and hyperglycemia. Antibodies to islet cells are detected by IF, while RIA or ELISA detects antibodies to insulin.

Immunoproliferative Disorders

Immunoproliferative disorders most frequently encountered in the clinical laboratory involve abnormalities of the B lymphocytes (precursors of antibody-producing plasma cells). These B cell malignancies are often accompanied by abnormal or excessive production of immunoglobulins (antibodies) that are monoclonal in nature (i.e., originating from a single genetically identical line or clone of cells). B cell malignancy can be diagnosed by determining the type of immunoglobulins that are produced by the abnormal B cell lineage. For example, detection of an increased amount of a single type of immunoglobulin, known as **monoclonal gammopathy,** is suggestive of a malignancy. Increase in total immunoglobulins (not in one specific cell clone) suggests a benign (harmless) response to a stimulus, known as *reactive cell proliferation.*

Plasma Cell Dyscrasias

Plasma cell dyscrasia is a generic term that describes any clinical disorder that is characterized by overproduction of a single type of immunoglobulin (Ig) that can be diagnosed and monitored by immunoelectrophoretic techniques (see Chapter 11).

Several related syndromes have been classified as plasma cell dyscrasias. Among these are:
- *Multiple myeloma (plasma cell myeloma):* This dyscrasia is characterized by *clonal proliferation of plasma cells*, resulting in an excessive production of a single type of immunoglobulin, known as *monoclonal immunoglobulin,* M protein (myeloma protein) or paraprotein, or by the production of a single light (L) or heavy (H) immunoglobulin chain (see Chapter 11). Free L chains of Ig molecule can be detected in the urine of multiple myeloma patients.
- *Waldenstrom's macroglobulinemia (WM):* This immunoproliferative disorder is characterized by malignant proliferation of lymphocytes (see Chapter 11). The large number of malignant lymphocytes (B cell lineage), sometimes referred to as *plasmacytoid lymphocytes,* produce large amounts of monoclonal IgM (19S), known as *macroglobulin* (paraprotein or M protein), which is responsible for an increase in serum viscosity.

Laboratory Detection of Plasma Cell Dyscrasias

Several test procedures are currently available to detect the existence of an immunoglobulin disorder and identify the disorder as monoclonal or polyclonal (more than one clone of cells). Of these procedures (Table 8-17), the most useful for characterization of immunoglobulins in serum, urine, or cerebrospinal fluid (CSF) are:
- *Protein electrophoresis:* Very useful screening procedure for establishing differential diagnosis in various clinical conditions. The diagnosis depends on evaluation of characteristic electrophoretic patterns for a distinct abnormality (see Chapter 11, Figure 11-5).

  For example, detection of a single sharp peak or band in the γ-globulin region of serum proteins on an electrophoretogram indicates presence of monoclonal immunoglobulins (see Figure 11-5).

- *Immunoelectrophoresis (IEP) or immunofixation electrophoresis (IFE):* These analytic procedures are essential for differentiation of monoclonal from polyclonal immunoglobulins and for detection of immunoglobulin fragments (i.e., heavy [H] chain or light [L] chain type of paraprotein in serum) or to detect an increase in γ-globulin (see Chapter 11).

   For example, it is possible to detect immunoglobulin light chains (free γ or λ L chains), known as *Bence Jones protein,* by IFE procedure in the urine of patients with light chain disease or in myeloma patients.

Immediate Hypersensitivity (Allergic Reactions)

Increased levels of immunoglobulin E (IgE) in a patient's serum may indicate the presence of an allergic disorder (see Chapter 7, type I hypersensitivity). This is because IgE, as a class of immunoglobulins, mediates a variety of hypersensitivity reactions such as hay fever, contact dermatitis, eczema, and asthma.

Laboratory Evaluation of Allergic Reactions

Although skin testing is a widely used technique for determining the type of allergic reaction, detection of an increased amount of allergen-specific IgE in serum indicates that an increased probability exists for experiencing symptoms associated with a particular allergic disorder.

High levels of total IgE may also be associated with other conditions, such as parasitic infections and aspergillosis. Differentiation between these conditions and specific allergic reactions is made by in vitro laboratory testing. The testing involves either quantifying antigen-specific IgE or total IgE in a serum sample by using the following methods:

- *Radioimmunosorbent test (RIST) or enzyme immunoassay (EIA):* Detects *total amount of IgE* in patient serum.

Table 8-17   LABORATORY EVALUATION OF PLASMA CELL DYSCRASIAS

Test	Indication for Testing
Protein electrophoresis	Differential diagnosis in various clinical conditions; detection of paraproteins
Immunoelectrophoresis or immunofixation electrophoresis	Differentiation of monoclonal from polyclonal immunoglobulins; detection of immunoglobulin light chains
Total protein quantitation	24 hr urine specimen
Nephelometric or radial immunodiffusion	Quantitation of immunoglobulins
DNA hybridization, DNA probing, and immunoblotting	Detection of abnormal gene, producing a particular class of monoclonal immunoglobulins

- *Radioallergosorbent test (RAST):* Widely accepted method for quantifying *antigen-specific IgE in patient serum,* using such common allergens (antigens) as ragweed, grasses, molds, animal dander, and milk. A modification of RAST includes the use of an enzyme or fluorimetric labels.

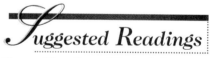

Suggested Readings

Henry JB, editor: *Clinical diagnosis and management by laboratory methods,* ed 19, Philadelphia, 1996, WB Saunders.

Ross NR, de Macario EC, Folds JP, Lane HC, Nakamura RM, editors: *Manual of clinical laboratory immunology,* ed 5, Washington, DC, 1997, American Society of Microbiology.

Review Questions

INDICATIONS FOR IMMUNOLOGIC TESTS

1. All conditions listed following are indications for immunologic testing, *except:*
   a. detection of immune response to parasitic infections
   b. detection of leukemia and lymphocytosis
   c. evaluation of immune competence
   d. monitoring treatment of an immune disorder

2. Select an example of hyperactivity of the immune system:
   a. autoimmunity
   b. plasma cell dyscrasias
   c. hypersensitivity
   d. all of the above

3. The most widely used immunologic tests for infectious disease are those that detect:
   a. recent or past infection
   b. antibody response to a specific microorganism
   c. components of the immune system
   d. all of the above

4. Recent infection can be demonstrated by comparing the antibody titer of current and convalescent serum samples and detecting one of the following titers:
   a. two-fold increase in antigen-specific IgG titer
   b. four-fold increase in antigen-specific IgG titer
   c. four-fold increase in antigen-specific IgM titer
   d. high titer of antigen-specific IgM

5. In congenital infection, fetal, cord, or newborn blood may contain several classes of immunoglobulins. Select the class that is of maternal origin:
   a. IgM
   b. IgG
   c. IgA
   d. all of the above

6. Immunologic procedure is the method of choice in diagnosis of a bacterial infection in one of the following situations:
   a. past infection
   b. most acute infections
   c. in the presence of a negative culture of microorganisms
   d. all of the above

7. TORCH Panel consists of selected methods for the detection of specific antibodies directed against all the following infectious agents, *except:*
   a. *Toxoplasma gondii*
   b. hepatitis virus
   c. cytomegalovirus
   d. rubella virus
   e. herpes simplex virus

8. Select the type of laboratory testing that should be performed to determine the effectiveness of immunization:
   a. evaluation of components of the immune system
   b. detection of antigen-specific antibodies
   c. evaluation of cell-mediated immune response
   d. all of the above

9. All of the following procedures are a part of the test panel used to evaluate immune competence, *except:*
   a. total T lymphocytes
   b. helper/suppressor T cell ratio
   c. phagocytosis
   d. natural killer cells

10-12. Match each test with the appropriate deficiency:

   _____ B cell deficiency
   _____ defective phagocytosis
   _____ deficiency in cell-mediated immune response

   a. test for neutrophil function
   b. test for antibody production
   c. evaluation of T cells

13. Select the method(s) used to quantify immunoglobulins:
   a. flow cytometry
   b. nephelometry
   c. radial immunoassay
   d. enzyme-linked immunosorbent assay

14. A tumor-specific marker is defined as:
   a. a gene product of a malignant cell
   b. antigenic molecule expressed on the surface of a tumor cell
   c. substance expressed by tumor cells and shed into body fluids
   d. all of the above

15. All of the following tumor markers are designated as tumor-specific, *except:*
   a. prostate-specific antigen (PSA)
   b. cancer antigen (CA 125)
   c. calcitonin
   d. carcinoembryonic antigen (CEA)

16. Tumor markers may be detected by all the laboratory procedures listed, *except:*
   a. molecular techniques
   b. cytotoxicity tests
   c. immunocytochemical techniques
   d. immunoassay procedures

17. In immunophenotyping for lymphocytic leukemias and lymphomas, which of the following antigens may be detected?
   a. nuclear antigens
   b. cytoplasmic antigens
   c. cell-surface antigens
   d. all of the above

18. Human leukocyte antigens (HLA) may be identified by all the following procedure(s), *except:*
   a. DNA analysis
   b. serologic tissue-typing procedure
   c. mixed lymphocyte method
   d. all of the above

19. A positive or incompatible crossmatch in pre-transplantation testing indicates that the potential recipient:
   a. has antibodies to the donor's human leukocyte antigens (HLA)
   b. is capable of rejecting the graft
   c. can mount an immune response to the graft
   d. all of the above

20-23. Match the type specimen required with the appropriate test:

   ____ HLA type
   ____ ABO/Rh type
   ____ HLA antibody screen
   ____ crossmatch

   a. patient and donor erythrocytes
   b. patient and donor T and B cells
   c. patient serum
   d. donor cells

24. Increased production of single type of immunoglobulin is referred to as:
   a. monoclonal gammopathy
   b. B cell malignancy
   c. abnormality of antibody-producing cell lineage
   d. all of the above

25-29. Match the following autoantibody specificity with the associated autoimmune disorder:

   ____ cells of the adrenal gland
   ____ receptors for thyroid-stimulating hormone (TSH)
   ____ glomerular basement membrane
   ____ intrinsic factor (IF)
   ____ ds-DNA molecule

   a. systemic lupus erythematosus
   b. Addison's disease
   c. Graves' disease
   d. Goodpasture's syndrome
   e. pernicious anemia

30. Detection of a single sharp peak in the gamma globulin region of a serum protein electrophoretogram is indicative of the presence of which one of the following disorders:
   a. light-chain disease
   b. monospecific immunoglobulin
   c. monoclonal gammopathy
   d. polyclonal gammopathy

31. Increase in total level of IgE may be associated with all of the following conditions, *except:*
    a. hay fever
    b. eczema
    c. parasitic infections
    d. fungal infections

32. Select a method used for detection of antigen-specific IgE in serum:
    a. radioimmunosorbent test
    b. latex agglutination technique
    c. radioallergosorbent test
    d. all of the above

CHAPTER 9

Laboratory Safety and Test Quality Assurance

Upon completion of Chapter 9, the student will be prepared to:

LABORATORY SAFETY

- Explain the main reason for enforcement of OSHA occupational exposure controls.
- List the major barrier and other protective measures to be used by laboratory practitioners, implemented under the Clinical Laboratory Improvement Act (CLIA '88).
- Define Universal Precautions.
- State three components of a written Exposure Control Plan, developed and implemented by each health care institution.
- List contents of the Safety Manual.
- Discuss the reason for implementing a Chemical Hygiene Plan.
- Describe the correct way of disposing of infectious waste.
- Define the following terms: biohazard, material safety data sheets (MSDS), Right-to-Know law.

PREPARATION FOR LABORATORY TESTING

- Calculate simple, compound, and serial dilutions.
- Define the following terms: *calibration, serial dilution and titer, solute, diluent.*
- Explain an acceptable protocol for method evaluation.
- Describe a procedure for method comparison used before implementation of any new technique.
- Differentiate between random and systematic error.
- Define correlation coefficient.

TEST QUALITY MANAGEMENT

- List components of a Quality Assurance Program.
- List government or private agencies that monitor performance accuracy of laboratories by using the Survey or Proficiency Testing Programs.
- Define the following terms: *performance standards, proficiency testing, quality control, quality assurance,* and *total quality performance.*

- Describe the issues defined under CLIA '88 Standards. Define the following terms: *test and diagnostic specificity, test and diagnostic sensitivity, predictive value, test efficiency.*
- Explain the significance of predictive test values.

Key Terms

accuracy - Extent to which the mean test result is close to the true value.

analyte - Refers to a molecule or substance that is being detected or analyzed.

biohazard - Usually appears as a "warning," signifying presence of contaminated waste or of supplies that have been contaminated with blood or other body fluids and which present a potential risk of exposure to infectious material.

controls - These specimens are obtained from large pools of serum, and are used to establish the test values for a particular analyte. They are also used in Quality Assurance Programs for establishing reliability (acceptability) of a patient's results.

error - Difference between a true or assigned value and the test result from an actual experiment.

monitor - Ongoing observation or survey of condition or situation as may occur in monitoring of laboratory performance or drug therapy.

precision - Reproducibility of test values (data) (i.e., consistency or agreement between replicate or series of test results).

proficiency testing - Also known as a **Survey Program.** It is provided by approved agencies or institutions for monitoring individual laboratory test performance accuracy. It is required for laboratory accreditation.

sample - Representative part (aliquot) of a specimen that is prepared for analysis.

sensitivity - **Method sensitivity** refers to the lowest amount of analyte that a particular test can detect, whereas **diagnostic sensitivity**

193

refers to the calculated frequency of positive test results detected by a particular method in patients with the disease.

specificity - Method specificity refers to the method's ability to detect only the antigen or antibody for which it has been designed, whereas **diagnostic specificity** refers to the calculated frequency of negative results in healthy individuals.

specimen - Refers to a representative aliquot or sample of the patient's specific tissue, cells, or body fluid (e.g., serum, whole blood, urine) that is collected for particular analysis. It is a representative part of the total.

statistics - Mathematics involved in estimation of deviation in test results from theoretically correct (reference) values.

titer - Refers to the highest dilution of serum in which antigen-specific antibodies are detectable. That highest serum dilution is reported as the titer.

quality assurance - Refers to a process or program that includes procedures and activities to achieve specified performance quality. It is an on-going effort to improve laboratory testing and provide reliable test results.

quality control - Component of a Quality Assurance Program designed to monitor the analytic phase (procedures) of laboratory testing to ensure overall reliability of test results.

Universal Precautions - Requirement that all personnel with a possible risk of exposure will handle all human blood or other potentially infectious materials as though they are contaminated with bloodborne pathogens and are potentially infectious.

LABORATORY SAFETY

INFECTION CONTROL

Laboratory practitioners, by the nature of their work, are at risk of exposure to infectious agents and hazardous chemicals. The most serious concern in laboratory safety is exposure to bloodborne viruses, such as the hepatitis virus and human immunodeficiency virus. This risk has prompted several government

agencies (Table 9-1) to develop a safety plan that would include strategies for prevention and management of exposure to infectious agents and biohazardous wastes (Box 9-1).

OSHA Standard

In addressing the need for prevention of accidental exposure of health care professionals to bloodborne pathogens, such as the hepatitis and immunodeficiency viruses, the U.S. Department of Labor, Occupational Safety and Health Administration (OSHA) published a Standard *(Federal Register)* entitled "Occupational Exposure to Bloodborne Pathogens: Final Rule." The Standard became effective in 1992 under the Clinical Laboratory Amendment '88 to the Clinical Laboratory Improvement Act (CLIA '88) of the Health Care Financing Administration (HCFA).

The regulations described under the OSHA Standard closely follow guidelines recommended by the Centers for Disease Control and Prevention (CDC) and are known as the Occupational Exposure Controls (Box 9-2).

Table **9-1**	REGULATORY GOVERNMENT AGENCIES FOR LABORATORY SAFETY
Government Agency	Regulatory Function
OSHA	Guidelines for safety issues regarding bloodborne pathogens
CDC	Safety standards for handling infectious agents
EPA	Management of biohazardous wastes
HCFA	Sponsor of CLIA '88
JCAHO	Overall quality of personnel, services, and laboratory testing
CAP	Improvement of services and test results

OSHA, Occupational Safety and Health Administration; *CDC,* Centers for Disease Control and Prevention; *EPA,* Environmental Protection Agency; *TB,* tubercle bacilli *(Mycobacterium tuberculosis); HCFA,* Health Care Financing Administration; *CLIA,* Clinical Laboratory Improvement Act; *CAP,* College of American Pathologists; *JCAHO,* Joint Commission on the Accreditation of Healthcare Organizations.

Box 9-1 PROTECTIVE MEASURES FOR LABORATORY PRACTITIONERS

Barrier Protection
- Vinyl or latex gloves worn when performing phlebotomy or handling blood, body fluids, or other laboratory specimens
- Protective equipment, such as gowns or laboratory coats
- Shields or masks and eye coverings, used as protection against splashes, sprays, or spattering

Preventive Measures
- Washing hands with soap and water immediately after removing gloves or other protective equipment
- Washing hands or any exposed area after accidental contact with potentially infectious material (blood, body fluids)
- No mouth pipeting or suctioning of blood or other potentially infectious material
- Decontaminating work surfaces after accidental spills or after completion of work with a solution such as hypochlorite (1:10 dilution of household bleach)
- Disposing of contaminated materials in appropriate biohazard bags or containers, according to established policies for infective waste
- No eating or drinking in the laboratory
- Washing hands and removing protective clothing before leaving the laboratory

Box 9-2 OCCUPATIONAL EXPOSURE CONTROLS*

Universal Precautions
- Work practice procedures
- Personal protective equipment
- Disposal and handling of contaminated waste
- Engineering
- Housekeeping practices
- Record keeping of exposures and follow-up
- Training and education
- Immunization

*Exposure Controls, defined under OSHA Bloodborne Pathogens Standard (Final Rule), published in the *Federal Register* 56:64175-29206, 1991; corrected and enforced in 1992 (*Federal Register 57* and 29CFR).

Universal Precautions
It is not always possible to verify that a patient's specimen (i.e., blood or other body fluids) is infected with a particular bloodborne pathogen. This fact emphasizes the importance of protecting oneself and others from a potential infection by adopting the following Universal Precautions rule:

"Handle all human blood or other potentially infectious materials as though they are contaminated with bloodborne pathogens and are potentially infectious."

The concept of Universal Precautions was first introduced by the Centers for Disease Control and Prevention (CDC) and subsequently was adopted under the U.S. Department of Labor, Occupational Safety and Health Administration (OSHA) Standards (see previously).

Basic Protective Measures
OSHA's requirements for implementing major protective measures (see Box 9-1), include the following components:
- Workplace hazard assessment
- Selection of protective equipment
- Availability of employee information and training

OCCUPATIONAL EXPOSURE

Occupational exposure of any health professional to bloodborne pathogens can occur through:

The intent of the OSHA Standard is to protect the health care practitioners from occupational exposure to blood and other potentially infectious materials (containing bloodborne pathogens) that may occur through cuts and abrasions, splashing or spraying into the eyes, nose, or mouth, and puncture wounds from contaminated needles or broken glass (sharps).

Although the standards specifically address hepatitis B virus (HBV) and human immunodeficiency virus (HIV), other pathogens, such as syphilis or malaria, present in human blood and capable of causing a disease, are also considered bloodborne pathogens.

- Cuts and abrasions
- Splashing or spraying into the eyes, nose, or mouth
- Puncture wounds from contaminated needles or broken glass (sharps)

Control of these sources of exposure may be achieved by implementing the Exposure Control Plan, following OSHA Exposure Controls (see Box 9-2).

Exposure Control Plan

Each health care institution is responsible for designing and implementing its own Exposure Control Plan (using published OSHA guidelines). The plan must include the following major components:

- Standard Operating Procedures (SOP) Manual
- Chemical Hygiene Plan (CHP)
- Education Program for laboratory personnel in safety procedures and policies

This written Control Plan must be readily available to all employees.

Standard Operating Procedures (SOP) Manual

The Standard Operating Procedures (SOP) Manual for Safety must include the following information and must be readily available to all laboratory personnel (i.e., technical, clerical, maintenance, environmental services, biomedical engineering):

- Listing of all laboratory tests and other associated procedures that present a potential for employee exposure to infectious agents
- Explanation of ways to control the risk of exposure
- Provision for personnel education (initial and periodic training programs), with a focus on preventing exposure to potentially infectious agents
- Signature of reviewer, date, and any updating of SOP review as regulations change (performed at least annually)

Chemical Hygiene Plan (CHP)

The Chemical Hygiene Plan is designed to help employees develop an awareness of potentially hazardous chemicals in the workplace and to provide a mechanism for training employees in safe working conditions. It includes written poli-

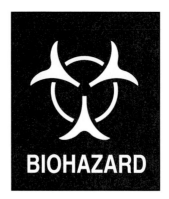

FIGURE **9-1** Universal biohazard symbol. This symbol is placed on any blood or body fluid–contaminated material, supplies, and waste as well as on blood, body fluids, and hazardous chemicals that require appropriate handling and disposal.

cies, procedures, and responsibilities to ensure that exposure to hazardous chemical materials is prevented or minimized. The Chemical Hygiene Plan is the essence of the OSHA Safety Standard.

OSHA document 29CFR 1910 and other chemical hazard legislation, such as the state "right-to-know" laws, establish standards for chemical hazard communication and the type of documentation that must be kept on file in the laboratory (e.g., yearly physical inventory of all hazardous chemicals and material safety data sheets [MSDSs]). Central location and good access to these documents are required.

In addition, OSHA recommends that all hazardous chemical materials be properly labeled with the biohazard symbol (Figure 9-1), rating of the severity of exposure (Table 9-2), and the content of these materials.

Material Safety Data Sheets (MSDS). These documents contain product information, obtained from the product manufacturer, that is used to determine whether a particular chemical is hazardous. The MSDSs must be kept on file within the laboratory where they are readily accessible to any employee.

chemical hazards. Certain chemicals used in the clinical immunology laboratory that are classified as hazardous may cause physical or health hazards to the laboratory practitioner because of their chemical composition:

- *Physical hazard:* The composition of certain chemicals may be explosive, flammable, or reactive and present a physical hazard.

- *Health hazard:* Certain chemicals that are carcinogenic, corrosive, or mutenogenic present a potential health hazard.

HAZARDOUS MATERIALS AND WASTE MANAGEMENT

Safety practices and waste management are implemented in laboratory practice to prevent exposure to hazardous materials, such as infectious (biologic), chemical, and radioactive waste.

Infectious Waste

Any waste that has been contaminated with blood or body fluids is considered a biohazard waste and should be treated with the same precautions as any blood and body fluid (see previous discussion). Contaminated waste includes such disposable supplies as test tubes, microtiter plates, sharps (needles, broken glass, and glass pipettes), disposable pipettes, and used gloves.

These contaminated supplies, as well as any blood or body fluids (liquids), must be discarded into appropriately labeled biohazard containers and incinerated or autoclaved (60 minutes at 121.5° C) before final disposal or removal from the laboratory or hospital facility. Each biohazard container must be labeled with the word "BIOHAZARD" or with the universal biohazard symbol (see Figure 9-1) and must be sturdy, leak-proof, and puncture resistant.

A current written contract is required between any trash (hazardous waste) disposal company and the laboratory or hospital facility, defining how the waste will be prepared for disposal and how it will be handled and discarded.

Chemical Waste

Hazardous chemical waste (i.e., any chemical [solids, liquids, and contained gases]) should be removed, transported, and discarded according to current EPA regulations and the Department of Transportation and local regulations, which track hazardous waste.

Radioactive Waste

The method of disposal of radioactive waste is regulated by the Nuclear Regulatory Commission (NRC). Radioactive waste generated from radioimmunoassays (RIA) may be disposed of

Table 9-2	LABELS FOR HAZARDOUS CHEMICALS	
Class*		Color of Label
Health hazard		Blue
Fire hazard		Red
Reactivity		Yellow
Special precautions		White

*Each class of hazardous chemicals is identified by a colored label and is rated on a scale of 1 to 4, according to the severity of exposure, (4 is the highest severity) as determined from the material safety data sheet (MSDS).

by storage in a locked, labeled room, until the radiation background count of ^{125}I, for example, is reduced to 10 half-lives.

PREPARATION FOR LABORATORY TESTING

METHOD EVALUATION

Typically, method evaluation is performed when there is a need for improving specificity, sensitivity, efficiency, or for reducing the cost of an existing method. Method evaluation is also performed to establish the adaptability of a particular procedure to the laboratory's need for the detection of a new or previously unavailable analyte (e.g., antigen-specific antibody).

Method Evaluation Procedure

A Method Evaluation Procedure consists of a different protocol or regimen (see following) than the one used in the routine Quality Assurance Program (discussed in subsequent sections of this chapter).

In performing method evaluation, it must be assumed that:

- The laboratory practitioner has the knowledge or familiarity with the particular procedure and required instrumentation through formal or practical education or training by the manufacturer
- Reagents, controls, and calibrating materials are being used according to the protocol included in the manufacturer's package insert
- Commercially prepared materials are being used before their expiration date to ensure their stability

- The method shows analytic linearity (linearity of response throughout the reportable or working range)

Most method evaluation outcomes and method performance information are documented and published. This eliminates the need for a complete method evaluation by an individual clinical laboratory. Particularly in view of the fact that a typical laboratory may lack the appropriate resources to perform a complete method evaluation, the evaluation should be limited to testing for "random errors" and to the performance of "comparison of methods" experiments to establish method acceptability before implementation.

Random and Systematic Error

Errors that affect the performance or reliability of a procedure are referred to as **random** and **systematic errors.**

Random Error (RE)

This error affects reproducibility of the test result and can be classified as related to precision, imprecision, reproducibility, or repeatability. Random error may be caused by factors or variability in any of the following:

- Temperature
- Reagents and calibrators
- Performance (e.g., pipeting, timing, mixing)
- Technologists' performance (technique)
- Instrument stability

Systematic Error (SE)

This type of error is consistently low or high and may be constant or proportional.

constant systematic error (CE). This error is consistently low or high by the same amount and is independent of the concentration. It may be caused by interfering substances (e.g., bacterial growth) or instrument malfunction. Each sample is affected in the same way.

proportional systematic error (PE). This is an error that is consistently low or high in proportion to the concentration of the analyte. It is most frequently caused by incorrect calibration (e.g., error in the reconstitution of control or calibrating solutions).

total error (TE). Total error may be present in a single measurement. This error is estimated by combing random and systematic error to determine the total error of a method being evaluated (test method).

Method Comparison

In method comparison, patient specimens (40 to 100 samples) are tested to determine systematic error of the method being evaluated (test method). The testing is performed using the test method and another method of highest accuracy and precision (reference method) or the method currently in use. The results of both methods are analyzed and compared (see following).

Statistical Analysis

Test and reference methods are performed at the same time, in duplicate. Test results (data) obtained from both methods are analyzed for systematic differences between the test and reference method, using the following statistical analyses:

- *Bias or t-test statistics.* Bias is the difference between the average result from the test method and the average result from the reference method and is indicative of the extent of the systematic error (see previously) between the two methods.
- *Correlation coefficient (r):* This most commonly cited statistic in method comparison studies is used to determine the degree of correlation between two methods (i.e., test and reference methods). If the *r* is equal to zero, there is no correlation observed, while an *r* value of +1 indicates a linear relationship, thus a perfect correlation between the methods compared.
- *Linear regression.* Linear regression is used to compare the test procedure and the reference method when a non-linear relationship exists between the two methods.

Detailed description and calculations of these statistical methods are not within the scope of this book.

SPECIMEN PREPARATION AND PROCESSING

A *specimen* is a representative aliquot of the patient's specific tissue, cells, or body fluid (e.g., serum, whole blood, and urine) that is collected for particular analysis.

Most immunologic procedures currently used to identify and/or quantify "free" or circulating antibodies require serum or plasma samples (clear portion of whole blood, after separation from cells).

However, depending on the type of analysis, specimens other than serum may be required (e.g., blood and tissue cells) for the detection of various cell markers and antigens.

General Preparation and Handling of Specimens

Universal Precautions must be followed at all stages of specimen procurement, processing, and handling (see laboratory safety discussed previously).

Collection of Test Samples

The integrity of a specimen depends largely on the appropriate blood collection method and the proper identification of a patient. In obtaining a blood sample, the following points must be considered:

- Blood sample should be collected into an appropriately evacuated test tube system, according to an established technique
- Care must be taken to avoid hemolysis (hemolysis may produce a false-positive test result)
- Collected sample must be correctly labeled with the patient name and ID number
- Sample transport should follow an established procedure

Preparation of Serum Specimens

When a serum specimen is required as a test sample, the collected blood specimen is prepared for testing in the following way:

- Blood specimen is allowed to clot at room temperature or at 4° C (refrigerator temperature) and then centrifuged
- Serum is promptly separated from the packed cell mass (at the bottom of test tube) by aspirating into another correctly labeled test tube
- The test tube with the serum specimen is then covered and may be frozen at −20° C if testing is not promptly performed
- Special preparation of the serum sample before testing may be required (see discussion following).

Specimen Transport and Storage

The specimen must be transported in a safe way to prevent contamination or biohazard exposure (see discussion of laboratory safety). To prevent leakage during transport from the blood collection site to the laboratory (should breakage occur), specimens should be placed in a carrier with a liner and delivered to the laboratory within 45 minutes of collection.

To mail a specimen in a frozen state (−70° C), dry ice (solid carbon dioxide) may be packed with the specimen into a styrofoam container. Courier services are provided for specimen transport by many reference laboratories (specialized or esoteric testing).

Specimens are never sent with attached needles or syringes.

Special Preparatory Techniques
Inactivation of Complement

Specimen preparation for procedures that involve absence of complement requires serum complement inactivation (i.e., inactivation of its activity). This is because the naturally occurring complement in a serum sample may interfere with certain tests. In a hemagglutination assay, for example, complement can become activated by an antigen-antibody interaction and cause lysis of the indicator cells, thus showing a false positive reaction. To avoid this type of interference, complement may be inactivated by heating the serum sample to 56° C for 30 minutes. Re-inactivation of the sample may be done at 56° C for 10 minutes if testing is not performed within 4 hours.

Preparation of Diluted Samples and Solutions

Dilution is an expression of the concentration or the amount of a sample (original solution) in a specified volume, contained in a total volume of sample and diluent. Diluent is a diluting solution (e.g., saline, distilled water) that is used for diluting the sample.

The following mathematical bases are used for determining and expressing dilution.

simple dilutions. These are performed when a certain amount of a specified dilution is required. A relationship between the sample and diluent is expressed as a fraction to enable calculation of the actual concentration of the diluted sample contained in the total volume. A dilution of ¼ (1:4) indicates a total volume of four, consisting of one volume (sample) plus three volumes (diluent).

The following examples illustrate this concept:

- *Example 1: To determine the volume of serum and diluent required to prepare 10 mL of 1/5 (1:5) dilution of patient serum, the following formula can be used (x = unknown volume):*

  1/dilution = volume of serum/total volume
  Therefore,

  1/5 dilution = x/10 mL total volume or 5x = 10

  x = 2 mL required sample (serum) volume
  And,
  10 mL total volume − 2 mL serum volume = 8 mL of required diluent

- *Example 2: To determine the amount of diluent necessary to prepare a 1:5 serum dilution using 0.1 mL of serum:*

  1/dilution = volume of serum/volume of diluent

  Therefore,
  1/5 = 0.1 mL/x or x = 0.5 mL total volume
  0.5 mL total volume − 0.1 mL original serum sample = 0.4 mL required volume of diluent

  The most commonly used equation in preparing any type of a simple dilution is as follows:
  Volume$_1$ × concentration$_1$ =
  volume$_2$ × concentration$_2$
  Or
  $V_1/V_2 = C_1/C_2$

compound dilutions. In preparing large dilutions, it is more efficient and accurate (and less expensive) to prepare dilutions in several steps, thus using smaller amounts of sample and diluent. In these dilutions, planning the amount and desired final dilution must be done before preparation of the dilution.

The following example illustrates this concept:

- *Example 1: To prepare a 1:200 dilution, the original serum sample can be diluted in three steps:*

(1) 1:10 dilution (stock solution):
0.1 mL serum + 0.9 mL diluent =
1/10 dilution

(2) 1:50 dilution:
0.1 mL of 1:10 dilution + 0.4 mL diluent =
1/5 dilution
Therefore,
1/10 dilution × 1/5 dilution = 1/50 dilution

(3) 1:200 dilution (working solution):
0.1 mL of 1:50 dilution + 0.3 mL diluent =
$^1/_4$ dilution
Therefore,
1/50 × $^1/_4$ = 1200 dilution

Dilutions in steps (compound dilutions) can be set up in any combination of dilutions and may include any number of steps and volumes but do require careful planning and calculation before performance.

serial dilutions. The concentration of the original solution (e.g., serum, urine, chemical solution) progressively decreases as the diluent (e.g., saline, distilled water) progressively increases. The variation between each dilution is in equal increments.

A serial dilution consists of a series of test tubes containing different concentrations of the same solution (Figure 9-2). The term "fold" is often used to describe a change in a dilution. For example, a serial dilution in which each succeeding dilution is twice that of the previous dilution (Box 9-3) is referred to as a two-fold dilution, expressed as a fraction (1/2, 1/4, 1/8, etc.). A series in which each dilution is four times that of the preceding dilution is a fourfold dilution (1/4, 1/16, 1/64, etc.).

calculations. See Box 9-3.

Let: x = dilution fold   *dil* = dilution
V = volume   *mL* = milliliter

Test Tube 1 (1:4 dil)

1.5 mL saline + 0.5 mL serum = 2 mL total volume
1/x = 0.5/2 or $^1/_4$ final serum dil

Test Tube 2 (1:8 dil)

1.0 mL saline + 1.0 mL from test tube 1
(1:4 dil) = 2.0 mL
1/x = 1.0/2.0 or $^1/_2$ test tube dilution

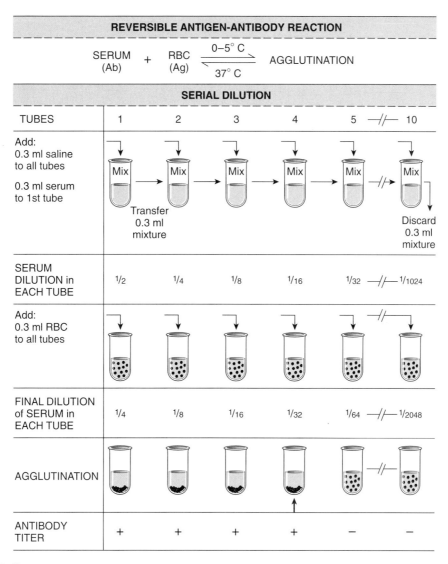

FIGURE **9-2**   **Antibody Titer.**   A two-fold serial dilution of patient serum is prepared *(see text)* using saline as diluent. After adding red blood cells (RBCs, type O) to serve as indicators, the mixture is incubated to allow for the antigen-antibody reaction to occur. The tubes are then evaluated (macroscopically) for presence of agglutination (clumping) of RBCs (see Chapter 12). The highest dilution or the last tube showing agglutination is the antibody titer. In this example, the cold agglutinins (non-specific antibodies) in serum react with the RBC cell surface and their titer is reported as positive in a 1/32 or 1:32 dilution. The 1:32 is the titer.

Therefore,
$\frac{1}{4}$ transfer dil × 1/2 test tube dil =
1/8 final serum dil

Test Tube 3 (1:16 dil)

1.0 mL saline + 1.0 mL from test tube 2
(1:8 dil) = 2.0 mL
1/x = 1.0/2.0 or $\frac{1}{2}$ test tube dilution

Therefore,
1/8 transfer dil × $\frac{1}{2}$ test tube dil =
1/16 final serum dil

Test Tube 4 (1:32 dil)

1.0 mL saline + 1.0 mL from test tube 3
(1:16 dil) = 2.0 mL
1/x = 1.0/2.0 or $\frac{1}{2}$ test tube dilution

Box 9-3 TWO-FOLD SERIAL DILUTIONS

Method

Test tubes	1	2	3	4	5	6	7	8	9	10
Saline (mL)	1.5	1.0	1.0	1.0	1.0	1.0	1.0	1.0	1.0	1.0
Serum (mL)	0.5	–	–	–	–	–	–	–	–	–
Transfer	1.0->	1.0->	1.0->	1.0->	1.0->	1.0->	1.0->	1.0->	1.0->	
Volume (ml) in test tube	1.0	1.0	1.0	1.0	1.0	1.0	1.0	1.0	1.0	1.0

Dilution

	1	2	3	4	5	6	7	8	9	10
Dilution in each test tube	1/4	1/2	1/2	1/2	1/2	1/2	1/2	1/2	1/2	1/2
Final dilution of serum in each test tube*	1/4	1/8	1/16	1/32	1/64	1/128	1/256	1/512	1/1024	

*Dilution in each tube is multiplied by the previous dilution (e.g., 1/4 × 1/2 = 1/8; 1/8 × 1/2 = 1/16; 1/16 × 1/2 = 1/32, etc.).

Therefore,

1/16 transfer × dil $\frac{1}{2}$ tube dil =
1/32 final serum dil

Test Tubes 5 to 10 (1:64 to 1:2048, in two-fold increments)

Calculations are continued as previously.

concept of titer. Antibody titer is an expression that refers to the concentration of antigen-specific antibodies in a particular serum dilution. It is reported as the highest (last) dilution in which the antibody is detectable by a selected laboratory method (e.g., antigen-antibody agglutination, see Figure 9-2).

To establish an antibody titer during an infection and/or to monitor its progress, blood samples are collected and tested by serial dilution method during the acute phase (or when first detected) and during the convalescent period of the infection (approximately 2 weeks later). Samples are saved for future reference.

The difference or change in antibody concentration or titer observed between the two samples (when tested concurrently) has a clinical significance in that a rise in the titer indicates presence of an increased concentration of antibodies and the existence of a current infection.

Typically, a four-fold increase in the patient's antibody titer (see Figure 9-2) over a period of several weeks is indicative of a current infection.

Cell Preparations
Certain laboratory procedures (e.g., cold agglutinin titer, see Figure 9-2) require addition of erythrocytes (red blood cells) in a specified concentration to serve as indicators in an antigen-antibody reaction. The following examples illustrate calculations used to determine the desired or available concentration of cells:

• *Example 1: To prepare a 2% suspension (solution) of erythrocytes in saline, when 0.5 mL packed cells (washed and centrifuged) are available, the following formula can be used (see Figure 9-3):*

packed cell volume × 100/desired % of cells =
final volume of cell suspension

Therefore,

0.5 mL of packed cells × 100/2% = 50/2 =
25 mL of 2% RBC cell suspension in saline (total volume)

• *Example 2: To determine the % of available cell suspension, using the previous example:*

% of cell suspension (x) = volume of
cells × 100/total volume

Therefore,

x = 0.5 mL packed cells × 100/25 mL total volume
x = 50/25 = 2% available cell suspension

Commercial Kits

Many immunologic methods use commercially prepared kits. These kits are a reliable, efficient, and simple way of detecting various antigen-specific antibodies.

Each kit contains the required reagents and materials, positive and negative controls, and a package insert that describes the protocol for performance of the procedure, guidelines for storage of reagents, a sample collection, and sample storage.

Results of Method Comparison studies (i.e., sensitivity, specificity, and reproducibility of the assay that provide the necessary information to establish kit reliability [acceptability of the method]) are also included in the manufacturer's package insert.

TEST QUALITY MANAGEMENT

QUALITY ASSURANCE AND QUALITY CONTROL

Quality is the most important parameter in laboratory testing. Therefore quality management must be a priority in the on-going efforts at improving laboratory testing processes and systems, so that reliable test results can be provided.

Quality Assurance (QA), according to the National Committee for Clinical Laboratory Standards (NCCLS), is defined as "the practice which encompasses all endeavors, procedures, formats, and activities directed toward ensuring that a specified quality or product is achieved and maintained."

Performance Standards

Desired Performance Standards for laboratory testing, also known as *analytic goals* or *outcome criteria,* are very powerful tools for maintaining quality laboratory testing. When activities associated with a well-defined (written) Quality Assurance Program are per-

formed with diligence, these desired goals or standards can be reached.

Several approaches have been proposed (since the 1960s) to define desirable laboratory performance standards. For example, a group of experts has proposed to set acceptability of analytic imprecision in laboratory testing based on biologic variations and clinical significance. This theoretic approach to setting performance standards, however, has failed to take into account state-of-the-art technology (proposed by another group), thus making performance standards difficult to achieve even though sophisticated techniques and equipment are available.

The first official proposal for setting analytic goals was made in 1976 by the College of American Pathologists (CAP), who recommended that analytic goals be defined in terms of the needs of patient care.

CLIA '88 Regulatory Requirements (Standards)

With the implementation of Clinical Laboratory Improvement Amendments of 1988 (CLIA '88), sponsored in 1992 by Health Care Financing Administration (HCFA), setting desirable performance goals became even more challenging.

CLIA '88 Standards place greatest emphasis on proficiency testing (PT). However, proficiency testing, quality control (QC), and personnel standards are all essential criteria required to obtain laboratory certification and to maintain laboratory accreditation.

Also defined under CLIA '88 Standards are such issues as fees, sanctions and enforcement practices, categories of tests classified by complexity (waived tests, moderate-complexity tests, and high-complexity tests), and the granting and withdrawal of deeming authority, which refers to HCFA-approved deemed status and equivalency with CLIA '88 Standards.

The intent of CLIA '88 implementation (1992) was to bring all laboratories that perform patient care activities (clinical, research, and physicians' office laboratories [POLs]) under federal regulation to ensure that quality laboratory tests (performed at a predictable standard of quality) would be available to all individuals.

Essentially, the CLIA '88 Standards combined Medicare, Medicaid, and Interstate Regu-

lations into one regulatory body and mandated that each laboratory (specialty and subspecialty) enroll in a Proficiency Testing Program (approved by Department of Health and Human Services [HHS]). Proficiency Testing (PT) providers such as the College of American Pathologists (CAP) are approved by HCFA.

Thus laboratories accredited by organizations with deemed status (e.g., CAP, Joint Commission on the Accreditation of Healthcare Organizations [JCAHO], and Commission of Office Laboratory Accreditation [COLA]) are considered to be in compliance with CLIA '88 Standards.

Quality Assurance Programs

Quality Assurance (QA) Programs may be designed according to the concept of total quality management (TQM), which includes such components as:

- *Quality control*
- *Policies and procedures*
- *Personnel training*
- *Inspections and audits*
- *Detection and correction of errors (corrective action)*

However, the success of any QA program depends on diligent attention and performance of all activities associated with these programs.

Concept of Total Quality Management (TQM)

TQM is a concept that involves monitoring of quality performance and encompasses all phases of laboratory performance (listed following) to ensure that the test results reported by the laboratory are correct. Typically, laboratory performance includes three stages or phases:

- *Preanalytic:* Ordering of laboratory tests
- *Analytic:* Accuracy and precision of method
- *Postanalytic:* Reporting and interpretation of test results

Quality Control (QC)

QC is a component of the Quality Assurance (QA) Program, which focuses on the analytic phase (procedures) of laboratory testing. It monitors the overall reliability of laboratory results, including accuracy and precision, according to previously specified test criteria.

quality control specimens. An effective QC program depends on specimens that are reproducible.

Most QC specimens currently in use are lyophilized (dehydrated) products that must be reconstituted (rehydrated), although liquid controls (not requiring rehydration) are also available. These specimens are obtained from large pools of serum from commercial suppliers and include previously established and specified test control values.

Control values for quantitative determinations are established by testing 20 to 25 QC specimens for a particular analyte, calculating the mean and standard deviation (SD) values, and determining an acceptable range for test results (i.e., ±2SD). Suppliers are encouraged to set known values close to the level that is acceptable for clinical decision-making.

Once control ranges are established for a particular analyte, the controls are expected to fall within the established ranges. Should a control test result be outside of the established range, a decision must be made regarding its validity (acceptance or rejection).

type of quality control specimens. Control specimens are analyzed each time a particular test is performed manually or with an appropriate instrument. The results of each control specimen must fall within the previously established reference range to determine if the patient's results are acceptable. Several types of controls (control specimens) are currently available:

positive and negative controls. In qualitative determinations (e.g., rubella), negative and positive controls are included with each test to check the reliability of test (analytic) results.

tri-level controls. In tests that produce quantitative results (e.g., prostate-specific antigen [PSA]), tri-level controls must be included. These controls are designated according to the known amount (concentration) of the analyte present:

- *Level 1 (A):* Low concentration of analyte
- *Level 2 (B):* Normal concentration of analyte
- *Level 3 (C):* High concentration of analyte

normal and abnormal controls. Certain quantitative tests, such as the ANA kit for anti-nuclear antibody detection, use only two controls:

- 1: Normal control
- 2: Abnormal control

These controls are useful in validating test results and can help to avoid the reporting of false positive or false negative results.

types of quality control programs. There are two major types of quality control (QC):

- *Internal or intralaboratory QC:* Monitors day-to-day performance (precision) of laboratory tests.
- *External or interlaboratory QC:* Monitors accuracy of laboratory tests by comparing test results with other laboratories that have analyzed the same specimen.

internal or intralaboratory quality control. The internal QC program monitors precision through a variety of statistical control techniques, such as control charts, calculated statistics, the mean and range techniques, trend analysis techniques, and analysis of variance techniques.

The ultimate goal of the internal QC program is to improve laboratory performance by developing uniform standards of performance throughout the laboratory and assessing the performance or precision of each of its specialty and subspecialty areas in relation to each other, identifying problems as they occur and documenting corrective action taken.

external or interlaboratory quality control. Currently, there are several major programs that allow large numbers of laboratories to monitor their *performance accuracy* by analyzing the same sample and comparing their analytic (test) results. These programs, also referred to as *Survey Programs* or *Proficiency Testing Programs (PT),* are available through such governmental and private agencies as:

- College of American Pathologists (CAP)
- Several state agencies
- Certain manufacturers

With the introduction of CLIA '88, satisfactory performance on proficiency testing (PT) became a requirement for laboratory accreditation.

All proficiency testing (PT) follows a similar protocol:

- All participating laboratories receive several specimens, several times per year for analysis.
- The test results are sent back for evaluation and written comments (report).
- The report includes a comparison of the reported test results with the mean value and SD (standard deviation) obtained by peer laboratories.
- Reported values that differ greatly from the group mean value are "flagged" to alert

the participant of a possible error (technical, analytic, or transcription).

- Alternatively, depending on the program, the reported test results are graded as "acceptable," "need improvement," or "unacceptable."

KEY FEATURES IN RELIABILITY OF TEST RESULTS

Currently, there are a multitude of immunologic tests available for diagnosis, monitoring, and treatment of a disease. However, these tests employ methods that have their own characteristic *inherent differences* in specificity, sensitivity, and predictive value that are the result of such factors as methodology, technical expertise, and the population tested. These differences must be given careful consideration before selecting and implementing a particular test procedure.

Sensitivity and Specificity
Sensitivity and specificity can be described in terms of the test method's analytic and diagnostic performance that shows its reliability in establishing an accurate diagnosis.

Assay or *test specificity and sensitivity* can be selected and adjusted to meet the needs of a clinician for the diagnosis and monitoring of a disease. This may be accomplished by changing the selection of the reference value (i.e., cut-off or upper limit of normal) for the particular test.

Analytic (Method) Sensitivity
The *analytic sensitivity of a method* refers to the lowest amount of an analyte that a particular test can detect or the lowest concentration of an antigen or antibody detectable by the method.

Analytic (Method) Specificity
The *analytic specificity of a method* may be defined as the particular method's ability to detect only the antigen or antibody for which it is designed. False positive results and decrease in analytic specificity may be caused by detection of cross-reactive substances.

Diagnostic Sensitivity
Diagnostic sensitivity of a method refers to the frequency (calculated) of positive test results

detected by a particular method in individuals with a particular disease.

Positive in disease:

$$\text{Sensitivity (\%)} = \frac{\text{\# of true positive results}}{\text{\# of true positive results} + \text{\# of false negative results}} \times 100$$

For example, a test showing 94% diagnostic sensitivity will detect 94 out of 100 individuals who have the particular disease (true positive result), whereas 6 out of 100 individuals with the disease will be negative (i.e., show false negative results).

Therefore the higher the test sensitivity (%), the higher is the number of positive results in diseased individuals.

Diagnostic Specificity

Diagnostic specificity of a method refers to the frequency (calculated) of negative test results detected by a particular method in individuals without the particular disease.

Negative in health:

$$\text{Specificity (\%)} = \frac{\text{\# of true negative results}}{\text{\# of true negative results} + \text{\# of false positive results}} \times 100$$

For example, a test with a diagnostic specificity of 94% will show negative results (true negative) in 94 out of 100 individuals tested without the particular disease but will show false positive results in 6 out of 100 who do not have the disease.

Therefore the higher the test specificity (%), the higher is the number of negative results in healthy individuals.

Predictive Values

In addition to technical quality, quality assurance (QA) must also encompass the concept of *predictive values* of tests. The importance of setting predictive values is to provide test results that are of diagnostic value.

The predictive value of a test is influenced by the prevalence of a disease in a particular population being tested and describes the performance of the test in that population.

Predictive Value of a Positive Test Result

The predictive value indicates the likelihood that a positive result represents a true positive for a particular disease. It is this *predictive value* of a positive test result that is of interest in a clinical setting, calculated as follows:

"True" positive result:

$$\text{Predictive value (\%)} = \frac{\text{\# of true positives}}{\text{\# of true positives} + \text{\# of false positives}} \times 100$$

Therefore the higher the prevalence of a particular disease, the higher is the predictive value of a positive result.

Predictive Value of a Negative Test Result

This value indicates the likelihood that a particular negative result is truly negative. The value may be calculated as follows:

"True" negative result:

$$\text{Predictive value (\%)} = \frac{\text{\# of true negatives}}{\text{\# of true negatives} + \text{\# of false negatives}} \times 100$$

Therefore the predictive value of a negative test result is higher in populations with a low prevalence of a particular disease than in populations with a higher prevalence of the particular disease.

Test Efficiency

Efficiency of a particular method (test) is a calculated percentage of individuals that are correctly classified as positive (diseased) or negative (non-diseased) for a particular disease, calculated as follows:

$$\text{Efficiency (\%)} = \frac{\text{\# of true positives} + \text{\# of true negatives}}{\begin{array}{c}\text{\# of true positives} + \text{\# of false positives} + \\ \text{\# of false negative} + \text{\# of true negatives}\end{array}} \times 100$$

Significance of Predictive Test Values

Predictive values are useful in classifying individuals as non-diseased (healthy) or diseased. A correct classification of an individual regarding a particular disease may be essential in avoiding adverse or detrimental psychologic and economic consequences, as described following:

high sensitivity. This is desired in situations where the suspected disease has serious consequences, is treatable, and false positive results do not produce adverse economic or psychologic consequences. For example, a false negative result cannot be tolerated in venereal disease.

high specificity. This is desired if the disease is serious but not curable or treatable. A false positive in this situation can lead to serious psychologic or economic consequences. For example, for multiple sclerosis or occult (hidden) cancers, the test must show the highest specificity. Thus sensitivity may be sacrificed.

high predictive value. The predictive value for a positive test result is essential where the treatment of a false positive may have serious consequences. For example, in the diagnosis of cancer, the predictive value for a positive result must be 100%.

high efficiency. A high efficiency is desired when the disease is serious and treatable and where the false positive and false negative test results have serious consequences (e.g., myocardial infarction, diabetes mellitus, lupus erythematosus).

✐ uggested Readings

Commission on Laboratory Evaluation: Commission of laboratory accreditation inspection checklist. In *Diagnostic immunology and syphilis serology,* section 6, Worthfield, IL, 1994, College of American Pathologists.

Henry JB, Kurec AS: The clinical laboratory: organization, purpose, and practice (pp 15-26). In Henry JB, editor: *Clinical diagnosis and management by laboratory methods,* ed 19, Philadelphia, 1996, WB Saunders.

Kringle RD: Statistical procedures (pp 384-453). In Burtis CA, Ashwood ER, editors: *Tietz textbook of clinical chemistry,* ed 2, Philadelphia, WB Saunders.

Pincus MR: Interpreting laboratory results: reference values and decision making (pp 74-77). In Henry JB, editor: *Clinical diagnosis and management by laboratory methods,* ed 19, Philadelphia, 1996, WB Saunders.

US Department of Labor, Occupational Safety and Health Administration (OSHA): Occupational exposure to blood-borne pathogens: Final rule (29 CFR Part 1910-1030), *Fed Regis* 56(235):64175-64182 (Rules and regulations), 1991.

US Department of Health and Human Resources, Medicare, Medicaid, and CLIA Program: Regulations implementing the clinical laboratory improvement amendments of 1988 (CLIA '88), *Fed Regis* 55:208991-20959 (Rules and Regulations), 1990; 57: 7156-7157, 1992.

Valenstein PL, Valenstein ML: Laboratory safety (pp 1213-1222). In Rose NR, et al, editors: *Manual of clinical laboratory immunology,* Washington, DC, 1997, American Society for Microbiology.

Vanderline RE, Hertz HZ, et al: Development of reference system for clinical laboratory. In *Clinical laboratory standards document* (NR SCL 2-A), vol 11, Villanova, PA, 1991, National Committee for Clinical Laboratory Standards.

Review Questions

LABORATORY SAFETY

1. All of the following regulatory agencies are involved in preparing safety guidelines, *except:*
   a. OSHA
   b. CAP
   c. CDC
   d. EPA

2. Control of occupational exposure to blood-borne pathogens can be achieved by implementing which of the following:
   a. employee education in safety procedures
   b. Safety Manual
   c. Chemical Hygiene Plan
   d. all of the above

3-6. Match the following government agencies with their regulatory functions:

   ____ improvement   a. CAP
        of services   b. HCFA
        and test   c. EPA
        results   d. OSHA
   ____ sponsor of
        CLIA '88
   ____ guidelines for
        safety issues
   ____ management
        of hazardous
        waste

7. Material Safety Data Sheets (MSDSs) are required to establish if a particular chemical is hazardous. The MSDSs are obtained from:
   a. OSHA
   b. product manufacturer
   c. EPA
   d. all of the above

8. Any waste contaminated with blood or body fluid is considered:
   a. biohazard waste
   b. chemical waste
   c. contaminated waste
   d. none of the above

9. All of the following phrases refer to the disposal of infectious waste, *except:*
   a. "biohazard"-labeled containers
   b. puncture-resistant containers
   c. incinerated or autoclaved bags
   d. hospital or laboratory general waste

10-15. Match the following statements with the appropriate term:

   a. precision
   b. accuracy
   c. method sensitivity
   d. quality control
   e. method specificity
   f. quality assurance

   ____ the extent to which the mean test result is close to the true value
   ____ reproducibility of test values in a series of test results
   ____ the lowest amount of analyte (e.g., antibody) that a particular test is able to detect
   ____ ability of a test procedure to detect only the antigen or antibody for which it has been designed
   ____ a program that includes procedures and activities necessary to improve and maintain reliable test results
   ____ monitors quality of laboratory procedures to ensure reliability of test results

PREPARATION FOR LABORATORY TESTING

16. Select the reason(s) for performing method evaluation in a clinical laboratory:
    a. improving specificity
    b. improving sensitivity
    c. reducing cost
    d. before implementing new method

17. Random error refers to reproducibility or repeatability of a test procedure. Select factors that may be responsible for this type of error:
    a. performance
    b. temperature
    c. instrument stability
    d. all of the above

18. An error that is consistently low or high by the same amount and is independent of concentration may be caused by:
    a. interfering substances
    b. incorrect calibration
    c. error in reconstitution of control
    d. none of the above

19. In method comparison, patient specimens are tested to determine:
    a. systematic error
    b. difference between the two methods compared
    c. degree of correlation between the two methods
    d. all of the above

20. Universal Precautions must be observed to prevent contamination or biohazard exposure during:
    a. specimen collection
    b. processing and handling of specimen
    c. transport and storage of specimen
    d. at all stages of laboratory testing

21. In preparing a serum specimen, if testing is not promptly performed, the specimen may be:
    a. stored at room temperature
    b. stored at 4° C (refrigerator temperature)
    c. frozen at $-20°$ C
    d. discarded

22. Perform the *following simple dilution problem:* determine the amount of saline required to prepare a 1:10 serum dilution using 0.2 mL of serum. _____

23. The highest dilution of serum in which an antibody is detectable in a serial dilution procedure is known as:
    a. two-fold increase
    b. antibody titer
    c. zone of equivalence
    d. all of the above

24. An increase in antibody concentration over a period of several weeks may be indicative of a current infection if the increase is:
    a. two-fold
    b. four-fold
    c. a reciprocal of the highest dilution
    d. all of the above

25. Calculate the final volume of 2% cell suspension that can be prepared when 0.2 mL packed cells are available. _____

TEST QUALITY MANAGEMENT

26. All of the following are essential criteria required to obtain laboratory certification and to maintain accreditation, *except:*
    a. proficiency testing
    b. quality control
    c. personnel standards
    d. state-of-the-art methods

27. To test the reliability of test results, controls are analyzed together with the patient's specimen. Results of control specimens must be:
    a. within set reference range
    b. reproducible
    c. ± 2SD from patient's test result
    d. acceptable for clinical diagnosis

28. Quality Control (QC) focuses on which of the following phases of laboratory testing:
    a. obtaining specimens
    b. accuracy and precision
    c. reporting and interpretation of test results
    d. all of the above

29. An internal Quality Control Program monitors laboratory performance through all of the following activities, *except:*
    a. day-to-day performance of laboratory tests
    b. comparison of test results with other laboratories that have analyzed the same specimen
    c. development of uniform standards of performance throughout the laboratory
    d. identifying and correcting problems as they occur

30-31. Match the following characteristics that define the method's analytic and diagnostic performance with the appropriate description:

____ lowest amount of analyte that the test can detect

____ method's ability to detect only the analyte for which it is designed

a. test sensitivity

b. test specificity

CHAPTER 10

Principles of Antigen-Antibody Reactions

Learning Objectives

Upon completion of Chapter 10, the student will be prepared to:

PRINCIPLES OF ANTIGEN-ANTIBODY INTERACTIONS
- Define the following terms: *cross-reactivity, particulate* and *soluble antigens, prozone* and *postzone phenomenon, zone of equivalence, specificity.*
- Name three factors that are essential for antigen-antibody binding.
- Describe events that occur during primary and secondary antigen-antibody interactions.
- Explain the importance of the *zone of equivalence* in antigen-antibody reactions.
- List five structural characteristics that affect antigen-antibody binding.
- Describe forces or energy that bind an antigen with its specific antibody in terms of affinity and avidity.

DETECTION OF ANTIGEN-ANTIBODY INTERACTIONS
- List methods that employ labels to evaluate the first phase of antigen-antibody interactions.
- Explain what is meant by the following terms: *antigen* or *antibody label, complement fixation, antigen-antibody complexes.*
- Name four methods used for detection of secondary manifestations of antigen-antibody reactions when soluble antigen is involved.

Key Terms

affinity - Force of attraction that exists between an antigen-binding site on an antibody molecule and its specific antigen.

agglutination - Formation of aggregates consisting of antigen-antibody complexes that form when a particulate antigen combines with its specific antibody.

antigen-binding site - Hypervariable region of an antibody molecule that is the location where binding a specific antigen takes place.

avidity - Overall strength of binding or attachment between an antigen and an antibody.

bivalent antigen - Antigen containing two identical epitopes.

complement fixation - Refers to binding of complement to an antibody of an antigen-antibody complex formed during detection of either an antigen or antibody.

cross-linking - Binding between several epitopes on a multivalent antigen and the antigen-binding sites of its complementary antibody molecule that results in formation of antigen-antibody complexes in the form of lattices.

cross-reactivity - Refers to an immunologic reaction in which specific antibodies react with two dissimilar antigens that share common epitopes. Cross-reactivity may also occur when antibodies with specificity to one epitope bind with another epitope with structural resemblance to the first epitope.

epitope - Antigenic determinant on an antigen that can trigger an immune response and is the site where binding with its specific antibody occurs.

hapten - Low molecular weight antigen.

immune complex - Antigen-antibody complex that results from in vivo binding between an antigen and its complementary antibody. Immune complexes may be found circulating in blood and/or deposited at various tissue sites.

multivalent antigen - Antigen containing two or more identical epitopes.

particulate antigens - Antigens located on the cell surface that, when bound to specific antibodies, form large cell aggregates (complexes) by an agglutination process.

postzone phenomenon - Occurs when an inappropriate proportion of antigens to antibodies (because of an excess concentration of antigen) prevents formation of antigen-antibody complexes.

precipitation - Reaction that occurs when an antibody (bivalent) cross-links with a soluble antigen to form an insoluble antigen-antibody complex that is detectable as a precipitin.

prozone phenomenon - Situation where presence of excess antibodies produces an inappropriate ratio of antigen-to-antibody molecules, thus creating a condition that prevents formation of antigen-antibody complexes (lattice formation).

soluble antigen - "Free" antigen, not fixed to any cell, that has the ability to diffuse in an appropriate medium, such as semi-solid agar.

specificity - Defined as an exact match or fit (complementarity) between an antigen and an antibody. It is the major factor promoting in vivo and in vitro antigen-antibody interaction. An antigen that induces the production of antigen-specific antibodies determines antibody specificity.

univalent antigen - Antigen that contains only one epitope.

zone of equivalence - Condition, shown as a discrete area on a precipitation curve, where optimal conditions (i.e., appropriate concentration or ratio of antigen to antibody) exist for formation of antigen-antibody complexes.

The use of antigen-antibody interactions as the basis for a variety of **immunologic** or **immunodiagnostic tests** (a more relevant name than *serologic tests*, which refers to an in vitro reaction between an antigen and serum antibodies) is based on the premise that maximal binding of antigen by an antibody will occur only in the presence of such conditions as:

- Complementarity (specificity) of the two interacting molecule
- Close proximity of antigen to its specific antibody
- High affinity and avidity of the antibody for the particular antigen
- Presence of approximately equal number of multivalent sites
- Appropriate concentration of antigens and antibodies (zone of equivalence)
- Appropriate environmental factors

Thus, when conditions that promote antigen-antibody interaction are present, binding of the antigen and antibody molecules will occur.

Evolution of immunologic methods that use the principle of antigen-antibody reactions made it possible to detect and quantify a variety of infectious and foreign antigens and the antibodies directed against these antigens (stimuli responsible for the specific antibody response).

PRINCIPLES OF ANTIGEN-ANTIBODY INTERACTIONS

Numerous immunologic methods that use the principles of antigen-antibody interactions are currently available for detection, identification, and quantification of unknown antigen and antibody molecules. These methods are based on the premise that binding of the interacting molecules (reactants) will not occur unless their specificity is the same (complementary).

Although specificity is fundamental to all of the methods based on antigen-antibody reactions, other factors (described following) also have a profound affect on antigen-antibody reaction, by either promoting or inhibiting binding of the two interacting molecules.

MECHANISM OF ANTIGEN-ANTIBODY INTERACTIONS

When antigen and antibody molecules interact, forming antigen-antibody complexes, it may be assumed that they are complementary to each other (i.e., show the same specificity).

The reaction may be represented as follows:

$$Ag + Ab \rightleftharpoons Ag/Ab$$

Where *Ag* represents an antigen, *Ab* is the antibody (immunoglobulin), *Ag/Ab* is the formed complex.

Thus, when the specificity of one reactant (antibody or antigen) is known, by definition, the other reactant of unknown specificity (antigen or antibody) must have the same specificity. *This is a fundamental concept used in antigen-antibody procedures that allows the detection and identification of unknown antigens and antibodies.*

Although complementary specificity between the interacting molecules and other factors (described following) are essential for binding of an antigen and its specific antibody, it is only when the two molecules are in close proximity to each other that the interactions and binding are able to occur.

Thus, when an antigen-antibody reaction occurs, it can be assumed that the reacting molecules are of the same specificity and that all other factors that support binding of an antigen with its specific antibody are appro-

priate for the reaction. This premise can be confirmed by detection of antigen-antibody binding and formation of complexes as well as by detection of antigen-antibody complexes that precipitate or agglutinate because of lattice formation (from cross-linking of antigen-antibody molecules) (Figure 10-1).

These antigen-antibody complexes are detectable by a variety of immunologic methods discussed in subsequent chapters.

Antigen-antibody reactions occur in two phases or stages (see Figure 10-1), each of which requires appropriate conditions for the reaction.

Primary Antigen-Antibody Interaction

Primary antigen-antibody interaction represents the first stage or the initial binding between an epitope (antigenic determinant) and the antigen-specific binding sites on an an-

tibody molecule (see Figure 10-1). The initial binding depends on various factors that include forces of attraction (affinity and avidity) between these molecules (see following).

These conditions and the presence of multiple binding sites on an antigen and antibody (responsible for a high level of forces of attraction) support maximal binding of the interacting molecules.

An approximately equal ratio of antigen and antibody molecules produces maximal conditions for binding of an antigen with its complementary antibody and is referred to as the *zone of equivalence* (Figure 10-2).

Secondary Antigen-Antibody Interaction

Secondary antigen-antibody interaction occurs between multivalent antigens (containing more than two identical epitopes) and antigen-

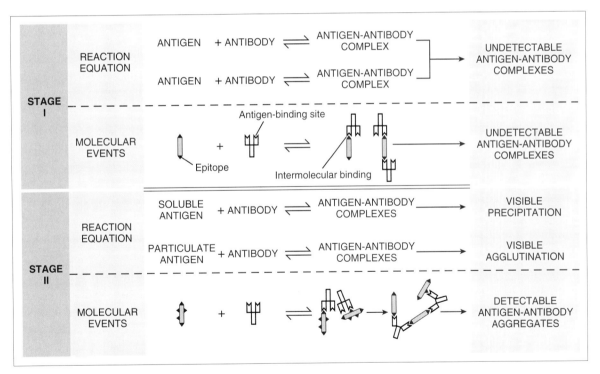

FIGURE **10-1** **Stages of Antigen-Antibody Interactions.** Antigen-antibody interaction occurs in two stages, as represented by *reaction equation* and by events that occur at the molecular level (i.e., *molecular events*). During *Stage I* of the reaction, the binding of the antigen and its specific antibody that occurs is not detectable unless one of the reactants (antigen or antibody) is labeled with visible signal or indicator (see Chapter 13). Events occurring during *Stage II* (secondary manifestation) culminate in large aggregates (antigen-antibody complexes) caused by cross-linking and lattice formation that occurs between a multivalent antigen and a bivalent antibody. These complexes are readily detectable by either precipitation or agglutination techniques (see also Figures 10-4 and 10-5).

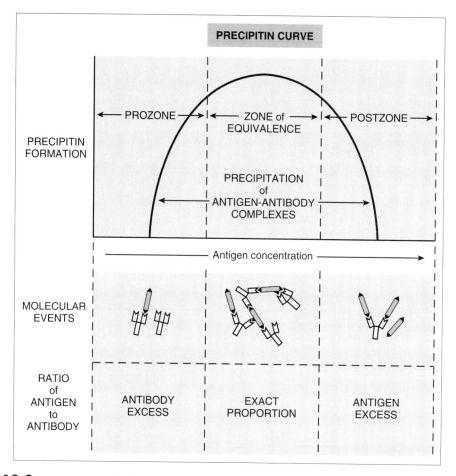

FIGURE **10-2** **Immunoprecipitin Formation.**   The classic *immunoprecipitin curve* shows the effect of antigen and antibody concentration (i.e., proportion of epitopes to antigen-binding sites, respectively) on the amount of precipitin formed during an antigen-antibody reaction when the antibody level is kept constant and the antigen concentration is progressively increased. The corresponding events that occur at the molecular level reflect the amount and type of complexes that form in presence of antibody excess *(prozone),* antigen excess *(postzone),* and when exact proportion of antigen to antibody exists *(zone of equivalence).*

specific antibodies. These interactions depend on **cross-linking** of various antigen molecules by specific antibodies (containing at least two antigen-binding sites) to produce lattices (aggregates) that can be visualized as precipitation or agglutination (see Figure 10-1).

FACTORS AFFECTING ANTIGEN-ANTIBODY INTERACTIONS

Formation of an antigen-antibody complex, when an antigen binds with its specific antibody, depends on a variety of structural and physicochemical factors that are briefly described following.

Structural Characteristics Affecting Antigen-Antibody Binding

As stated previously, structural complementarity (exact match or fit) between an antigen and an antibody is the fundamental requirement for formation of antigen-antibody complexes. Other structural factors, important in the formation of antigen-antibody complexes, are described following.

Specificity of Antigen-Binding Sites

Because an immune response is triggered by an encounter of the immune system with a particular epitope (antigenic determinant) of an antigen, the immunoglobulins (antibodies) pro-

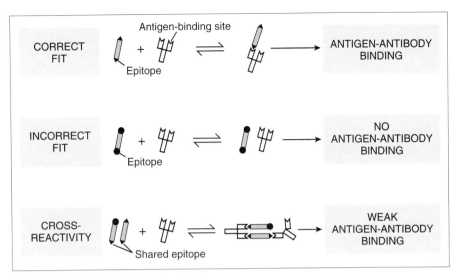

FIGURE **10-3** **Effect of Specificity on Formation of Antigen-Antibody Complexes (at the Molecular Level).** When the antigen and antibody are complementary to each other (i.e., show the same specificity), binding and formation of complexes occurs because of the exact or correct fit ("lock and key" concept) between these molecules. No binding occurs when the antigen and antibody show different or dissimilar specificities (incorrect fit). However, in the presence of shared epitopes on different antigens, binding of antibody may occur between an antigen of different specificity (showing shared epitopes). This type of binding is weaker because of *cross-reactivity* or *cross-reaction* (in the test procedure).

duced during this response show specificity of their antigen-binding sites for that particular stimulating antigen. The antigen and antibody are said to be *complementary* to each other (show complementarity).

Thus antibody specificity is established by the particular antigen and is a function of the sequence of amino acids that are located within the antigen-binding sites on an antibody molecule. It is this sequence of amino acids that determines whether the binding of an antigen (epitope) with its specific antibody will take place.

As shown through experimental fragmentation of an antibody molecule (see Figure 5-11), **antigen-binding sites** are located within the hypervariable segments of the variable region (V_L and V_H) on the Fab fragment of an antibody molecule. These hypervariable regions (complementarity-determining regions [CDRs]) form protruding loops of amino acid sequences on the surface of an antibody molecule that facilitate a close contact with the specific antigen. Any change in the hypervariable regions of an antibody may alter its specificity.

The concept of specificity or "exact fit" of the two molecules has been compared to a "lock and key fit," where the "lock" refers to

the antigen binding-site (antibody) and the "key" to the epitope on an antigen (Figure 10-3).

cross-reactivity. This refers to an immunologic reaction in which specific antibodies react with the following:

- Two dissimilar antigens that share common epitopes.
- An epitope with a structural resemblance to the epitope that stimulated their production.
- Heterophil antigen (from other species such as animals, microorganisms, plants) that is structurally identical or closely related. Specific antibodies that cross-react with heterophil antigens are known as *heterophil antibodies*.

Antigen Accessibility
Although binding of an antigen to an antibody requires complementarity (specificity) between the particular epitope and the antigen-binding site, the particular epitope must also be **accessible** to the antigen-specific binding site.

The antigen accessibility and its subsequent binding by an antibody is affected by the structural characteristics of the antibody molecule, such as the arrangement of segments of the constant region and the presence of a hinge region (see Figure 5-11). These characteristics render flexibility to the antibody molecule that allows it to approach and bind with the specific epitope.

Structure of Immunoglobulins

The numbers of antigen-binding sites on an antibody molecule have a direct effect on the size of antigen-antibody complexes. The number of available units depends on the immunoglobulin class.

Each antibody molecule consists of two or more identical monomeric units (see Figure 5-7). Thus an IgA class with two identical units in its structure (dimer) has four antigen-binding sites and is able to bind with four identical epitopes on an antigen. IgM class molecules (pentamers) will bind with ten identical epitopes. *Therefore, the greater the number of*

binding sites, the larger is the resulting antigen-antibody complex (Figure 10-4).

Valence of Antigen

Two or more identical epitopes on a particular antigen define it as a **multivalent antigen.** As a multivalent antigen interacts with an antigen-specific antibody, antibody molecules cross-link with the antigen to produce large three-dimensional lattices (antigen-antibody complexes) that can readily precipitate in vitro (see Figure 10-1). This reaction serves as a foundation for various immunologic methods that use precipitation for detecting antigen-antibody complexes, referred to as *precipitins (visible insoluble complexes that form as a soluble antigen binds with its specific antibody).*

The binding between an antibody and a multivalent antigen is much stronger (has

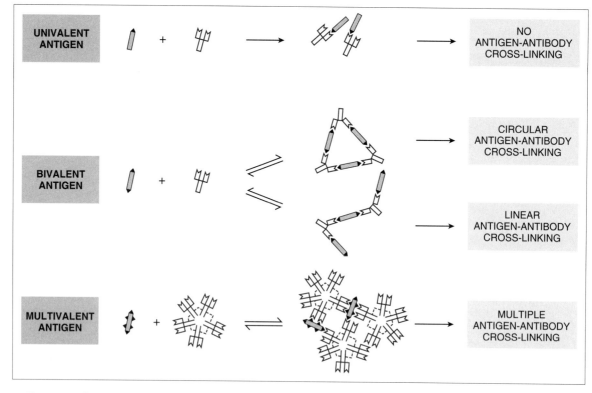

FIGURE **10-4**   **Effect of Antigen and Antibody Structure on Cross-Linking and Formation of Complexes.** The number of epitopes (antigen) and antigen-binding sites (antibody) affect the size of an antigen-antibody complex (amount of cross-linking) that forms during an antigen-antibody interaction. Note the different types of cross-linking that occur in the presence of univalent, bivalent, and multivalent antigens and their corresponding antibodies.

greater avidity) than the binding between an antibody and a single epitope. For example, an IgM molecule (a pentamer) can bind with ten identical epitopes on a multivalent antigen with a greater avidity than does an IgA molecule (a dimer), which binds with only four identical epitopes.

When an antibody interacts with a bivalent antigen, only linear chains or circular complexes are produced. When only one epitope is available, cross-linking cannot occur (see Figure 10-4).

Thus the size of an antigen-antibody complex depends largely on the valence of an antigen.

Concentration of Antigens and Antibodies

In addition to the previously described factors, relative molar concentration (quantity) of antigen and antibody molecules (i.e., the number of epitopes [antigenic determinants] and the number of antigen-binding sites, respectively) also significantly influences the formation of antigen-antibody complexes (three-dimensional lattices or aggregates).

precipitin zones. An *appropriate proportion* (molar concentration) of antigen to the antibody will promote cross-linking of a multivalent antigen by its specific antibodies. Three situations, referred to as **precipitin zones** (see Figure 10-2), either promote or inhibit formation of antigen-antibody complexes.

zone of equivalence. The zone of equivalence is defined by a narrow range on the precipitin curve (see Figure 10-2), which represents the **exact proportion** (ratio of antigen-to-antibody molar concentration) at which cross-linking of a multivalent antigens by their specific antibodies will occur. The resulting antigen-antibody aggregates (complexes) are manifested in vitro as a precipitin.

Precipitin (visible insoluble complexes that form as a soluble antigen binds with its specific antibody) is detectable by a variety of laboratory techniques that use precipitation as the basis for identification and quantitation of unknown antigens and antibodies.

prozone. In the presence of **excess antibodies** to the available identical antigenic determinants during an antigen-antibody reaction, complexes do not form. This condition is referred to as the **prozone phenomenon** (see

Figure 10-2). Reduction of antibodies is required to produce conditions that promote formation of antigen-antibody complexes. In many immunologic procedures, dilution of serum is included to reduce the number of antibodies present (see Chapter 8), if necessary, to bring the reaction to the zone of equivalence.

postzone. In the presence of an **excess amount of antigen** (number of identical epitopes) in proportion to the available antibodies (antigen-binding sites), antigen-antibody complexes do not form. This condition is known as **postzone phenomenon** and requires reduction of antigen concentration to produce conditions that promote formation of antigen-antibody complexes (see Figure 10-2).

Physicochemical Factors Affecting Antigen-Antibody Binding

The stability of an antigen-antibody complex that forms as an antibody interacts with its specific antigen depends to a great degree on forces or binding energy (described following) that exist between the two molecules.

Affinity and Avidity

Forces or binding energy between an antigen and antibody that give stability to the antigen-antibody complex can be calculated (see following) and may be described by the terms:

- *Affinity:* The term refers to an intrinsic force of attraction or association between an antibody (antigen-binding site) and one epitope on a corresponding antigen (univalent antigen), usually a hapten (Figure 10-5).
- *Avidity:* When the antigen consists of several repeating and identical epitopes (definition of multivalent antigen), the affinity between an antigen and an antibody is the sum of the affinities involved (i.e., affinity between each epitope and its corresponding antibody). This overall binding energy between antibodies and multivalent antigens, known as **avidity** (see Figure 10-5), is a measure of the stability of an antigen-antibody complex.

Binding Forces (Energy)

Forces that bind antigens with antibodies are non-covalent and relatively weak (see discussion following). This allows dissociation of the formed antigen-antibody complexes (making

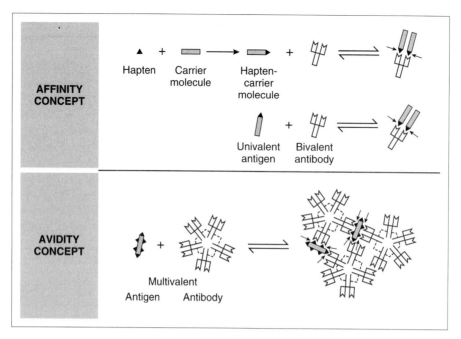

FIGURE **10-5** **Affinity vs. avidity.** Binding energy (forces of attraction) between an antigen and an antigen-specific antibody is defined by the affinity and avidity concept, which depends on the number of bonds that can be formed between the interacting molecules and the amount of binding force or energy (see arrows [→]) that exists. *Affinity* refers to binding between the univalent antigen (usually a hapten) and the bivalent antibody, which has a lesser amount of binding energy. *Avidity* refers to binding between a multivalent antigen (more than two epitopes of the same specificity) and a multivalent antibody (a molecule with more than two antigen-binding sites) that is characterized by more binding energy (total bonding) and the production of a larger and more stable antigen-antibody complex (see Figure 10-4).

the interaction reversible) when such conditions as agitation (stirring), high or low pH, or high salt concentration are present.

The effectiveness of the binding forces depends on a close proximity of the interacting molecules. Thus the closer the antigenic determinant (epitope) is to the binding site on an antibody surface, the greater is the probability of interaction and binding of the antigen and antibody molecules (formation of complexes) by binding forces described following:

- *Ionic interactions (charge complementarity):* Ionic bonds form as oppositely charged portions of the molecules are attracted to each other (e.g., $CO_2^-.NH_3^+$).
- *Hydrogen bonds:* Hydrogen bonds form between negatively charged atoms of polar molecules (COO−) and the positively charged H + ions (H^+), which are attracted by the polar molecules.

- *Hydrophobic bonds:* These bonds form between nonpolar molecules as they come together, eliminating water molecules during the process.
- *Van der Waals forces:* Weak forces of attraction between molecules that depend on an interaction between external electron clouds. These very weak and nonspecific forces become stronger as the epitope comes closer to the antigen-binding site.

Kinetics of Antigen-Antibody Reactions

As discussed previously, bonds formed during an antigen-antibody reaction (**association**) are relatively weak (non-covalent bonds), thus allowing the formed antigen-antibody complexes to **dissociate** in presence of certain conditions (e.g., deviation from optimum temperature).

The kinetics of association and dissociation of antigen-antibody reactions follows the **Law** of Mass Action (as applicable to chemical reactions) and may be represented by the following equation:

$$Ag + Ab \underset{k_2}{\overset{k_1}{\rightleftharpoons}} Ag/Ab$$

Where K_1 is association rate constant (equilibrium constant) for the forward reaction and K_2 is a dissociation rate constant for the reverse reaction, *Ag* is an antigen, *Ab* is an antibody, *Ag Ab* is an antigen-antibody complex.

association or affinity constant (K). The constant for the previous antigen-antibody reaction may be calculated according to the following equation: At equilibrium:

$$K = K_1/K_2 = [Ag/Ab]/[Ab][Ag]$$

Where K_1 is the rate of association, K_2 is the rate of dissociation, [*Ag/Ab*] is the concentration of antigen-antibody complex, and [*Ag*][*Ab*] is the concentration of antigen and antibody, respectively. Both concentrations are expressed in mol/L.

The association constant *(K)* for multiple antigen and antibody reactions is a measure of **avidity,** whereas binding of one epitope (antigen, usually a hapten) to one antigen-binding site (antibody) measures **affinity** between the interacting molecules (see Figure 10-5).

Environmental Factors

In addition to the previously described factors, the following factors also affect antigen-antibody interactions.

Hydrogen Ion Concentration (pH)

Changes in pH of the environment (reaction media) may cause ionization of amino acids (antibody proteins contain ionization groups [$-NH_3$ and $-OOH$]), which can ionize (donate H ion) as the pH changes. Ionization may lead to conformational changes in antibody and/or antigen and modify the affinity constant, described previously.

Temperature

Antibodies, such as IgG, require warm temperatures (and energy) to form stable antigen-antibody complexes. Temperatures above 40° C, however, affect both the antigen and the antibody molecules by altering their conformation and/or denaturing their protein. A denatured antibody may no longer have its antigen-binding sites. Increasing temperature decreases stability of the antigen-antibody complex and promotes its dissociation.

Salt Concentration (Ionic Strength)

Low salt concentrations promote specific antigen-antibody binding. This observation led to the development of laboratory methods that use products with low ionic strength or low salt concentration (particularly in blood banking) to promote formation of antigen-antibody complexes.

With high salt concentrations, however, loss (neutralization) of active sites on the interacting molecules (i.e., antigen and antibody) may occur, causing reduction in affinity between an antigen and its specific antibody and inhibition of binding. Therefore, in methods that employ antigen-antibody reactions, evaporation of samples must be avoided to prevent increase in salt concentration.

Zeta Potential

An electrical charge may be present on the surface of certain particulate antigens, and, when these antigens (e.g., antigens on erythrocytes or red blood cells) are suspended in saline solution (reaction media), an electrical potential forms between the particles that prevents them from coming in close proximity to each other. This electrical potential is referred to as the *zeta potential.*

Zeta potential may produce difficulty in agglutinating red blood cells (negatively charged) by IgG (antibodies) in certain blood bank procedures. This is caused by the fact that the Fab portion of IgG is too short to span the zeta potential between two red cells. Antibodies against human IgG (anti-immunoglobulins) have been developed in rabbits that, when added to the reaction media, can form bridges (cross-link) between red cells, causing them to agglutinate. The inclusion of anti-immunoglobulin in the procedure (see Indirect Antiglobulin Test in Chapter 12) has successfully overcome this difficulty.

An IgM molecule (a pentamer) is better able to bridge the distance between cells, created by the zeta potential and is, therefore, a more effective agglutinating antibody.

DETECTION OF ANTIGEN-ANTIBODY INTERACTIONS

Development of methods that employ antigen-antibody reactions with a detectable end-product or outcome (i.e., antigen-antibody complex) has greatly facilitated the detection and identification of unknown antigens and antibodies.

Because antigen-antibody reactions occur in two phases or stages (discussed previously), two types of manifestations or end-products of the reaction may be detected (one at the end of each stage). These end-products are known as **primary** and **secondary manifestations** of an antigen-antibody interaction (see Figure 10-1):

- *Primary manifestations (formation of antigen-antibody complexes):* During **the first stage** of the antigen-antibody reaction, bonds form between an antigen and antigen-specific antibody to produce antigen-antibody complexes. The interaction occurs when the antigen and antibody show the same specificity (recognition and binding stage). *The reaction is specific and reversible.*
- *Secondary manifestations (lattice formation resulting in precipitation or agglutination):* End-products or manifestations (precipitins, aggregates), which occur during the second stage of an antigen-antibody reaction, are caused by cross-linking and formation of lattices between the multivalent antigen and antigen-specific antibody. *The reaction is not reversible and the formed end-products are insoluble.*

USE OF MONOCLONAL ANTIBODIES

Most laboratory procedures that use reagent antibodies depend on the ability of the antibody to bind with an antigen showing the same specificity, thus forming an antigen-antibody complex that can be detected by various methods, discussed in subsequent chapters.

With the availability of current technology for the production of large numbers of monoclonal antibodies (see Chapter 14), showing specificity for a known and predetermined antigenic determinant (epitope), use of monoclonal

antibodies as reagents has become highly accessible and useful for:

- Detection of antigens and antibodies by methods using antigen-antibody reactions
- Detection of various antigens
- Cell population studies

Detection of Antigen-Antibody Reactions

Initially, antigen/antibody complexes were detectable in body fluids by observing light scattering or collecting the antigen/antibody complexes by *centrifugation* or *precipitation* with a variety of chemical reagents.

The development of gel media for supporting diffusion of antigens and antibodies and detecting a "precipitin line" at the site of antigen/antibody complex formation (precipitation), provided information on antigen concentration and inferred structural differences or similarities of antigens, based on the position of the precipitin line (see Immunodiffusion Techniques, Chapter 11).

Subsequently, as *immunoelectrophoresis* became available, using the principle of electrophoresis and immunodiffusion, reagent antibodies, directed against each Ig class (monovalent antisera) or against total immunoglobulins (polyvalent antisera), were used to identify antibody molecules in serum or urine.

This was accomplished by first separating antibodies (serving as antigens in this protocol) from body fluids (serum or urine) by electrophoresis and then allowing the separated antibody molecules to diffuse in gel toward a trough filled with antisera (reagent antibodies). As the antibodies and antisera diffused toward each other, characteristic arcs were formed that permitted identification of antibody in the body fluid.

These and other earlier methods described in subsequent chapters have now been replaced by more sophisticated procedures that use stationary (immobilized) antigens or antibodies (e.g., *enzyme-linked immunosorbent assay [ELISA]*) to detect and/or quantify antigens or antibodies in the patient sample.

Detection of Antigens in Tissues (Cell Surface Antigens)

In procedures that detect antigens in tissues (i.e., labeled immunoassays, Chapter 13), the *reagent antibodies* are labeled (tagged) with a substance that can be visualized, such as fluorescent dye that is detectable with fluorescent microscopy or flow cytometry. Thus, when a specific antigen-antibody complex forms, it is detectable by the presence of the particular labeled antibody, serving as an indicator of antigen-antibody binding.

An example of this method is its use in demonstrating antigens in tissue, referred to as *immunohistochemistry* (see following). The procedure is mainly applied to the study of neoplasms (new or abnormal growths, tumors) with various currently available commercially prepared reagent antibodies and kits that detect specific tumor markers (antigenic determinants or epitopes) expressed on the cell surface.

Study of Cell Populations

The most commonly used procedure to identify surface molecules on a variety of cells (e.g., lymphocyte subpopulations and hematopoietic cells [developing blood cells]) is by the use of *labeled monoclonal antibodies (mAbs)* directed against the specific cell surface marker (e.g., CD marker) and detection of the product formed by flow cytometry. This procedure is known as *immunophenotyping by flow cytometry* (see Chapter 14).

Fluorescein-labeled mAbs specifically bind with cell surface antigens, producing an antigen/antibody complex that can be detected as a characteristic fluorescent signal when a single cell passes through a light source of a flow cytometer.

For example, in the diagnosis and classification of hematopoietic neoplasia (e.g., leukemia and lymphoma), a leukemia/lymphoma immunophenotyping panel (panel of monoclonal antibodies directed against HLA-DR and various CD markers) is used to classify these neoplasms by flow cytometry.

METHODS BASED ON PRIMARY MANIFESTATIONS OF ANTIGEN-ANTIBODY INTERACTIONS

Binding of an antigen with its specific (complementary) antibody to produce an antigen-antibody complex is a primary manifestation of an antigen-antibody interaction (see Figure 10-1). These complexes are not readily detectable by precipitation or agglutination reactions because of their small size or low concentration. Labeling techniques, therefore, were developed to detect these complexes.

Techniques Employing Labels

In a technique that uses a label, a known antigen or a known reagent antibody is labeled or tagged (conjugated) with a visible label such as an enzyme (e.g., alkaline phosphatase), a dye (e.g., fluorescein), or a radioactive isotope (e.g., ^{125}I). The label serves as a detectable "signal" or "flag" that indicates the presence of a labeled, known antigen or antibody in the antigen-antibody complex and identifies the unknown reactant (antigen or antibody) with the same or complementary specificity.

A labeled (known) antigen is used to detect an unknown antibody. A labeled (known) antibody detects an unknown antigen. Thus, of the two reactants in an antigen-antibody interaction, one is the test reagent (of known specificity) while the other is the unknown reactant (unknown specificity).

The methods employing labels are extremely reliable, sensitive, and the most versatile of the diagnostic laboratory procedures. The following procedures use labels in their protocols (see Chapter 13 for a more detailed discussion).

Fluorescent Immunoassays (FIA)

These assays are based on labeling reactants (antigen or antibody) with a fluorescent label or probe, an alternative to radioimmunoassays and enzyme immunoassays. They are commonly used in clinical laboratories to detect and quantify antibodies, proteins, peptides, drugs, and hormones in body fluids, such as serum. The fluorescent immunoassays (FIA) include:

- Heterogenous or homogenous FIA
- Antibody or ligand-labeled FIA
- Competitive or non-competitive FIA
- Solid phase or non-solid phase FIA

Immunohistochemical Techniques

These methods, also referred to as *cytochemical techniques,* are used to detect and localize antigens in cells or tissues. Antigen-specific antibodies are tagged (conjugated) with substances, such as fluorescein, biotin (Biotin/

Avidin System), or enzyme, which serve as a tracer or signal when a particular cell or tissue antigen is present.

Chemiluminescent Immunoassays

These assays are used to evaluate antigen-antibody complexes by tagging one of the reactants that participates in the reaction. The substance used for labeling the reactant has the ability for chemiluminescence (e.g., acredium esters, luminol). As the labeling substance oxidizes during an antigen-antibody reaction that includes hydrogen peroxide and an enzyme (catalyst), energy is produced as a product of a chemical reaction and is emitted as a visible light (detectable by a specific instrument).

Radioimmunoassays (RIA)

RIA uses a known amount of reactant (i.e., antigen or antibody) that has been labeled with selected radioactive isotope. The unknown reactant (antigen or antibody) can be determined by measuring emitted radioactivity.

Enzyme Immunoassays (EIA)

These tests use a selected enzyme (e.g., alkaline phosphatase, horseradish peroxidase) as a label that is linked to a substance that will be measured, i.e., either an antibody or a ligand (molecule that binds with another complementary molecule). The enzyme catalyzes certain biochemical reactions in the presence of an appropriate substrate to produce a measurable end-product (e.g., color).

Fluorescence-Activated Cell Sorting Analysis (FACS)

Using fluorescein-labeled reagent antibodies that show specificity for various cell-surface antigens, FACS makes possible a rapid and accurate identification of cell populations according to the differential molecules (CDs) expressed on their surface.

Techniques Employing Complement Fixation

Fixation of complement occurs during binding of antigen with its complementary antibody. Thus, during an antigen-antibody reaction that occurs when an unknown antigen or antibody, a known reactant (antigen or antibody), and a defined amount of complement are combined (reaction components), the complement is "consumed" or bound (fixed) to the resulting antigen-antibody complex. The remaining complement is measured by the amount of its lytic (hemolytic) effect on subsequently added erythrocytes. By performing a hemolytic assay that includes a titration, it is possible to determine the amount of antigen or antibody present in the initial reaction (see Chapter 14).

Although complement fixation tests have been applied both in research and in clinical laboratory practice, they are very complex and cumbersome, particularly the newer and more sensitive microcomplement techniques.

METHODS BASED ON SECONDARY MANIFESTATIONS OF ANTIGEN-ANTIBODY INTERACTIONS

Precipitins or aggregates form as the end-products of antigen-antibody reactions that occur when an antigen binds with its corresponding antibody to form a complex that is characterized by formation of lattices, as an outcome of cross-linking of an antigen (must be multivalent) and its specific antibodies. Precipitation and agglutination reactions are methods used to detect these end-products (i.e., precipitins and aggregates, respectively).

Immunoprecipitation Techniques

These antigen-antibody reactions occur when a *soluble antigen* and its corresponding antibody cross-link to form a lattice that produces an insoluble aggregate *(precipitin)*. Detection of precipitin is the most simple method of detecting antigen-antibody reactions (see Chapters 11, 13, and 14) and includes such methods as the following.

Turbidimetry

This immunoturbidimetric technique detects turbidity or cloudiness of a solution when antigen and antibody are mixed in a fluid. Turbidity is followed by precipitation. A detection device measures the amount of reduction in light intensity caused by absorption of light in proportion to the size, concentration, or shape of the molecules present in the solution.

Nephelometry

This immunonephelometric technique measures the amount of light scatter (at an angle from incident beam) as it passes through the solution. The amount of light scatter is a measure of concentration of the antigen or antibody measured (e.g., quantification of serum immunoglobulins, C3 and C4 complement components, C-reactive protein).

Immunodiffusion Techniques (Single, Double, Radial Immunodiffusion)

These techniques use support medium, such as agar or agarose, to detect formed antigen-antibody complexes by the process of diffusion in one direction (single diffusion), diffusion of antigen and antibody (independently) through a medium in two directions (double diffusion), or by radial diffusion (modified single diffusion).

Electrophoretic Techniques (Immunoelectrophoresis, Rocket and Countercurrent Immunoelectrophoresis, Immunofixation Electrophoresis)

These techniques use a combination of diffusion (single and double) and separation of molecules in an electric field, according to their size, by the process of electrophoresis. The current that is applied to the gel causes antigen and/or antibody to migrate (diffuse) and form detectable precipitin bands (antigen-antibody complexes).

Agglutination Techniques

Cross-linking and production of aggregates or clumping (antigen-antibody complexes) occur when an antibody reacts with a *particulate* (insoluble) multivalent antigen. The particulate antigen may be an insoluble native (unprocessed) antigen, cells expressing antigens (e.g., group AB erythrocytes), or antigen-coated particles (e.g., latex particles).

Agglutination reactions have a high degree of sensitivity and their end point can be detected visually. The methods that use agglutination reactions (see Chapter 12) to detect a variety of analytes (reactants) are classified as follows.

Direct Agglutination

Direct agglutination of antigen with its specific antibody is used when the antigen is naturally located on a particle, such as in bacteria or erythrocytes.

Passive Agglutination

Carrier particles (available in commercially prepared kits), such as latex, bentonite, and charcoal, are coated with antigens that are not naturally located on their surface. These antigen-coated particles are used to detect antibodies (e.g., antibodies to group A streptococcus).

Reverse Passive Agglutination

The carrier particles are coated with a known antibody, rather than an antigen, and are used to detect antigens, such as *Staphyloccocus aureus,* group A streptococcus, and *Candida albicans.*

Agglutination Inhibition

The procedure is based on competition between soluble and particulate antigens for a limited number of antigen-binding sites on an antibody molecule. Lack of agglutination during an antigen-antibody reaction is an indication of a positive result (opposite of other agglutination reactions). An example of agglutination inhibition technique is testing for presence of human chorionic gonodotropin (hCG) hormone as an indication of pregnancy.

Formation of Immune Complexes

Immune complexes are antigen-antibody complexes that form in vivo and may be detected in tissues or in blood circulation.

Detection of circulating immune complexes in serum involves binding of the complex to a variety of complement components, whereas detection of immune complexes in various tissues uses antigen-specific antibodies, known as *specific antisera.* The latter is an immuno-histochemical technique.

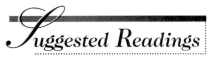

Suggested Readings

Henry JB, editor: *Clinical diagnosis and management by laboratory methods,* ed 19, Philadelphia, 1996, WB Saunders.

Rose NR, et al, editors: *Manual of clinical laboratory immunology,* ed 4, 1997, American Society for Microbiology.

Review Questions

PRINCIPLES OF ANTIGEN-ANTIBODY INTERACTIONS

1-3. Match the following terms with the appropriate definition:

_____ avidity
_____ affinity
_____ specificity

    a. the strength of interaction between a single antigenic determinant (epitope) and an antigen-binding site on an immunoglobulin molecule
    b. an exact or correct fit between an antigen and an antibody molecule
    c. the total (cumulative) strength of an interaction between epitopes of a multivalent antigen and their corresponding binding sites on an immunoglobulin molecule
    d. an electrostatic attraction between two molecules

4. Equal ratio of antigen and antibody molecules produces maximal conditions for binding of antigen with its complementary antibody. The zone on an immunoprecipitin curve that represents this condition is the:
    a. postzone
    b. zone of maximal binding
    c. zone of equivalence
    d. prozone

5-8. Match each listed characteristic with the antigen-antibody interaction that it defines:

    a. primary antigen-antibody interaction
    b. secondary antigen-antibody interaction

_____ an interaction that involves binding between an antigen-binding site on an antibody with its specific antigen (epitope)
_____ an interaction between a complex (multivalent) antigen and antibodies showing the same specificity

_____ interaction that results in cross-linking and lattice formation
_____ interaction that is characterized by precipitation, agglutination, and complement activation

9-12. Match listed forces of attraction between an antigen and its corresponding antibody with their related statements:

_____ ionic interactions
_____ hydrogen bonds
_____ hydrophobic bonds
_____ Van der Waals bonds

    a. caused by attraction of oppositely charged groups on interacting molecules (e.g., NH_3^+ and COO^-)
    b. attraction between negatively (COO^-) and positively (H^+) charged ions
    c. these bonds form as non-polar molecules come together, expelling water molecules in the process
    d. weak forces of attraction that become stronger as a specific antigen approaches an antibody

13. All of the following environmental factors have an effect on an antigen-antibody reaction, *except*:
    a. temperature
    b. salt concentration
    c. hydrogen ion concentration (pH)
    d. concentration of antigen and antibody

14. Antibody specificity or its "exact fit" is determined by:
    a. specific epitope on an antigen
    b. antigen-stimulated immune response
    c. antigen-binding sites on an antibody
    d. all of the above

15. All terms listed following refer to the kinetics of association and dissociation of antigen-antibody reaction, *except*:
    a. Van der Waals forces
    b. Law of Mass Action
    c. affinity constant
    d. avidity

DETECTION OF ANTIGEN-ANTIBODY INTERACTIONS

16. A known antigen or known antibody can be tagged with a visible label to identify the presence of an unknown antibody or antigen detectable in a formed antigen-antibody complex, thus identifying the unknown antigen or antibody. All labels listed following may be used for this purpose, *except:*
    a. selected enzymes
    b. selected radioisotopes
    c. vital stains
    d. fluorescent probes

17. Secondary manifestations that occur during an antigen-antibody interaction can be detected by the following method(s):
    a. agglutination
    b. precipitation
    c. complement fixation
    d. all of the above

18. All of the following procedures use labels for detection of antigen-antibody complexes, *except:*
    a. fluorescent immunoassays
    b. radioimmunoassays
    c. complement activation
    d. enzyme immunoassays

19. Immunoprecipitation reactions are used to detect aggregates (precipitins) formed during an antigen-antibody interaction. The antigen involved in the interaction is a:
    a. particulate antigen
    b. soluble antigen
    c. univalent epitope
    d. none of the above

20. All of the following methods use agglutination reactions to detect an antigen-antibody interaction, *except:*
    a. direct agglutination
    b. passive agglutination
    c. agglutination inhibition
    d. indirect agglutination

CHAPTER 11

Precipitation Techniques

Learning Objectives

Upon completion of Chapter 11, the student will be prepared to:

IMMUNODIFFUSION TECHNIQUES

- Define the following terms: *immunoprecipitation, zone of equivalence, precipitin curve, precipitin rings,* and *precipitin bands.*
- Describe two phases in formation of immunoprecipitin.
- List methods that use immunoprecipitation as the basis for identifying and quantifying antigen or antibody molecules.
- State the main difference between immunodiffusion and immunoelectrophoresis techniques.
- Describe three different precipitin patterns as they relate to the specificity of antigens being compared by immunodiffusion.
- Compare the end-point method with the kinetic method used in radial immunodiffusion assay for determining the concentration of an antigen.
- List three clinical applications of radial immunodiffusion.

IMMUNOELECTROPHORETIC TECHNIQUES

- Describe the principle of electrophoretic separation of a complex mixture of molecules such as protein.
- List five normal protein fractions as separated by electrophoresis.
- Explain the difference between polyclonal and monoclonal increase in immunoglobulins, according to their immunoelectrophoretic patterns.
- State the reason for preference of immunofixation electrophoresis over immunoelectrophoresis when characterizing monoclonal immunoglobulins.

LIGHT SCATTERING IMMUNOASSAYS

- Explain the main difference between turbidimetric and nephelometric method of detecting light scattered by immunoprecipitins.
- State the reason for selecting the end-point method for quantifying antigens by light scatter instruments.

Key Terms

analyte - Refers to any protein, glycoprotein, or lipoprotein molecules present in biologic fluids (serum, urine, and cerebrospinal fluid), which serves as an antigen that can be measured in an antigen-antibody reaction, when the antigen-specific reagent antibodies are available.

antisera - Commercially prepared antibodies with known specificity that serve as a reagent or as one of the reactants in an immunology assay using antigen-antibody reaction.

cross-reactivity - Occurs when an antibody with specificity for one antigen reacts with another that is structurally similar.

immunodiffusion - Refers to the movement of antigen molecules, antibody molecules, or both in a support medium by the process of diffusion (spreading or distribution).

immunoprecipitin - Insoluble (stable) complex, consisting of antigen-antibody lattices, that forms when a soluble antigen reacts with an antibody of the same specificity (i.e., antigen-specific antibody).

gammopathy - Abnormality associated with a specified class of immunoglobulins.

light scatter - Refers to bending of light at various angles to the original path of light by particles suspended in a solution.

monospecific antiserum - Reagent antibody showing specificity for one particular epitope (antigenic determinant).

paraprotein - Single immunoglobulin fraction seen in lymphoproliferative disorders, characterized by increased proliferation of a single malignant clone of B cells.

polyspecific antiserum - Reagent antibodies with more than one antigen (epitope) specificity, referred to as *multispecific antibodies.*

precipitin lines or bands - Refers to a point on a support medium where the antigen and its specific antibody meet to form antigen-antibody complexes, visible as precipitins.

reactant - Term that describes an analyte or a reagent antibody. Refers to molecules participating in a particular reaction (antigen-antibody).

reaction medium - Also referred to as support medium, provides necessary environment for development of an antigen-antibody interaction.

reagent antibody or antigen - Commercially prepared antigens or antibodies with known specificity that are used in identifying or quantifying the analyte (antigen or antibody) in a sample.

turnaround time - Total time required to provide laboratory results on a given sample, from the time of obtaining the specimen to the time the interpreted data (result) is reported.

zone of equivalence - Point of optimal formation of antigen-antibody complexes, where the antigen concentration is approximately equal to the antibody concentration of the same specificity in a reaction medium. More specifically, the number of epitopes is equal to the number of antigen-binding sites.

—·—·—•—●—•—·—·—

*I*mmunoprecipitation is the formation of insoluble (stable) antigen-antibody complexes (Ag-Ab), known as *precipitins*, when a *soluble* antigen is mixed with its corresponding (specific) antibody (Figure 11-1). Formation of these visible, non-reversible precipitins occurs at the *zone of equivalence*, when the antigen concentration (number of available multivalent antigen sites or epitopes) and the antibody concentration (number of antigen-binding sites on the specific antibodies) are approximately equal (see Chapter 10 and Figure 10-2).

Immunoprecipitin occurs only when an antigen and an antibody are of the same specificity. The process involves two phases. During the *primary phase*, the antigen binds with its specific antibody. This is followed by a *secondary phase* of the antigen-antibody reaction, during which an optimal formation of insoluble antigen-antibody lattices occurs at the zone of equivalence. These lattices are visible as precipitins (see Figure 10-2).

In immunoprecipitation, as in any antigen-antibody interaction, the formation of antigen-antibody complexes depends on the complementary or corresponding specificity of the two reactants (antigen and antibody), known as *complementarity* (see Chapter 5). *This funda-*

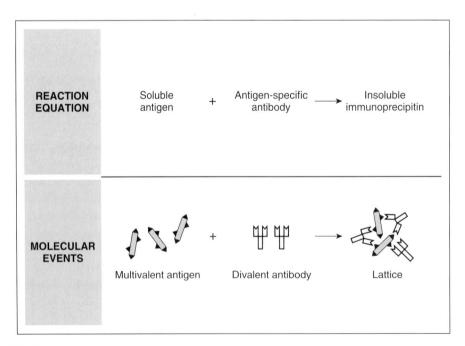

FIGURE **11-1** **Immunoprecipitation.** Events occurring at the molecular level during a precipitation reaction. The reaction involves binding of a multivalent antigen with a divalent antibody of corresponding specificity (antigen-specific antibody) to produce an insoluble antigen-antibody complex that is visible in a support medium (solution) as a precipitin.

mental concept allows identification and quantification of one reactant (unknown antigen or antibody, often known as an analyte) when the specificity of the other reactant (reagent antigen or antibody) is known.

Thus immunoprecipitation is the basis for many qualitative and quantitative immunologic methods frequently used in the laboratory to identify and quantify antigens or antibodies. These methods include:

- Immunodiffusion techniques (passive immunodiffusion)
- Immunoelectrophoretic techniques (immunodiffusion/electrophoresis)
- Light scattering measurements (turbidimetry)

The following factors must be considered when implementing any immunoprecipitation procedure (see Chapter 10):

- *Relative concentration of antigen and antibody (reactants)*
- *Hydrogen ion concentration (pH)*
- *Ionic strength of solution (reaction medium)*
- *Antibody affinity and avidity*

IMMUNODIFFUSION TECHNIQUES

Immunodiffusion involves movement of antibody and/or antigen molecules (reactants) within a selected support medium (e.g., solution or agarose) by the process of diffusion. When the reacting molecules diffuse, without any other enhancement (e.g., electric current), the reaction is referred to as **passive immunodiffusion.**

As the two reactants of the same specificity diffuse and meet, insoluble antigen-antibody complexes are formed. This reaction is referred to as **immunoprecipitation** and the complexes formed that are visible are known as **precipitin bands or lines.** These precipitin bands remain stationary within the support medium at the site where the precipitation has occurred (Figure 11-2).

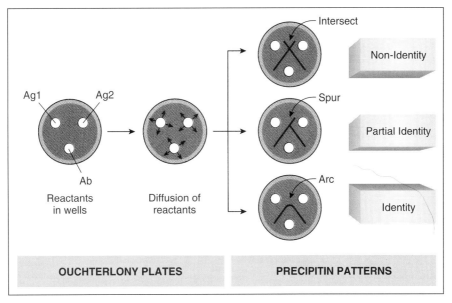

FIGURE **11-2** **Double Immunodiffusion (Ouchterlony Technique).** Diagrammatic representation of three characteristic positions of precipitin bands (patterns) that form when antigens (Ag1, Ag2) of unknown specificity and a polyspecific antibody (Ab) are allowed to diffuse from their wells and bind at the site where they meet in the support medium. The positions where precipitin bands form are designated as **identity, partial identity,** or **non-identity patterns,** depending on the specificity of the epitopes on the antigens being analyzed. *Pattern of identity:* Continuous precipitin line that forms an arc, indicating that the antigens have common (shared) epitopes and are identical. *Pattern of partial identity:* Precipitin line of identity between shared epitopes on antigens being compared and an extended precipitin line (spur) produced between the more complex antigen containing an epitope not common to both antigens. *Pattern of non-identity:* Two separate precipitin bands that cross (intersect) each other, indicating dissimilarity of the epitopes on both antigens.

Immunodiffusion procedures have been classified according to the direction of the diffusion and the number of reactants (i.e., antigens and antibodies) that are involved in the process as follows:

- *Single immunodiffusion*
- *Double immunodiffusion*
- *Radial immunodiffusion*

The addition of an electric current to immunodiffusion technique, as means of increasing the diffusion process of the reactants, constitutes the basis for **immunoelectrophoresis** (see discussion that follows).

MEDIA SUPPORTING IMMUNOPRECIPITIN FORMATION

Immunoprecipitin Formation in Solution

A random cross-linking between soluble multivalent antigen and its complementary divalent antibody molecules results in formation of a lattice or network of antigen-antibody complexes in a liquid medium (solution). As the size of these complexes increases, the complexes lose their solubility and precipitate out of the solution. This reaction is represented by a **precipitin curve,** constructed by plotting the amount of precipitin that forms against the amount of antigen that has been added to the solution (Figure 11-3).

Immunoprecipitin Formation in Semi-Solid Medium

Production of antigen-antibody complexes (immunoprecipitins) in such semi-solid media as agar gel (polysaccharide from seaweed) or agarose (purified agar) depends on diffusion of soluble antigens and antibodies (reactants) in tubes or in plates containing semi-solid medium. The rate at which the reactants diffuse may be affected by such factors as their concentration, molecular size, molecular shape, temperature, gel viscosity, and interaction between the gel and the reactants.

As the reactants meet, they bind to each other and form cross-links (antigen-antibody complexes) that remain at the site of their formation and are visible as *precipitin lines* within the agarose (see Figure 11-2). Agarose is the preferred medium because of its neutral charge and transparency.

SINGLE IMMUNODIFFUSION TECHNIQUE

In this infrequently used immunologic procedure, which forms the basis for radial immunodiffusion (see following), either the antigen or the antibody remain fixed within the support medium, while the other reactant is allowed to move toward the fixed reactant, binding and forming stable complexes (precipitin band) at the point of contact. Thus, in this technique, also known as *diffusion technique of Oudin,* only one of the reactants travels,

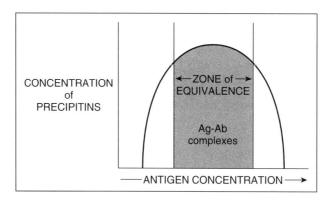

FIGURE **11-3** **Precipitin Curve.** The curve depicts production of antigen-antibody (Ag-Ab) complexes within the zone of equivalence, when the antibody concentration remains the same while the concentration of antigen increases. At a point where both reactants (antigen and antibody) are approximately equal (zone of equivalence), they bind, form lattices, and precipitate.

while the other remains stationary within the medium.

DOUBLE IMMUNODIFFUSION TECHNIQUE

General Concept

Double immunodiffusion procedure, also known as *Ouchterlony technique,* is a semi-quantitative method based on the premise that when both of the reactants (i.e., an *unknown* antigen and polyspecific antibody molecules) are allowed to diffuse outward and toward each other within a selected support medium, the point where the reactants meet and form stable antigen-antibody complexes can be seen as a *precipitin band* or *line* (see Figure 11-2).

This procedure allows for a comparison of unknown antigens on the basis of their epitopes. Thus the antigens being compared may have epitopes that have the same, partial, or different specificity. Accordingly, the position of the precipitin pattern formed as a particular antigen binds with an antibody that shows the same specificity is designated as either a *pattern of identity, partial identity,* or *non-identity* (described following).

Procedure

Briefly, Ouchterlony plates (commercially available immunodiffusion plates) containing agarose medium are prepared by placing poly-specific antiserum (antibodies) within the central well and unknown antigens within the surrounding wells on the plate. The plate is then incubated (12 to 48 hours) to allow diffusion of the antigens and antibodies within the medium.

Evaluation of Results

The location and size of the precipitin bands formed at the point where the two reactants meet depends on various factors, such as the rate of diffusion and the concentration of both of the reactants (i.e., the antigen and antibody).

The patterns of precipitin bands *(precipitin patterns)* formed between the antigen and antibody wells are determined by the specificity of the antigens being compared, thus allowing for determination of their relationship.

Precipitin Patterns

The following precipitin patterns may be visible, depending on the specificity of antigens being compared (see Figure 11-2).

Pattern of Identity

Antigens forming this pattern have a common epitope (antigenic determinant). As the antigens diffuse toward the antibodies, continuous precipitin lines that merge and form an *arc* indicate that the antibodies are precipitating identical epitopes of the antigens being compared.

Pattern of Partial Identity

This reflects the fusion of two precipitin bands and the formation of an additional *spur.* Fusion of precipitin lines indicates that the antibody is precipitating epitopes present on both antigens (i.e., epitopes that are common to both antigens). Presence of a spur (extended precipitin line) indicates that the antibody is also precipitating an additional epitope that is not common to both antigens (i.e., the epitope present on the more complex antigen).

Pattern of Non-Identity

When different epitopes are present on the antigens being compared and no common epitopes are shared, two separate precipitin bands will form and cross *(intersect)* each other. This reaction pattern indicates that the antibody is precipitating two separate (not identical) epitopes on antigens that are of different specificities.

Comments

Clinical Application

Double immunodiffusion method may be used to identify antibodies, such as extractable nuclear antigen (ENA), in such conditions as:

- Mixed connective tissue disease (MCTD)
- Systemic lupus erythematosus (SLE)

Technical Errors

Possible technical errors associated with the method include:

- Alteration of precipitin pattern by excessive condensation in wells, improper filling of wells, or failure to incubate in horizontal position
- False results because of improper identification of wells

- False negative results because of insufficient incubation
- Incorrect interpretation of precipitin patterns
- Reliability of test standards or controls (see discussion of quality control in Chapter 9) with known antigen concentration that must be analyzed concurrently with the patient sample (unknown or analyte) to check the reliability of test results

RADIAL IMMUNODIFFUSION

General Concept
Radial immunodiffusion technique is based on the same principle as single immunodiffusion (i.e., one of the reacting molecules [antibody] is evenly distributed within the support medium and the other [antigen] is allowed to diffuse out from a central well cut within the medium). As the antigen diffuses, the proportion of antigen-to-antibody concentration changes until an equivalence point is reached.

The diameter of the visible precipitin ring, formed around the well at the zone of equivalence (Figure 11-4), is proportional to the concentration of the available antigen, so that *ring diameter = concentration.*

Procedure
Briefly, the patient's *serum sample* containing test antigens of *unknown concentration* (e.g., specific proteins, such as IgA, IgG, IgM and complement components, such as C3, C4, and Factor B) and *commercially obtained standards (controls containing known concentration of test antigens in mg/dL)* are added to appropriate wells in agarose medium that contains *monospecific antiserum* (anti-immunoglobulin of known antigen-specificity).

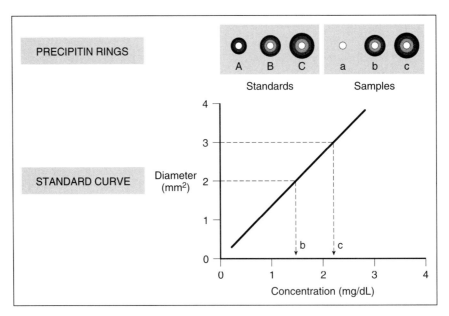

FIGURE **11-4   Radial Immunodiffusion.**   Patient samples (unknowns) and standards (known quantities of antigens) are allowed to diffuse out of wells cut within gel containing known monospecific antibodies. As diffusion occurs, antigens and antibodies meet, bind, and form immunoprecipitins (antigen-antibody complexes) in varied quantities until a zone of equivalence is reached. The immunoprecipitins form a visible ring. The diameter of the ring is proportional to the antigen concentration, thus allowing for the determination of antigen concentration of unknown **samples b** and **c,** by interpolating from a standard curve. Note that **sample a** (unknown antigen) shows no precipitin formation because of its specificity that differs from antibodies within the support medium. The standard curve is constructed by plotting known concentration of the **A, B,** and **C standards** (mg/dL) vs. the diameter of the precipitin ring (mm^2) formed by these standards.

As the *unknown (patient sample)* and *standards (control samples)* diffuse from wells within the agar during a specified incubation period (see discussion following), antigen-antibody complexes form at the point where the diffusing antigen and the stationary antibody meet within the medium. The complexes are visible as precipitin rings surrounding the wells. The diameters of the precipitin rings (unknown and standard samples) are measured in millimeters (mm) and used in constructing a standard curve (see Figure 11-4).

There are two methods of determining the concentration of antigens using the radial immunodiffusion assay.

End-Point Method (Mancini)

In this method, the antigen is allowed to diffuse to completion (approximately 24 hours), forming precipitins with the antibody in the support medium until the point (zone) of equivalence is reached (see Figure 11-4) and no additional precipitation occurs (ring diameter remains the same). The ring diameter is directly proportional to the antigen concentration.

In this method, a standard curve is constructed on a graph by plotting concentration *(x-axis)* vs. ring diameter squared *(y-axis)* of the analyzed standards (controls). Concentration of unknown antigen *(ring diameter)* is interpolated from the constructed standard curve (see Figure 11-4).

The end-point method is used by many manufacturers in preparation of immunodiffusion plates.

Kinetic Method (Fahey and McKelvey)

This method differs from the method of *Mancini* in that the measurement of precipitin diameter is made (at an established time of approximately 18 hrs) before the zone of equivalence is reached.

A standard curve is constructed on a semilog paper by plotting antigen concentration *(log axis)* vs. precipitin diameter *(arithmetic axis)*. The *ring diameter* (D^2) is proportional to the log of antigen concentration.

Evaluation of Results

The ring diameter of the precipitate formed around the well containing the patient sample (unknown) is measured in millimeters (mm) and is used to determine or derive (interpolate) antigen concentration in the patient sample from the constructed standard curve (see Figure 11-4).

This derivation is possible because the size of the diameter (D^2) of the formed precipitin is proportional to the antigen concentration of the unknown antigen (e.g., specific immunoglobulin class in serum).

Comments

Reference sera (standards), with known concentrations, must be tested simultaneously with the patient sample (unknown).

Clinical Application

The clinical application includes:
- Identification and quantification of proteins found in serum and other body fluids in such conditions as mixed connective tissue disease (MCTD).
- Quantifying C5 complement component when increased susceptibility to infections exists.
- Quantifying immunoglobulins in suspected hypogammaglobulinemia or hypergammaglobulinemia.

The radial immunodiffusion procedure is based on quantification of antigens. However, it is also possible to apply this procedure to quantify antibodies by reversing the process (i.e., using antibodies as standards to construct a standard curve and using the medium that contains stationary antigen). The antibody concentration in this reverse process is interpolated from the standard curve (antibody standards).

Technical Errors

Technical errors associated with the method include:
- Incorrect filling of wells, specimen contamination, inappropriate support medium (e.g., outdated gel), or failure to incubate the plate in a horizontal position
- Calculation error: since final concentration of a diluted sample (unknown) is obtained by multiplying results by an appropriate dilution factor

IMMUNOELECTROPHORETIC TECHNIQUES

Electrophoresis has been introduced into the clinical laboratory as a way of *separating protein mixtures* that have been found too complex for separation and identification by a simple diffusion or precipitation technique. Thus, by applying voltage through the support medium (paper, agarose, or cellulose acetate strips) that stabilizes the molecules, it is possible to separate complex protein mixtures.

The movement of molecules in an electric field depends mainly on their surface charge, which is determined by the pH of the support medium used (Figure 11-5). As the protein molecules become ionized, they separate by moving toward the oppositely charged electrode (i.e., either to the cathode [negative electrode] or to the anode [positive electrode]), depending on the charge of the molecule. This principle of electrophoretic separation of complex mixtures of molecules has allowed the development of other immunologic techniques that require higher resolution for proper characterization of the separated molecules. Thus protein electrophoresis has been adopted for separation of mixed molecules in such methods as:

- Immunoelectrophoresis
- Immunofixation electrophoresis
- Countercurrent immunoelectrophoresis
- Electroimmunodiffusion (Rocket electrophoresis)
- Isoelectric focusing

ELECTROPHORESIS

General Concept

Serum protein electrophoresis procedure (SPEP) separates serum proteins into five fractions (albumin, α_1, α_2, β, and γ globulins), which appear on selected gel medium as *bands* and show a characteristic pattern of mobility (see Figure 11-5). The components of serum globulin fractions are presented in Table 11-1.

Migration of the protein molecules in an electric field occurs primarily on the basis of their surface charge in a support medium, although molecular weight and size of the molecule, the characteristics of the medium and buffer (e.g., pH), and the physical conditions (e.g., temperature) also affect the separation process.

FIGURE 11-5   **A, Protein electrophoresis gel (membrane),** containing five bands according to their characteristic patterns of mobility: albumin (alb) and four globulin fractions (alpha$_1$ (α_1)-globulin, alpha$_2$ (α_2)-globulin, beta (β)-globulin, gamma (γ)-globulin). Lanes 2 through 10 depict normal and abnormal amounts of serum protein fractions. An increase or a decrease in a particular fraction is visible as a greater or lesser intensity of stain (respectively) and indicates presence of a particular abnormality. **B, Electrophoretic scans,** showing conversion of each band (see gel) into its characteristic peak: band 6 = normal pattern of serum protein fractions; bands 2 and 7 = pattern seen in monoclonal gammopathy; bands 3 and 8 = pattern seen in polyclonal gammopathy; bands 4 and 9 = pattern seen in chronic inflammation; bands 5 and 10 = pattern seen in cirrhosis of the liver. Size of each peak is proportional to the intensity of the corresponding band on gel. (**A,** courtesy Monmouth Medical Center, New Jersey.)

Densitometric scanning of the separated and stained serum protein fractions, which appear as discrete bands on gel, converts each band pattern into its characteristic peak (see Figure 11-5). This allows quantification of each of the protein fractions. The intensity of staining (thickness) of a band determines the size of its peak and, therefore, the concentration of the protein fraction in grams per deciliter (g/dL).

*Thus separation of a mixture of proteins by electrophoresis, also referred to as **protein** or **zone electrophoresis**, makes it possible to identify and quantify discrete protein molecules. However, other tests, such as immunoelectrophoresis or immunofixation, are used as a follow-up procedure to characterize or identify any monoclonal component.*

Procedure

Briefly, serum, urine, or a cerebrospinal fluid (CSF) specimen and an appropriate standard are placed at the origin of the selected support medium (e.g., agarose gel) and an electric current is applied to separate the protein molecules within the sample. As the molecules migrate to the anode (positive electrode) accord-

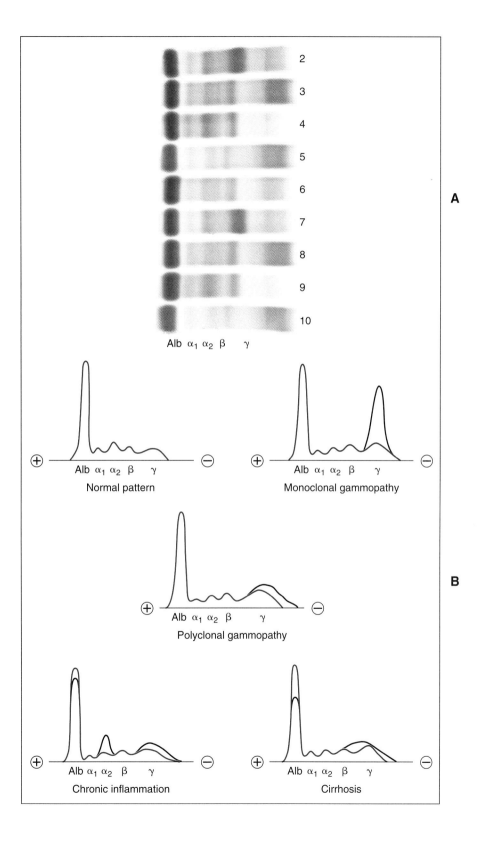

Alb α_1 α_2 β γ

$\oplus$ Alb α_1 α_2 β γ $\ominus$
Normal pattern

$\oplus$ Alb α_1 α_2 β γ $\ominus$
Monoclonal gammopathy

$\oplus$ Alb α_1 α_2 β γ $\ominus$
Polyclonal gammopathy

$\oplus$ Alb α_1 α_2 β γ $\ominus$
Chronic inflammation

$\oplus$ Alb α_1 α_2 β γ $\ominus$
Cirrhosis

A

B

Table 11-1	MAJOR COMPONENTS OF SERUM GLOBULIN FRACTIONS*	
Protein Fraction	**Components**
Albumin	
Alpha (α_1) globulin	α_1-Acid glycoprotein
	α_1-Antitrypsin
	α-Lipoprotein
Alpha (α_2) globulin	α_2-Macroglobulin
	α_2-Antitrypsin
	Haptoglobin
Beta (β) globulin	β-lipoprotein
	Fibrinogen
	Transferrin
	Complement
	Immunoglobulin A (IgA)
Gamma (γ) globulin	Other immunoglobulins
	(IgG, IgM, IgD, IgE)
	C-reactive protein

*Electrophoretically separated.

ing to their electrophoretic mobility (i.e., negative charge in an alkaline buffer solution on gel), they separate, forming bands that are promptly stained. The stained bands are then visualized for their characteristic position on the gel.

To quantify each protein fraction, the stained bands are scanned with a densitometer, which converts them into the characteristic serum protein peaks (i.e., albumin, α_1-globulin, α_2-globulin, β-globulin, and γ-globulin [see Figure 11-5]).

Evaluation of Results

Results obtained from the patient's serum protein electrophoresis are interpreted on the basis of bands produced by each separated protein fraction in gel and on the size of the corresponding peak obtained from the densitometric scanning of bands in gel.

Patient's serum proteins and the normal control, separated in gel by electrophoresis into five protein fractions and scanned with a densitometer, are quantified. The quantity of each protein fraction can be expressed either as a percent (%) of total serum protein concentration or as grams per deciliter (g/dL). Patient's total serum protein concentration and control is required for these calculations.

The normal control is included to verify both the separation and the staining procedures. The protein fractions originating from the control specimen must be within the previously established normal range for the sample results to be acceptable (see Figure 11-5).

Abnormal serum protein electrophoretic patterns are of greatest value in the diagnosis of monoclonal and polyclonal gammopathies. *Of these, polyclonal gammopathies are the most commonly encountered protein abnormality.*

Monoclonal Gammopathies

A sharp spike or peak, usually in the γ globulin region of the electrophoretogram, is suggestive of the presence of monoclonal paraprotein (see Figure 11-5) although monoclonal components can be seen in the β-globulin through γ-globulin regions.

Monoclonal components are derived from an uncontrolled proliferation of a *single clone of B lymphocytes* that have differentiated into monoclonal antibody-producing plasma cells, at the expense of other B cell clones. The stimulus for the proliferation is not known but it is probably not antigenic. For example, an increase in a monoclonal component, such as IgM, is seen in a condition known as Waldenstrom's macroglobulinemia (One Step Further Box 11-1).

Certain molecules, such as C-reactive protein, fibrinogen, C3 variant, and hemoglobin-haptoglobin complexes that are present in a hemolyzed specimen, may appear in the same region of the electrophoretogram as the monoclonal components. These molecules can be characterized and differentiated from monoclonal components by immunofixation or immunoelectrophoresis (described following).

Polyclonal Gammopathies

Polyclonal gammopathies are characterized by a broad, diffuse, and intensely staining band in the γ region of the serum protein electrophoretic pattern, representing an increase in the quantity of polyclonal immunoglobulins.

Polyclonal serum immunoglobulins (i.e., increase in various classes of immunoglobulins) are a product of various plasma cells, seen most frequently in response to an antigenic stimulation by infectious agents. Thus a polyclonal increase reflects a common protein abnormality that may be associated with such conditions as

Box 11-1

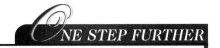

Waldenstrom's Macroglobulinemia

Classification

Waldenstrom's macroglobulinemia (WM) (primary macroglobulinemia) is classified under monoclonal gammopathies as a malignant lymphoproliferative disorder.

Monoclonal gammopathies are a group of disorders, also referred to as *plasma cell dyscrasias*, that are characterized by an uncontrolled proliferation of a single clone or line of plasma cells (antibody-producing cells of the B cell lineage). These cells produce a homogenous (similar in structure) monoclonal (M-) protein at the expense of other clones.

The *M-protein* represents an overproduction of a normal protein, such as the IgM in Waldenstrom's macroglobulinemia. Although M-proteins are referred to as "abnormal" because of their homogeneity that appears as a spike on an electrophoretogram, nevertheless, they are only an excessive quantity of immunoglobulins that occur normally. Thus presence of M-protein requires a specific assay, such as immunofixation electrophoresis (IFE) or immunoelectrophoresis (IEP) for identification of the heavy-chain class and light-chain type in order to characterize the "abnormal" immunoglobulin.

Mechanism of Disease

Although the cause of WM is not known, genetic predisposition may play a role (based on observation of certain relatives of patients with the disorder).

The WM disorder, found mainly in older individuals, is characterized by a malignant proliferation of the B cell line with an increased number of antibody-secreting plasma cells. The resulting abnormally high amounts of IgM class produced are responsible for the accumulation of IgM in plasma (intravenous accumulation). Thus patients with WM exhibit a feeling of weakness and fatigue, bleeding from the nose, gums, gastrointestinal tract, and other locations (leading to anemia) as well as an increased occurrence of infections, weight loss, and an increase in blood viscosity (hyperviscosity). Hyperviscosity may result in neurologic disturbances and cardiac and vascular insufficiency.

Laboratory Findings

When screening for suspected Waldenstrom's macroglobulinemia (Figure 11-6), presence of the M-protein on the electrophoretogram requires characterization of the M-protein by immunofixation (IFE) or immunoelectrophoresis (IEP) assays and quantification of the IgM in serum is performed using nephelometry. Urine sample is evaluated by IEP or IFE (method of choice) for presence of M-protein.

For example (see Figure 11-6), a patient's serum may show a characteristic monoclonal peak on the electrophoretic scan that is identified by immunofixation electrophoresis (see Figures 11-5 and 11-7) as IgM heavy chains and κ light chains (IgAκ). IFE performed on a urine sample shows free κ light chains also known as Bence Jones protein. Nephelometric measurements quantify the IgM and κ light chains, thus confirming the existence of a monoclonal gammopathy, suggestive of Waldenstrom's macroglobulinemia. When no monoclonal band is found on SPEP, no further testing is indicated.

ELECTROPHORESIS RESULTS

A sharp spike is observed in the gamma globulin region of an electrophoretogram although the abnormal spike may also appear in the β-through γ-globulin regions, suggesting presence of monoclonal immunoglobulins (see Figure 11-5).

IMMUNOELECTROPHORESIS RESULTS

Although IEP is less sensitive and more difficult to interpret than the immunofixation procedure, the IEP procedure can be used for evaluation of monoclonal protein (M-protein) by characterizing specific light and heavy chain components of the M-protein (see Figure 11-7).

IMMUNOFIXATION RESULTS

Currently IFE is the method of choice for specific identification of abnormal proteins. The procedure is quicker, more sensitive, and easier to interpret than immunoelectrophoresis.

An example of immunofixation results, from a serum sample to which an anti-IgM, κ and λ (antisera) has been applied, is the appearance of localized (distinct) IgM band and a similar kappa band, indicating the presence of IgMκ monoclonal protein (Figure 11-8).

QUANTIFICATION RESULTS

The quantity of monoclonal protein (M-protein) present in a patient's sample is reported in mg/dL when a nephelometric procedure is employed. In this example, anti-IgM (antiserum) is used in the nephelometric procedure to quantify IgM, according to the established protocol.

Continued

Box 11-1—cont'd

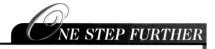

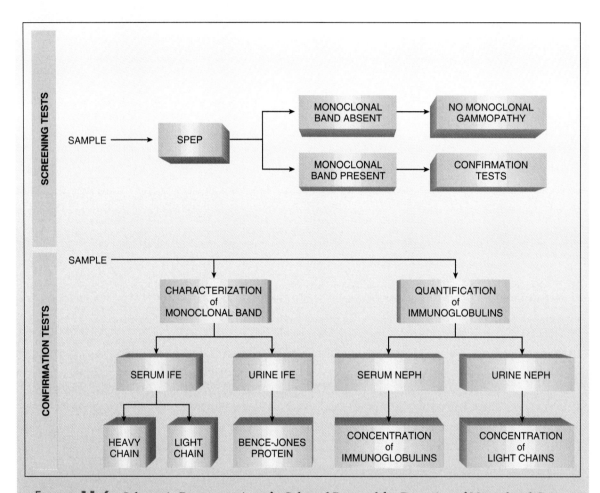

FIGURE **11-6** **Schematic Representation of a Selected Protocol for Detection of Monoclonal Gammopathies.** Monoclonal gammopathies such as Waldenstrom's macroglobulinemia can be detected by *screening of serum for monoclonal immunoglobulins* by serum protein electrophoresis (SPEP) and (2) by *confirmation testing* using immunofixation electrophoresis (IFE) to characterize the abnormal immunoglobulin (Ig) as γ, α, μ, ϵ or δ (heavy chain) and κ or λ (light chain). Detected mIg can be quantified in mg/dL by nephelometry. *SPEP,* serum protein electrophoresis; *IFE,* immunofixation electrophoresis; *Neph,* nephelometry.

Box 11-1—cont'd

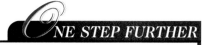

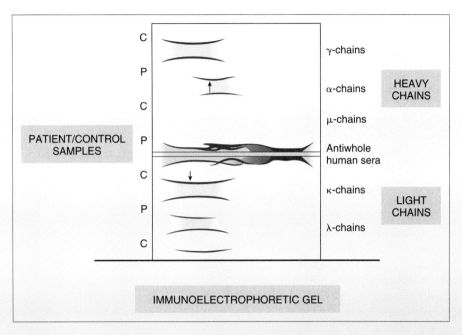

FIGURE **11-7** **Immunoelectrophoretic Gel (Membrane) Showing Monoclonal Immunoglobulin Pattern.** Characterization of an abnormal monoclonal immunoglobulin (mIg) is made by comparison of arcs formed by patient and control serum immunoglobulins (Igs) on the gel. Note presence of a denser precipitin arc *(arrows)* at the site where the patient's γ heavy chain and κ light chain interact with their specific antisera (anti-IgA, anti-κ). *These patterns indicate presence of monoclonal gammopathy of IgA(κ) specificity (IgA heavy chain, κ light chain).* γ, gamma (IgG); α, alpha (IgA); μ, mu (IgM); κ, kappa chain; λ, lambda Ig; *C,* normal control (pooled human serum); *P,* patient serum.

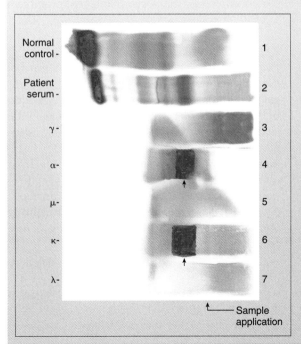

FIGURE **11-8** **Characterization of Monoclonal Gammopathies by Immunofixation Electrophoresis (IFE).** Deeply stained bands (see *arrows* pointing to α and κ chains in lanes 4 and 6, respectively) are readily visible on IFE gel (membrane) and indicate the presence of IgA(κ) monoclonal immunoglobulin. (See also text.) *Ig,* immunoglobulin; α, alpha Ig (IgA); γ, gamma Ig (IgG); μ, mu Ig (IgM), κ, kappa Ig, λ, lambda Ig. (Courtesy Monmouth Medical Center, New Jersey.)

chronic infections, inflammation, or chronic liver disease.

Comments

Clinical Application

Clinical application of protein electrophoresis includes its use as a presumptive screening test for serum protein abnormalities. For example:

- In *paraprotein disorders,* such as multiple myeloma and Waldenström's macroglobulinemia (see One Step Further Box 11-1), a protein spike (abnormal peak) is seen in the γ-globulin region of the electrophoretogram (see Figure 11-5).
- Appearance of oligoclonal bands within the γ region of the patient's cerebrospinal fluid (CSF) protein electrophoresis is suggestive of the presence of *multiple sclerosis (MS)* (One Step Further Box 11-2).

Although protein electrophoresis serves as a valuable tool in screening for protein abnormalities, definitive diagnosis must be made on the basis of other more sensitive methods (e.g., immunoelectrophoresis or immunofixation electrophoresis), which provide information on the identity of a particular protein.

Technical Errors

Technical errors have an effect on the quality and interpretation of electrophoretic results. For example:

- *Artifacts* may form in a hemolyzed sample, which has been improperly stored or processed, and can be mistaken for the monoclonal component in the α_2-globulin and β-globulin regions of the electrophoretogram.
- Poor or excessive migration of protein molecules, caused by insufficient or increased time, or as a result of the amount of voltage applied to gel, or because of improper preparation of the buffer, may cause abnormal results.
- *Overfilling wells* in gel will increase the quantity of proteins within the sample and may cause cross-contamination of the samples.
- A sharp peak in the β region (patient on anticoagulation therapy) may be the result of fibrinogen and can be mistaken for IgA.

IMMUNOELECTROPHORESIS

General Concept

Immunoelectrophoresis (IEP) is typically performed as a confirmation procedure when a monoclonal component (M-protein or paraprotein) is detected on protein electrophoresis (see Figure 11-5). IEP procedure allows characterization of monoclonal proteins by identifying specific heavy-chain (H chain) class and light-chain (L chain) immunoglobulin components, seen on the electrophoretogram (scan) as a sharp spike in the γ-globulin or β-globulin through γ-region (see Figure 11-5). The procedure is used to differentiate polyclonal from monoclonal increase in immunoglobulins.

The IEP is a two-step process that combines electrophoresis and immunodiffusion, as follows:

- *Electrophoresis* is used to separate proteins in serum or urine (as described previously).
- *Immunodiffusion/precipitation* involves diffusion of separated proteins (antigens) and reagent antibody molecules (antiserum) of known specificity in gel. Subsequent precipitation of the antigen and antibody molecules occurs at the point where the two reactants (antigen, antibody) meet and form antigen-antibody complexes that are visible as precipitin lines in gel.

Procedure

Briefly, serum or urine samples and a normal control are placed in antigen wells in the test gel and their protein molecules are separated by electrophoresis. Antiserum (monospecific reagent antibodies) (i.e., anti-alpha [α], anti-gamma [γ], and anti-mu [μ] heavy chains and anti-kappa [κ] and anti-lambda [λ] light chains) are then placed in troughs also prepared in test gels. As the antigens and antibodies diffuse toward each other, antigen-antibody complexes form, producing a precipitin at the point where they meet (see Figure 11-7).

The free (unbound) proteins in gel are then removed by rinsing, and the remaining precipitated antigen-antibody complexes (precipitin arcs) are stained for evaluation. The test samples are compared with precipitin arcs

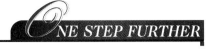

Box 11-2

Multiple Sclerosis

Mechanism of Disease

Although the cause of multiple sclerosis (MS) is not known, it is believed that a combination of genetic and environmental factors is responsible for the development of the disease. Inheritance of histocompatibility (HLA) DRw15 and DQw6 has also been associated with MS. Further, it has been proposed that an inflammatory response of the immune system to bacteria or viruses may be responsible for triggering the autoimmune response seen in MS.

Immunoglobulin G (IgG), produced in the cerebrospinal fluid (CSF) of approximately 80% of patients with MS, is directed mainly against the basic protein of the myelin sheath of an axon. Thus destruction of the myelin sheath (demyelination) results in formation of lesions, known as *plaques,* in the white matter of the brain and spinal cord. This damage to the tissues of the central nervous system can result in various sensory abnormalities, such as visual disturbances and lack of locomotor (movement) coordination.

The degree of disease activity can be assessed by performing an assay for myelin basic protein (MBP), a component of the myelin sheath. Presence of MBP in CSF is indicative of an active demyelinating process as seen in MS.

Laboratory Findings

Because of the fact that proteins have the ability to cross the blood-brain barrier and that patients with inflammatory diseases of the central nervous system, such as MS, show an increase in gamma globulin synthesized within their CSF (local synthesis), it is important to ascertain the source of the IgG present in the CSF. The question to be answered is: are these IgG molecules synthesized in the CSF or do they originate from the serum?

There are no characteristic autoantibodies that can be detected in MS. However, two assays are currently commonly used in the laboratory to establish the source of the IgGs in the CSF, thus providing useful information to support the diagnosis of MS. These methods include oligoclonal banding and the CSF IgG index (see following).

OLIGOCLONAL BANDING

Synthesis and normal distribution of IgG (electrophoretic pattern [see Figure 11-5]) in a normal serum sample reflects the function of a variety of plasma cells. In MS, however, the CSF *electrophoretic pattern* shows multiple bands in the γ region, instead of the normal distribution of gamma globulins.

Separation of protein molecules by *isoelectric focusing* in CSF and serum samples of a patient with possible MS produces a band pattern (oligoclonal bands) in the γ region of the CSF but not in the serum sample (Figure 11-9). Therefore, appearance of oligoclonal bands in CSF but not in the serum sample indicates a positive test for neurologic abnormality and is suggestive of MS disease.

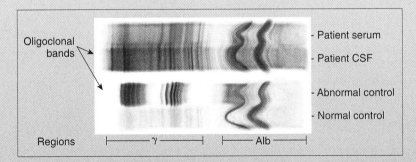

FIGURE **11-9 Isoelectric Focusing Band Pattern.** Band pattern produced in γ and albumin regions on gel, representing separated protein molecules in patient's serum and cerebrospinal fluid (CSF) and in a normal and abnormal samples used as controls (all four samples are analyzed simultaneously). Note presence of bands *(oligoclonal bands)* in the CSF γ region but not in the serum, indicating local (brain) production of IgG *(positive test for a neurologic abnormality, such as multiple sclerosis).* (Courtesy Monmouth Medical Center, New Jersey.)

Continued

Box 11-2—cont'd

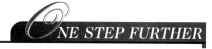

ONE STEP FURTHER

CSF IgG INDEX
In addition to oligoclonal banding, determination of a CSF IgG index (IgG/albumin ratio) can also provide information regarding the origin of the increase in CSF IgG. The index is calculated by the equation that follows, using the CSF and serum concentration of albumin and IgG values obtained by nephelometric procedure.

$$CSF\ IgG\ index = \frac{IgG_{CSF}/albumin_{CSF}}{IgG_{serum}/albumin_{serum}}$$

The CSF IgG index can be interpreted as follows:
• The CSF index remains within the normal range (0.0 to 0.77 mg/dL) when the increase in IgG is caused by an increased permeability of blood-brain barrier.
• An abnormally high index indicates an increase in CSF IgG produced by increased local synthesis.

formed by individual proteins in the normal serum sample (control).

Evaluation of Results
Analysis of the gel for immunoprecipitin bands obtained from a patient test sample may show an increase in the quantity of precipitin formed and suggests an abnormal production of antibodies, seen in such conditions as monoclonal gammopathy described in One Step Further Box 11-1. Absence of precipitin lines is suggestive of an immunodeficiency state.

Comments
Technical Errors
Technical errors that will produce inaccurate results include the following:
• *Improper storage:* Serum, urine, and cerebrospinal fluid samples must be stored in a frozen state to preserve antigens if the assay is delayed for more than a day.
• *Poor technical performance of IEP:* This includes electrophoretic separation of proteins, concentration of specimens and antisera, immunodiffusion step, and staining and photographic procedures.

IMMUNOFIXATION ELECTROPHORESIS

General Concept
Immunofixation electrophoresis (IFE) procedure is used as an alternative to immunoelectrophoresis (IEP) technique for characterization of protein fractions in monoclonal gammopathies in terms of:
• Antigen specificity
• Electrophoretic mobility

• Quantity of each protein fraction
• Ratio of one protein to other protein fractions

Both immunofixation and immunoelectrophoresis contain a two-step process, in which protein electrophoresis is the first step and immunoprecipitation is the second. However, the IFE procedure differs from IEP (described previously) in that during the second step of IFE, monospecific antisera are applied (overlayed) directly over the gel and allowed to bind with the antigens of corresponding specificity to form a band if a monoclonal protein is present.

Procedure
Briefly, the patient's serum sample and the normal control are electrophoresed as described in the discussion of serum protein electrophoresis. Specific antibodies are applied directly to the supporting gel. As antigen-antibody complexes form between the two reactants (antigens, antibodies) of the corresponding specificity, immunoprecipitin bands can be seen in gel. The non-precipitated proteins are then washed out of the gel. Only the precipitated antigen-antibody complexes (bands) remain in the gel for staining to facilitate their visualization.

Evaluation of Results
Gels are evaluated for typical patterns of staining characteristic for monoclonal immunoglobulins in monoclonal gammopathies. These monoclonal immunoglobulins show narrow, deeply stained bands, which differentiate them from polyclonal immunoglobulins, which show broad, diffusely stained areas or patterns in gel (see Figure 11-8).

Table **11-2**	**SELECTED CHARACTERISTICS OF IMMUNOELECTROPHORESIS AND IMMUNOFIXATION ELECTROPHORESIS**	
Characteristics of Electrophoresis	Immunoelectrophoresis	Immunofixation Electrophoresis
Sensitivity	Less sensitive than IFE	Can characterize any monoclonal band separated on SPE
Resolution	Some paraproteins (mAbs) cannot be separated	Separates monoclonal bands showing close electrophoretic mobility
Ease of interpretation	More difficult to interpret than IFE (Slight deviation in shape of precipitin arc)	Results easier to interpret than IEP (precipitin patterns correspond to SPE pattern)
Turn-around time	Longer than IFE (overnight incubation)	½ to 2 hours
Labor and cost	Relative ease of performance and less costly than IFE	Labor-intensive and costly

SPE, serum protein electrophoresis; IFE, immunofixation electrophoresis, IEP, immunoelectrophoresis; mAbs, monoclonal antibodies (immunoglobulins).

Comments

Immunofixation electrophoresis is currently the method of choice in many diagnostic laboratories for characterization (typing) of monoclonal immunoglobulins and is replacing the traditional immunoelectrophoresis procedure because of the attributes of IFE described in Table 11-2.

ELECTROIMMUNODIFFUSION

In the previously described immunodiffusion electrophoresis (i.e., immunoelectrophoresis) and immunofixation electrophoresis procedures, an electric current is employed for the separation of proteins (antigens). The diffusion of antigen and antibody molecules toward one another and formation of precipitin lines (antigen-antibody complexes), however, is a passive process that may be enhanced by an electromotive force. Therefore it is possible to drive the antigen and antibody toward each other more quickly by applying voltage (electric current) to gel containing the separated proteins, thus reducing the time required for formation of antigen-antibody complex when both reactants are of the same specificity.

Countercurrent Electrophoresis
General Concept

The principle of countercurrent electrophoresis procedure is similar to that of double immunodiffusion (described previously) with the addition of an electric current for separation of antigen proteins. However, selected pH of the support medium must be able to produce a different surface charge of the antigen and antibody molecules, thus allowing these molecules to move toward each other at the selected pH.

For example, at pH 8.0 the antibody is positively charged and moves to the negative pole, while the negatively charged antigen moves toward the positive pole in an electric field. As the two reactants meet, precipitin bands or lines will form, when the antibody and antigen show the same specificity.

The identity of an antigen or an antibody can be determined according to the formation of precipitin lines, described in the discussion of immunoelectrophoresis and in Figure 11-7.

Electroimmunoassay (Rocket Electrophoresis)
General Concept

The procedure depends on creation of different charges of the antibody and antigen molecules at a selected pH of the support medium (gel, agarose, or cellulose acetate). The pH of the gel is chosen so that the antibodies distributed within the support medium maintain a neutral charge, remaining stationary within the gel, whereas the antigen at the selected pH becomes negatively charged, thus moving (diffusing) toward the positive pole (anode) when an electric current is applied to the antibody-containing gel.

As the antigens move through gel in an electric field, several precipitin bands appear in the antibody-containing gel. The height of each band, referred to as "rocket," is proportional to the antigen concentration of the sample.

Standards containing various concentrations of antigen are processed together with the patient's sample and a graph is constructed, by using the height of each standard as its concentration. The concentration of the test sample is interpolated from the constructed curve.

The procedure may be applied to any protein (antigen) that has a different electrophoretic mobility than the antibody incorporated within the support medium. However, the electroimmunoassay procedure is not used routinely for analysis of immunoglobulins because special treatment is required to increase the migration of immunoglobulins to the positive pole.

ISOELECTRIC FOCUSING

Isoelectric focusing (IEF) is another procedure that is used to separate a mixture of proteins. The separation of protein molecules in the IEF procedure depends on very small differences that exist between their isoelectric points. Although the procedure has mainly been used in the clinical laboratory for detecting certain serum enzymes and for hemoglobin separation, it is now also performed to detect oligoclonal immunoglobulin bands in cerebrospinal fluid (CSF) and to assist with diagnosis of multiple sclerosis (see One Step Further Box 11-2) and other diseases affecting the central nervous system.

General Concept

Immunoglobulins are protein molecules, composed of amino acids, which can be either negatively or positively charged. Such molecules are known as amphoteric molecules because of their ability to behave as an acid or a base, depending on the pH of the medium in which they are suspended.

By creating a pH gradient within the medium in which proteins are suspended, the protein molecules will move in an electrophoretic system to a point where their *isoelectric point (pI) is equal to the pH of the medium.* At this point, their mobility is interrupted and the band patterns produced in gel represent separated protein molecules according to their isoelectric points.

The pH gradient in gel is produced by addition of carrier ampholytes (amphoteric compounds that have their isoelectric point over a broad range of pH).

Thus the basis for the isoelectric focusing procedure is the electrophoretic separation of immunoglobulins according to their isoelectric point in a pH gradient (see Figure 11-9).

Procedure

Briefly, the patient's serum and CSF IgG are quantified, and the IgG concentration of the serum sample is adjusted by diluting the sample to equal that of the CSF IgG. Conversely, the CSF can be concentrated to equal the amount of IgG present in serum.

A sample of CSF and an appropriately diluted serum sample from the same patient are placed into adjacent wells located within commercially prepared agarose gel. The samples are allowed to diffuse into the gel, which is then placed in the IEF unit (prepared according to manufacturer's instructions) for separation of protein molecules.

Electrophoresis of the gel containing diffused molecules consists of migration of charged molecules to oppositely charged poles (electrodes) through a pH gradient. The pH gradient between the two electrodes (anode and cathode) is created by the presence of ampholytes (solution of macromolecules showing different isoelectric points).

As the migrating molecules reach a point where the pH of the gel is equal to the pI of each migrating protein molecule, their net charge becomes zero (no charge) and their migration stops. At this point, a band pattern is produced in gel representing each separated protein molecule (see Figure 11-9). The bands are fixed and stained with silver stain for visualization.

Evaluation of Results

Test results of the serum and cerebrospinal fluid (CSF) samples are evaluated for the presence of 2 to 15 discrete (sharp) oligoclonal bands (IgG class) in the gel at pH 7.0 to 9.3 (see One Step Further Box 11-2). These bands appear in the IgG region of the electrophoretogram and have been identified as IgG class by immunofixation electrophoresis.

Patients with no neurologic disease have an IgG concentration of less than 10% of their total CSF proteins. However, in neurologic abnormalities, such as multiple sclerosis (MS), the patients typically show IgG concentration of 11% to 35% of their total CSF proteins (see One Step Further Box 11-2).

Although the interpretation of oligoclonal bands is subjective, the following guidelines may be helpful in evaluating the test results:

- Banding present in CSF sample but not present in the serum sample indicates local (CSF) production of IgG (positive test result).
- Identical banding present in both the CSF and serum samples indicates passage of IgG from blood into the CSF through the blood-brain barrier because of increased permeability.
- Abnormal and normal control samples should be included with the patient's sample. Normal samples (CSF and serum) show diffuse bands.
- Two calculations, based on CSF and serum IgG and albumin concentrations, have been found useful for evaluation of local (CSF) production of IgG. These are the *IgG index* and *IgG synthesis rate*.

Comments

Although the isoelectric focusing (IEF) shows sensitivity to multiple sclerosis (MS), the procedure is not specific for MS. Other neurologic disorders, such as viral encephalitis, psychoneurosis, and cerebral infarction also produce oligoclonal banding. Results of a more recent study indicate that patients with acquired immunodeficiency syndrome (AIDS) also have a high incidence of oligoclonal bands in their cerebrospinal fluid (CSF). In view of these findings, interpretation of oligoclonal bands in the CSF of a patient suspected of having MS should be considered as an adjunct to the clinical evaluation and correlation and other diagnostic procedures [e.g., CSF index and presence of myelin basic protein (MBP)] that are used in the diagnosis of MS (see One Step Further Box 11-2).

LIGHT SCATTERING IMMUNOASSAYS

Biologic and drug molecules (soluble antigen), —often referred to as *analytes* (Box 11-3)—are detectable in biologic fluid samples such as serum, urine, and cerebrospinal fluid. When the analyte molecule interacts with its corresponding antibody (high affinity reagent antibody of the same specificity as the antigen), the resulting antigen-antibody complexes produce aggregates that increase in size and eventually form immunoprecipitins.

The formed immunoprecipitins have the ability to scatter a beam of light as it passes through a sample. Thus the concentration of immunoprecipitins in a solution (liquid support medium) can be determined by measuring light scatter (Figure 11-10) with an appropriate instrument either as an antigen-antibody interaction occurs *(rate assay)* or as the interaction reaches an equilibrium *(end-point assay)*. The methods capable of measuring the light scatter are known as:

- *Turbidimetry:* Photometric determination of the reduction of light that passes through a solution or detection of a forward light scatter (turbidity).
- *Nephelometry:* Detection of light scatter at a 90° angle.

These *methods differ* from each other primarily by the type of instrument that is used

Box 11-3	SELECTED BIOLOGIC AND DRUG ANALYTE MOLECULES DETECTABLE BY IMMUNOLOGIC ASSAYS
Biologic Molecules	**Drug Molecules**
Immunoglobulins (IgG, IgA, IgM, IgD, IgE)	Drugs of abuse, Antibiotics
Protein hormones	Hormones (e.g., steroid)
Complement components (C3, C4, factor B)	Prostaglandins
Lipoprotein	Anticonvulsant drugs
Coagulation factors (Factor VIII, fibrinogen)	Digoxin/Digitonin

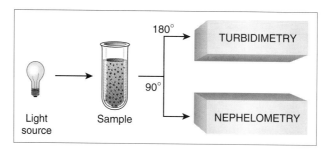

FIGURE **11-10** **Light Scatter Measurements.** Two types of optical arrangements are shown for measuring light scatter by immunoglobulins: *turbidimetry,* detecting reduction of forward light scatter (180°) by antigen/antibody complexes formed in a solution; *nephelometry,* measuring the light scattered by particles at an 90° angle.

to measure the light scattered by antigen-antibody complexes formed in the liquid medium. The two *methods* are *similar* in their ability to measure light scatter (see Figure 11-10) as the antigen-antibody reaction occurs (rate assay) or as the reaction reaches a point of equivalence (equilibrium, see Figure 11-3). In addition, both methods can be automated, thus quickly providing results that enable a fast "turnaround" time.

IMMUNOTURBIDIMETRIC METHODS

General Concept

In the immunoturbidimetric procedure, the quantity of an antigen-antibody complex formed in a liquid medium (solution) can be determined by the degree of turbidity or cloudiness that is produced in the solution, thus an instrument with an appropriate detector, such as an automated chemistry analyzer, is able to detect the amount of **light absorbed (optical density),** not the amount of **light scattered,** by the formed antigen-antibody complexes, as does a nephelometer (see following).

In turbidimetry, when an instrument containing an appropriate light detection device (detector) is placed in a direct line with the incident light (original path of light), the detector measures the light reduced by absorption as it passes through the sample. The *reduction in light intensity is measured in absorbance units (optical density),* which represent the ratio of incident light to the transmitted light, and is proportional to the size, shape, and concentration of the antigen-

antibody complexes formed in the measured sample (see Figure 11-10).

The measurement may be performed either as an *end-point* or as the *rate* of an antigen-antibody reaction. In clinical chemistry, however, a widely used measurement of turbidity is a two-point technique (for explanation, refer to any clinical chemistry textbook).

Evaluation of Results

In a turbidemitric determination of light scatter, a linear relationship exists between the concentration of an analyte in the sample and the optical density (OD) reading. Thus, a standard curve can be constructed using optical density vs. antigen (e.g., protein) concentration. *The concentration of the analyte (antigen) in the sample can be interpolated from the standard curve.*

IMMUNONEPHELOMETRIC METHOD

General Concept

As in the immunoturbidimetric procedure, the antigen-antibody complexes formed in a liquid medium can be quantified by measuring the light that has passed through the sample. However, in the nephelometric method, the *amount of light that is **scattered** at a particular angle* (e.g., 90°) from the incident beam of light as it passes through the sample is measured by the nephelometer, equipped with an appropriate detector (see Figure 11-10). The *amount of light scattered* is an index of the concentration of the antigen-antibody complexes in the sample.

In addition, as in the turbidimetric method, the nephelometric method has the capability of measuring the kinetic (rate of reaction) and end-point reaction for quantifying antigens (e.g., serum proteins). However, the end-point method, being a simpler procedure and requiring less sophisticated instruments, is the method of choice.

Evaluation of Results

In nephelometry, *the constructed standard curve is non-linear* and needs inclusion of calibrators and other curve-fitting routines as well as inclusion of quality control materials (commercial source) with each analytic "run" before interpolating the results.

Comments

General Comments

Commercially prepared kits are currently available for light scatter immunoassays and include appropriate standards with assigned values for the included analytes (antigens). Small antigen molecules such as a drugs (see Table 11-3) must be linked (conjugated) to a large carrier molecule (protein) to increase the size of the antigen before reacting to a specific reagent antibody.

Nephelometry is the method of choice for quantification of plasma proteins.

Technical Errors

The following measures and considerations can reduce technical errors:

- Reagent antibody must be in excess for valid quantification of the analyte when using these methods, thus avoiding falsely low precipitin formation.
- The reagent antibody must be of high affinity and titer and must contribute only a minimal amount of background light scatter.
- Lipidemia causes high background light scatter and must be avoided.
- End-point methods are influenced by colored solutions and are factors requiring attention.
- Reliability of the rate method depends on formation of uniform particles (aggregates). The method requires constant mixing during the formation of antigen-antibody complexes.
- False negatives (low levels) can be caused by prozone reaction, such as occurs when an excess of antibodies is present. In such situations, dilution of the serum sample is required.

Suggested Readings

Duc J, B Morel, Petrequin R, Frei PC: Identification of monoclonal gammopathies: a comparison of immunofixation, immunoelectrophoresis, and measurements of kappa- and lambda-immunoglobulin levels, *J Clin Lab Immunol* 26:141-146, 1988.

Henry JB: *Clinical diagnosis and management by laboratory methods,* ed 19, Philadelphia, 1996, WB Saunders.

Ross NR, et al, editors: *Manual of clinical laboratory immunology,* ed 5, Washington, DC, 1997, American Society of Microbiology.

Review Questions

IMMUNODIFFUSION TECHNIQUES

1. Optimum precipitin formation is seen in which of the following zones on a precipitin curve:
   a. postzone
   b. prozone
   c. zone of equivalence
   d. zone of antibody excess

2. Select the factor(s) that have an effect on an immunoprecipitation assay:
   a. concentration of reacting antigen and antibody molecules
   b. hydrogen ion concentration (pH)
   c. antibody affinity and avidity
   d. all of the above

3. Immunodiffusion procedures have been classified according to:
   a. direction of the diffusing molecules
   b. number of reacting molecules
   c. direction of the electric current
   d. none of the above

4. The antigen-antibody reaction may be represented by a precipitin curve, which is constructed by plotting:
   a. amount of antibodies that have been added against the precipitin that forms
   b. amount of precipitin formed against amount of added antigen
   c. amount of antigen added against amount of detectable antibodies
   d. amount of antibodies added against amount of unknown antigen

5. Agarose is the preferred medium used in immunodiffusion because of its:
   a. ability to support antigen-antibody complexes in place
   b. neutral charge and transparency
   c. charge that is the same as the reacting molecules (antigen and antibody)
   d. all of the above

6. An immunodiffusion technique known as *Ouchterlony technique* is also known as:
   a. single immunodiffusion
   b. double immunodiffusion
   c. radial immunodiffusion
   d. none of the above

7. All of the following statements are true for double immunodiffusion procedure, *except:*
   a. antigen-antibody complexes formed may be seen as precipitin bands
   b. procedure allows for comparison of unknown antigens
   c. the location and size of precipitin formed depends on the concentration of antigen and antibody molecules
   d. the precipitin pattern is determined by the concentration of an antigen and an antibody

8-10. Match each precipitin pattern with its description:

   ___ pattern of identity
   ___ pattern of non-identity
   ___ pattern of partial identity

   a. visible spur or extended precipitin line
   b. continuous lines that merge, forming an arc
   c. two separate lines intersecting each other

11. Select statement(s) that are *not true* for the end-point method of measuring antigen concentration by radial immunodiffusion assay:
   a. the reading of ring diameter is performed at the point of equivalence
   b. precipitin diameter is measured before the zone of equivalence
   c. concentration of an unknown antigen is interpolated from a standard curve
   d. method uses support medium containing stationary reagent antibodies

IMMUNOELECTROPHORETIC TECHNIQUES

12. Select the most commonly used method in a clinical laboratory for separating protein mixtures:
    a. isoelectric focusing
    b. double immunodiffusion
    c. electrophoresis
    d. electroimmunodiffusion

13. Movement of molecules in an electric field depends mainly on:
    a. surface charge of the molecules in a support medium
    b. concentration of the molecules
    c. type of support medium
    d. all of the above

14. Scanning of stained protein fractions (bands) separated by electrophoresis in gel allows:
    a. identification of immunoglobulin heavy and light chains
    b. quantification of discrete protein molecules
    c. conversion of stained bands into appropriate optical density units
    d. all of the above

15. Select a protein abnormality that is most commonly encountered when performing electrophoresis assay:
    a. multiple myeloma
    b. polyclonal gammopathy
    c. monoclonal gammopathy
    d. monoclonal paraprotein

16. The clinical application of immunoelectrophoresis is to:
    a. identify heavy and light chain immunoglobulin components
    b. differentiate polyclonal from monoclonal increase in immunoglobulins
    c. characterize monoclonal proteins
    d. all of the above

17. One of the statements below is true for immunofixation electrophoresis but *not* for immunoelectrophoresis:
    a. electrophoresis is performed after diffusion
    b. antibody is directly overlayed on the gel
    c. antibody is placed into the trough in gel
    d. the method is used mainly for antigen characterization

18. The following characteristic(s) of various protein fractions, in monoclonal gammopathies, can be determined by serum electrophoresis:
    a. antigen specificity
    b. electrophoretic mobility
    c. quantity of each protein fraction
    d. all of the above

19. Immunofixation electrophoresis (IFE) is currently the method of choice for characterization of monoclonal immunoglobulins and is rapidly replacing:
    a. double immunodiffusion procedure
    b. radial immunodiffusion procedure
    c. immunoelectrophoresis procedure
    d. electrophoresis procedure

20. Antigen and antibody molecules can be driven toward each other by applying electric current to gel containing these molecules, to hasten formation of antigen-antibody complexes, in a procedure known as:
    a. electrophoresis
    b. immunoelectrophoresis
    c. countercurrent electrophoresis
    d. electroimmunodiffusion

21. The principle of countercurrent electrophoresis is similar to:
    a. radial immunodiffusion
    b. double immunodiffusion
    c. electroimmunodiffusion
    d. immunoelectrophoresis

22. A procedure currently used to detect oligoclonal immunoglobulin bands in cerebrospinal fluid (CSF) in diseases affecting the central nervous system, such as multiple sclerosis, is:
    a. electroimmunoassay
    b. isoelectric focusing
    c. electroimmunodiffusion
    d. immunoelectrophoresis

LIGHT SCATTERING IMMUNOASSAYS

23. Concentration of formed immunoprecipitins in a liquid medium is determined by:
    a. photometric determination of reduction of light that passes through a solution
    b. detection of forward light scatter
    c. detection of light scattered at a 90° angle
    d. all of the above

24. Select statement(s) listed following that apply to rate nephelometry:
    a. measurements are time dependent
    b. the method is more sensitive than the turbidimetric method
    c. readings are taken before the zone of equivalence
    d. all of the above

25. Measurements of reduction of light intensity in optical density units, because of light absorption by formed antigen-antibody complexes in a sample, are performed by:
    a. immunonephelometry
    b. immunoturbidimetry
    c. isoelectric focusing
    d. all of the above

26-29. Match the following methods with their
corresponding characteristics:

_____ radial immunodiffusion (RID)
_____ turbidimetry
_____ rocket electrophoresis
_____ nephelometry

a. concentration is directly
   proportional to the ring diameter^2
b. combines RID method with
   electrophoresis
c. readings indicate the ratio of
   incident light to transmitted light
d. detects light scattered at a angle

Agglutination Techniques

Upon completion of Chapter 12, the student will be prepared to:

MECHANISM OF AGGLUTINATION

- Define the following terms: *particulate antigens, carrier particle, lattices, aggregates, in vivo* and *in vitro reactions, sensitization,* and *end-point of agglutination reaction.*
- State the main purpose for performing an agglutination reaction.
- Describe the two phases occurring in an agglutination reaction.
- Name six ways that lattice formation can be enhanced.
- Explain the effect that the following factors have on agglutination reaction: class of antibodies, zeta potential, number of epitopes, concentration of reactants (antigen, antibody), mixing and incubation time.

METHODS

- Describe the major differences between direct and indirect agglutination.
- Define the following terms: *hemagglutination, agglutinin, agglutinogen,* and *titer.*
- List the currently available carrier particles in methods that use agglutination reactions.
- State the main difference between passive (indirect) agglutination and reverse passive agglutination.
- Describe the mechanism involved in agglutination-inhibition reaction.
- Indicate the reason for using a second antibody in antiglobulin procedures.
- Explain the difference between in vivo and in vitro sensitization of red blood cells.
- State the clinical application for direct and indirect Coombs' tests.

Key Terms

adsorption - Attachment of an antigen or antibody onto the surface of a particle, such as a red blood cell or latex particle.

agglutination - Visible end-point of an antigen-antibody reaction, caused by formation of aggregates when particulate antigens are used in the reaction.

aggregates - Clumping or aggregation of particles, such as red blood cells, bacteria, or inert particles, as a result of formation of lattices (cross-linking) between the particles.

antiglobulin - Anti-human globulin (antibodies produced in animals against human globulin) that is used in antiglobulin tests (Coombs' tests) as a second antibody that bridges the space between red blood cells, thus facilitating formation of lattices.

carrier particle - Refers to red blood cells and certain inert particles, such as latex, that are coated (usually commercially) with either a multivalent antigen or with a divalent antibody. Carrier particles are used as reagents in agglutination reactions.

cross-linking - Refers to binding that occurs between an antigen and an antibody showing a corresponding specificity, resulting in lattice formation.

hemagglutination - An agglutination of red blood cells.

lattices - Structural arrangement that forms as antigens bind (cross-link) to specific antibody molecules, resulting in formation of antigen-antibody complexes.

monospecific antiserum - Reagent antibodies with known antigen specificity that will react with an antigen of the same specificity. For example, anti-IgG (reagent antibody) will bind only with an IgG (antigen).

particulate antigens - Antigens that occur naturally on the surface of cells (red blood cells or bacteria) or have been attached (coated) onto the surface of inert particles (latex, charcoal, or bentonite) and are used in agglutination reactions to produce a visible end-point when reacted with an antigen-specific antibody.

polyspecific antiserum - Reagent antibodies produced in animals against human globulin and containing a variety of antigen-binding sites of known specificities.

reactant - Refers to antigens or antibodies that are allowed to react with each other in an antigen-antibody reaction.

sensitization - Refers to the first stage of an antigen-antibody reaction during which an antibody attaches to a particulate antigen.

— · ✦ ● ✦ · —

Agglutination reactions occur when particulate antigens, such as cells or inert carrier particles with multiple epitopes on their surface bind with bivalent antigen-specific antibody molecules to form stable cross-linked lattices (Figure 12-1). These lattices (antigen-antibody complexes) are visible as aggregates (clumping), which may settle out of a solution when their molecular weight becomes sufficiently high. Particulate antigens, also known as *insoluble antigens*, may occur naturally on red blood cells (RBCs) or bacterial surfaces or they may consist of commercially prepared antigen-coated particles or RBCs (reagent antigens). A reagent antigen is prepared by adsorbing (attaching) antigen of known specificity onto the surface of the carrier particles to be used for detecting and quantifying unknown antibodies.

When performing an agglutination reaction, it is essential that a particulate antigen be used to react with its specific antibody when a visible agglutination (antigen-antibody complexes) is expected. The particulate antigen may serve either as the unknown antigen or as the reagent antigen, depending on the purpose of the procedure. When the carrier particle is an RBC, the agglutination reaction is known as hemagglutination.

Thus it is possible to use agglutination reactions in the following situations:

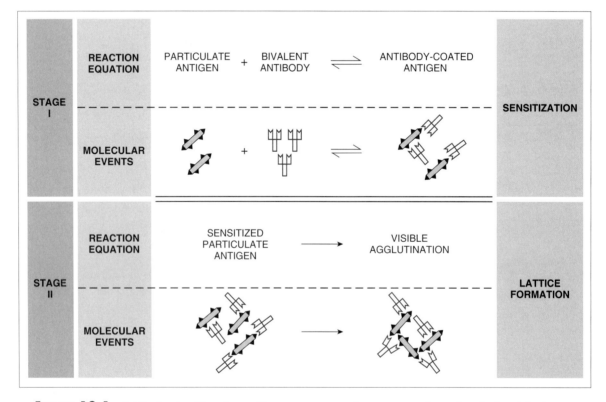

FIGURE **12-1**   **Agglutination Reaction.**   Shown are events that occur at the molecular level during the two stages of an agglutination reaction. **Stage I** illustrates events that occur as bivalent antibodies bind to multivalent particulate antigens, thus sensitizing (coating) these antigens, without producing a visible reaction. Formation of antigen-antibody complexes (lattices) is shown in **Stage II** as the sensitized particles rearrange to form visible agglutination. These events serve as the basis for various types of agglutination reactions.

- Detecting circulating (free) antibodies in plasma, using particulate antigens with known specificity (reagent antigen).
- Detecting naturally occurring antigens on the surface of RBCs and bacteria (unknown antigen), using known antisera (reagent antibodies).
- Detecting soluble antigens (unattached) by a method known as *reverse passive agglutination,* using commercial antibody-coated particles.

Agglutination reactions form the basis for many immunologic methods currently used in the clinical laboratory, which have been classified as follows:

- *Direct agglutination*
- *Indirect or passive agglutination*
- *Antibody-mediated agglutination*

Although these methods are only semiquantitative, other factors such as high sensitivity, versatility, relative ease of performance, and the method of evaluation (i.e., visual observation), make agglutination procedures a desirable choice for the detection or quantification of antibodies directed against a variety of particulate antigens.

MECHANISM OF AGGLUTINATION

The mechanism by which agglutination of particles occurs consists of a two-step process (see Figure 12-1).

- **Sensitization:** Affects antigenic particles and may occur in vivo (within the body) or in vitro (in a test tube). This reversible process involves the first stage of the antigen-antibody reaction, during which the antigen-binding site on an antibody molecule binds with a single epitope on the surface of the multi-epitope antigen. The reaction (sensitization) is not detectable, unless one of the reacting molecules is "tagged" with a substance that makes the molecule visible (see types of labels, Chapter 13).
- **Aggregate formation:** During the second stage of the reaction, cross-linking occurs between free epitopes and their corresponding antigen-binding sites of an antibody molecule, resulting in lattice formation. These lattices are detectable either

microscopically or macroscopically as aggregates or clumping.

AGGLUTINATION ENHANCEMENT TECHNIQUES

Enhancement of lattice formation (agglutination) may be performed by altering various factors, such as:

- Reducing ionic strength of the suspending medium by addition of low ionic strength saline (LISS)
- Decreasing particle surface charge by addition of albumin (5% to 30%)
- Increasing viscosity by adding such substances as dextran
- Reducing surface charge on red blood cells (RBC) and exposure of additional epitopes by adding enzymes (bromelin, papain, and ficin)
- Increasing contact between the reactants (antigen and antibody) by mixing (agitation) and centrifugation
- Maintaining appropriate temperature during the reaction; for example, IgG molecules react best at 30° to 37°C, while IgM molecules can agglutinate best at 4° to 27°C.
- Maintaining appropriate pH (6.7 to 7.2) because most reactions produce best results at this pH, except when IgM is involved

Antigen-antibody complexes formed during the agglutination reaction (described previously), particularly when IgM molecules are involved, have the ability to activate the complement system (see Figure 4-2), thus causing red blood cell lysis (hemolysis). This phase of agglutination is sometimes referred to as *tertiary reaction* (third step of agglutination reaction) because it requires an addition of complement to produce cell lysis (see complement-dependent procedures, Chapter 14). The resulting hemolysis is an indicator of an end-point of various procedures, particularly those used in blood banking.

FACTORS AFFECTING AGGLUTINATION TECHNIQUES

The effects of structural and environmental factors on the antigen-antibody reactions were previously discussed (see Chapter 10). The factors discussed following have also been shown to specifically affect agglutination reactions:

- *Class of antibody:* Multivalent antibodies (e.g., IgM class) are larger molecules that contain multiple antigen-binding sites and, therefore, are more effective than IgG in bridging the space (cross-linking) between the particulate antigens (e.g., RBCs) to form lattices (antigen-antibody complexes).
- *Charge of the "carrier" particles:* Such particles as bacteria, RBCs, and inert particles carry a negative surface charge, known as *zeta potential* (electrostatic potential or charge around the surface of a particle or RBC, discussed in Chapter 10). The density of this charge (i.e., zeta potential) can be reduced by the addition of low ionic strength saline (LISS), thus diminishing the gap between the reactants (antigen, antibody) and facilitating cross-linking.
- *Number of epitopes (antigenic determinants):* The number, location, and distribution of epitopes on a particular antigen affects the agglutination reaction. Thus antigens containing multiple epitopes (see Chapter 10, Figure 10-4) that are densely distributed will facilitate cross-linking between the epitope and the antigen-binding site on the antibody molecule.
- *Concentration of reactants:* Generally, the antigen-antibody reaction is more rapid at a higher concentration of the reactants. However, the concept of the zone of equivalence, postzone, and prozone phenomena (see Figure 10-2) discussed in Chapter 10 also applies to agglutination.
- *Environmental factors:* Agitation or mixing, centrifugation, temperature (depends on antigen-antibody system), and appropriate incubation time can enhance agglutination reaction.

METHODS

DIRECT AGGLUTINATION

Direct agglutination may be used for detection of naturally occurring *unknown antigens* (particulate antigens) by using known antigen-specific reagent antibodies. The procedure may

also be used to detect and quantify *unknown antibodies* by using known particulate reagent antigens with the same specificity.

General Concept

Antigens that naturally occur on a particle (particulate antigens), such as red blood cells (RBCs) or various microorganisms, can be directly agglutinated by an antigen-specific antibody. The agglutination reaction proceeds according to the two-stage process, as discussed previously.

Classic examples of a direct agglutination procedure are the identification of various types of bacteria (e.g., *Salmonella* species) and the detection of ABO blood group antigens present on the surface of red blood cells by a technique known as *blood group typing,* commonly used in blood banking.

Procedures
Slide and Test Tube Procedures

In identifying specific bacteria by direct agglutination, a cell suspension of an unknown bacterial sample is combined in a test tube with commercially prepared antiserum (antibodies with known antigen-specificity), and the reaction is read either immediately or after an appropriate incubation period. A positive agglutination reaction is indicated by clouding of the suspension, thus identifying the specific bacterial species.

Blood typing for ABO blood group antigens may be performed by a slide or a test tube method. Reagent antibodies (commercially prepared antiserum with known specificity for A or B antigen (i.e., anti-A or anti-B) are mixed with a suspension of the patient's red blood cells (unknown surface antigens) in saline, or in the patient's own serum and are checked for hemagglutination (agglutination of RBCs). Formation of hemagglutination (end-point of the reaction) indicates the presence of a blood group antigen on the RBC surface with the same specificity as the antiserum (Figure 12-2). Lack of hemagglutination indicates absence of that antigen. The agglutination reaction endpoint is graded according to the presence or absence of aggregates (clumps of particles or red cells). The strength of the reaction in most procedures is graded by the size of the aggregates (Figure 12-3).

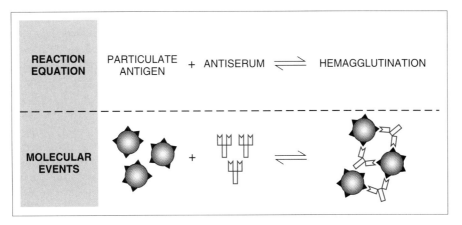

FIGURE **12-2** **Hemagglutination Reaction.**   Red blood cells (RBCs) with naturally occurring surface antigens, serving as particulate antigens, are reacted with antibodies of known specificity (antiserum). The visible lattices formed consist of agglutinated RBCs bound by their surface antigens of the same specificity as the reagent antibodies (antiserum).

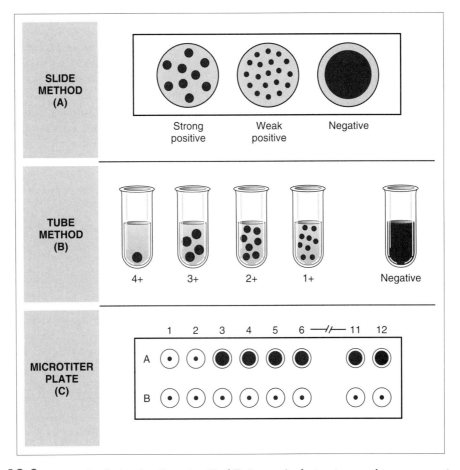

FIGURE **12-3** **Direct Agglutination Reaction End-Points.**   Agglutination can be macroscopically detected as presented in the slide method **(A)**, tube method **(B)**, or microtiter plate **(C)** techniques. Presence or absence of aggregates (clumping) of a particulate antigen. (e.g., red blood cells or latex particles) shows the reaction end-point. The grading (strength) of the reaction depends on the size of the aggregates. For example, the microtiter plate **(C)** shows positive hemagglutination in rows A 3 through 12 and no hemagglutination (negative reaction) in rows B 1 through 12.

Semiquantitative Procedure

A semiquantitative direct agglutination procedure may be performed by preparing serial dilutions of the patient's serum (antibody) in tubes or on microtiter plates and reacting it with a known particulate antigen (e.g., red blood cells). End-point of the agglutination reaction is reported as a titer.

The titer is the highest dilution giving visible agglutination and reflects the concentration of antibodies in serum with specificity for the known antigen.

Comments
Clinical Application
The following are clinical applications of direct agglutination technique:
- Detect antibodies to such organisms as *Salmonella,* a causative agent of typhoid fever, or to detect heterophil antibodies in infectious mononucleosis.
- Detect the amount of antibodies during an acute phase of a microbial infection that rises significantly with time, which is an important finding in the diagnosis and monitoring of an infection.
- Detection of an antibody titer, which must differ by at least a two-fold dilution (two tubes) between samples in order to be clinically significant (see Figure 9-2).
- Identify various antigens naturally occurring on the surface of red blood cells in blood banking practice.

Technical Considerations
The following are significant technical considerations:
- Manufacturer's directions must be carefully followed when using commercially prepared reagents.
- Positive and negative controls must be included with each group of tests.

INDIRECT (PASSIVE) AGGLUTINATION
General Concept
Passive or indirect agglutination reactions use carrier particles that have been coated with antigens not normally present on their surface. Among the carrier particles currently used are red blood cells (RBC) from humans, sheep, and turkeys, and such inert particles as polystyrene latex, charcoal, and bentonite.

Procedure
Indirect agglutination procedure (Figure 12-4, *A*) is similar to direct agglutination, except that the indirect procedure requires reagent antigen preparation (i.e., coating) before reacting with its specific antibody.

Comments
Clinical Application
Indirect agglutination procedure may be used as a screening tool for the detection of various antibodies such as antibodies directed against group A streptococcus, rheumatoid factor (IgM directed against IgG in rheumatoid arthritis), and rubella-specific antibodies (One Step Further Box 12-1).

Technical Considerations
Technical considerations include the following:
- Most passive (indirect) agglutination procedures use commercially prepared kits.
- A prozone phenomenon may be responsible for producing a false negative agglutination reaction in antibody excess. Performance of serial dilution procedure eliminates this phenomenon.
- Presence of high concentration of IgM, with high agglutinating efficiency, may affect agglutination results of other classes of antibodies.
- Commercially prepared antigen-coated particles are available for detection of total immunoglobulin molecules (IgG and IgM) and, specifically, for IgM molecules.

REVERSE PASSIVE AGGLUTINATION
General Concept
The main difference between passive agglutination (described previously) and reverse passive agglutination procedures is that in the passive agglutination procedure the *antigen* is attached to a carrier particle while in the reverse passive agglutination procedure, the *antibody* is attached to the carrier particle (see Figure 12-4).

Procedure
In a reverse passive agglutination procedure, the reagent antibody is attached (adsorbed) onto the surface of a carrier particle (commercially prepared RBC or inert particle) in such a way that the antigen-binding sites of the anti-

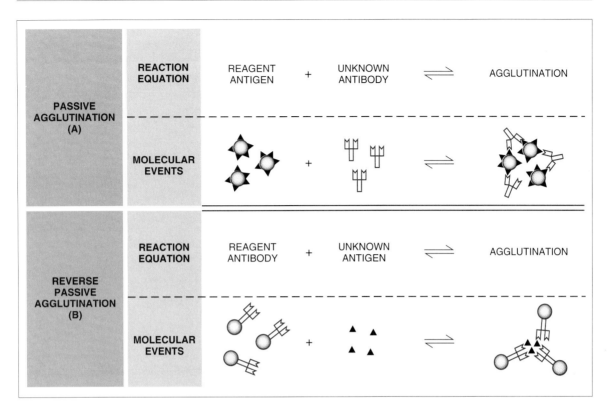

FIGURE **12-4**   **Indirect Agglutination Reactions.**   **A,** Indirect (passive) agglutination. Commercially prepared reagent antigen (carrier particle coated with soluble antigen of known specificity) and an unknown antibody (patient's serum) are reacted and produce a visible agglutination (antigen-antibody complex) when both reactants are of the same specificity. **B,** Reverse indirect (passive) agglutination. This reaction is the same as presented in **A.** However, commercially prepared *reagent antibody* is a carrier particle, coated with a known antibody. The reagent antibody is used to detect an unknown antigen, a *reverse concept* of **A.**

body molecule are free to bind with an antigen (see Figure 12-4, *B*).

When these antibody-coated particles (reagent antibodies) are reacted with the patient sample containing the suspected antigen, agglutination of the particles will occur (if the specificity of the antigen and the antibodies is the same), thus providing the identity of the microorganism.

In procedures that use red blood cells as the carrier particles, the procedure is referred to as *reverse passive hemagglutination.*

Comments
Clinical Application
Many currently available commercial kits use reverse passive agglutination procedure for a rapid identification of antigens produced by a variety of bacterial and fungal microorganisms, particularly those that are difficult to grow in the laboratory (e.g., *Mycoplasma pneumoniae* and *Candida albicans*).

Technical Considerations
Technical considerations involve the following:

- Commercial kits show fairly high sensitivity and specificity and reduce the possibility for cross-reactivity by using monoclonal antibodies.
- Most kits use latex particles as carriers.

AGGLUTINATION-INHIBITION

General Concept
Agglutination inhibition or hemagglutination inhibition (HI) is a two-step procedure. It is based on competition between a reagent

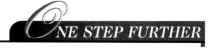

Box 12-1

ONE STEP FURTHER

Rubella Infection

Infection with Rubella Virus
Congenital rubella and *acute rubella (German measles) infections* are caused by a rubella virus and, in spite of on-going attempts to eliminate the infection through vaccination, rubella virus continues to infect humans. Its occurrence and severity, however, have been dramatically reduced by vaccination.

ACUTE RUBELLA INFECTION (GERMAN MEASLES)
Rubella infection is a benign and self-limiting infection, occurring mainly in children and young adults. The infective microorganism (i.e., single-stranded RNA rubella virus) enters the body through the upper respiratory tract by direct or droplet contact with the nasopharyngeal secretions from an infected individual.

Rubella infection is characterized by a mild fever, upper respiratory symptoms, transient rash, and enlarged lymph glands. Although in pregnant women only minor symptoms may be produced, the infection is a *serious risk to the fetus in early pregnancy,* causing serious consequences (see following).

Thus testing of pregnant women for their immune status (immune response) to rubella and other congenital infections, collectively referred to as TORCH (*toxo*plasma, *rubella*, *cytomegalovirus*, and *herpes* simplex) should be performed during the first prenatal visit.

CONGENITAL RUBELLA INFECTION (TRANSPLACENTAL INFECTION)
The major concern in maternal rubella infection is its potential to affect the fetus as the infection passes from mother to fetus through the placenta.

Rubella and other congenital infections transmitted to a fetus can be fatal or have very severe consequences (e.g., ocular and brain damage, deafness, hepatitis, and cardiac malformations). This is because the fetal immune system is not yet fully effective in protecting the fetus/newborn against foreign antigens, such as the rubella virus.

However, as a result of pediatric vaccination and prenatal screening (see following), maternal transmission of the infection and its severe effect on the fetus are now very rare.

Immunologic Testing
Several methods are currently available for the detection and quantification of rubella-specific antibodies (IgM and IgG class). The most widely used procedures are the indirect fluorescent antibody (IFA) technique, enzyme-linked immunosorbent assay (ELISA), passive hemagglutination (PHA), and hemagglutination inhibition (HI). Commercially prepared kits, based on available procedures, are the most commonly used screening tests for rubella infection.

Immunologic testing for rubella-specific antibodies is performed to determine:
- Immunity to rubella virus
- Presence of congenital rubella
- Presence of acute (postnatal) infection

DETECTION OF IMMUNITY TO RUBELLA VIRUS
Screening for the presence of rubella-specific antibodies (IgG) can be performed by commercially pre-

antigen (antigen-coated carrier) and a soluble test antigen in the patient's sample for the same antigen-combining sites on the reagent antibody (Figure 12-5).

Procedure
During the *first phase of the agglutination reaction* (Stage 1), the patient's sample is allowed to react with the reagent antibody. When the suspected test antigen is present in the patient sample, it binds with the reagent antibody and forms antigen-antibody complexes, thus blocking the antigen-combining sites on the reagent antibody.

In the *second phase of the agglutination reaction* (Stage II), antigen-coated particles (re-

agent antigen), showing the same specificity as the reagent antigen, are added to the reaction and allowed to react with the reagent antibody. If the suspected antigen (test antigen with same specificity as the reagent antibody) has already reacted with the reagent antibody during the first phase, it is unavailable for subsequent binding with a particulate reagent antigen in the second phase.

Evaluation of Results
Results can be evaluated as follows:
- *Positive reaction (absence of agglutination):* When the suspected soluble test antigen is present in the patient sample, it will react with the reagent antibody (first

Box 12-1—cont'd

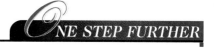

pared hemagglutination or latex fixation procedures (kits), thus establishing the presence of immunity to rubella infections.

Presence of rubella virus–specific IgM antibodies in the patient's serum indicates infection with rubella virus and a probable immunity to rubella. Absence of antibodies to rubella indicates that the patient is susceptible to the infection. This finding is of particular importance in women of child-bearing age.

DIAGNOSIS OF CONGENITAL RUBELLA

Demonstration of rubella virus–specific IgM class antibodies in an infant's serum or presence of virus-specific antibodies during the first 6 months after birth is very suggestive of congenital (transplacental) rubella infection. A four-fold rise in IgG antibody titer confirms the diagnosis of infection. Methods most commonly used for diagnosis of congenital rubella include hemagglutination inhibition and ELISA.

DIAGNOSIS OF ACUTE RUBELLA INFECTION (GERMAN MEASLES)

The antibodies that initially appear during an acute infection may be of the IgM and IgG class. A four-fold rise in IgM titer within 5 days is diagnostic of a recent infection, while IgG persist throughout life (indicator of lifetime immunity). Although reinfection with rubella virus can occur, it is asymptomatic and is only detectable by a rise in the IgG class antibod-

ies. Procedures used to detect both IgG and IgM class of rubella-specific antibodies are the HI, ELISA, and PHA procedures.

Preventive Measures

VACCINATION

Attenuated (non-virulent) rubella virus is a component of a pediatric vaccine that is collectively referred to as *MMR* (mumps, measles and rubella). The vaccine induces production of IgM and IgG classes of antibodies that are similar to the immune response in acute infection.

PRENATAL TESTING

Immunologic testing is performed on serum of pregnant women to detect presence of rubella virus–specific antibodies (IgG), thus establishing immunity to rubella virus.

Vaccines are not administered to pregnant women even if no virus-specific antibodies are demonstrated.

Testing for rubella virus–specific IgM class of antibodies should follow exposure to rubella virus during pregnancy. A positive result may be confirmed by a serial dilution test. A four-fold or greater rise in IgM titer 5 days later is diagnostic of a recent infection (acute rubella infection).

stage of reaction), leaving no antigen-binding sites for binding with the indicator particles (agglutination inhibition, see Figure 12-5).

• *Negative reaction (visible agglutination):* When the suspected test antigen is not present in the sample, the reagent antibody remains free to react with the reagent antigen during the second phase of the reaction, producing visible agglutination of the particles.

*Thus lack of agglutination (agglutination inhibition) indicates presence of a soluble test antigen (**positive reaction**). A visible agglutination indicates absence of a soluble test antigen (**negative reaction**).*

Comments
Clinical Application
Clinical application includes the following:

• Agglutination-inhibition procedure may be used to detect the presence of soluble antigen in a patient sample.
• The procedure may also be used to quantify a soluble antigen in the patient sample by the serial dilution method (see Figure 9-2).

Technical Considerations
It is important to carefully control the concentration of reagent antigen and antibody in order to avoid antibody excess (false negative reaction).

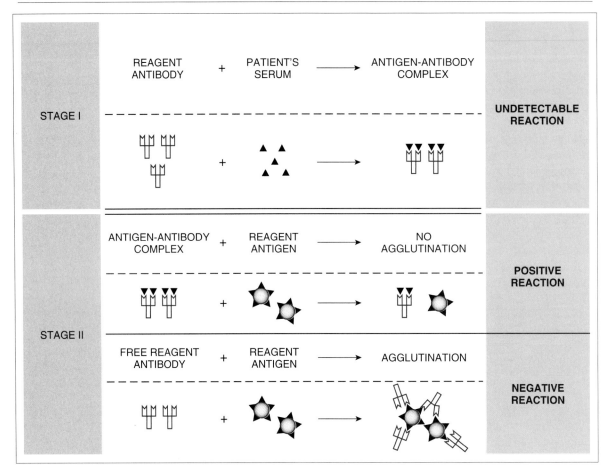

FIGURE **12-5** **Agglutination Inhibition Reaction.** This two-stage procedure can be used to detect a soluble antigen in patient's serum. In **Stage I,** if the unknown antigen shows the same specificity as the reagent antibody, the antigen will bind to the reagent antibody, forming undetectable antigen-antibody complexes. This blocks the available antigen-binding sites on the antibody, making then unavailable for subsequent binding with the reagent antigen. In **Stage II,** absence of agglutination indicates a positive reaction, while appearance of a visible agglutination is indicative of a negative reaction (absence of suspected soluble antigen in serum).

ANTIBODY-MEDIATED AGGLUTINATION

Antiglobulin Tests (Coombs' Tests)

An antiglobulin test, also known as *Coombs' test,* is an example of antibody-mediated agglutination. It is a procedure that is commonly used in blood banking for the detection of antibodies (previously known as "incomplete antibodies"), such as IgG, that are not able to span the distance between red blood cells (RBCs) to form antigen-antibody complexes (lattices).

In these situations, a second antibody, known as *anti-human globulin* (reagent antibody produced in animals against human globulin) is added to facilitate formation of lattices. The anti-human globulin will bind with the protruding Fc portion of the IgG molecules

previously attached to the red blood cell surface, thus bridging the space between red blood cells. This will allow formation of antigen-antibody complexes that are visible as aggregates of red blood cells, known as **hemagglutination.** The intensity of the hemagglutination reaction (see Figure 12-3) is proportional to the amount of the antibodies that are coating the red blood cells.

There are two types of antiglobulin tests, each of which is used for a different purpose:

1. *Direct antiglobulin test (DAT).* Applications of the test include:
   - Detection of autoantibodies
   - Investigation of hemolytic disease of the newborn

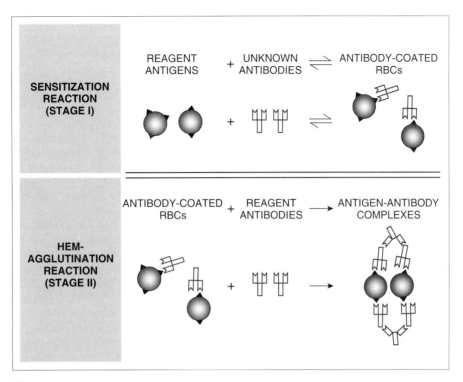

FIGURE **12-6**   **Indirect Antiglobulin Test.**   During **Stage I** of this procedure, coating (sensitization) of reagent red blood cells (RBCs panel, containing known antigens) with serum antibodies (IgG) takes place, if both the serum antibodies and reagent antigen (RBCs) are of the same specificity. During **Stage II,** reagent anti-human globulin (anti-IgG) is reacted with the antibodies coating the reagent RBCs to form lattices, known as **hemagglutination** (clumping of RBCs).

- Detection of medication-induced antibodies
- Investigation of hemolytic transfusion reaction
2. *Indirect antiglobulin test.* Applications of this test include:
   - Typing of red blood cell (RBC) antigens
   - Crossmatching (compatibility testing) before administration of donor blood
   - Detecting and identifying RBC antibodies in serum

Direct Antiglobulin Test (DAT)

general concept. Direct antiglobulin test is used to detect antibodies or complement components that have been adsorbed (attached) in vivo onto the surface of the patient's red blood cells. This type of in vivo antibody adsorption, known as *RBC sensitization,* has been associated with such conditions as hemolytic disease of the newborn (One Step Further Box 12-2), autoimmune hemolytic anemia, and transfusion reactions.

procedure. Briefly, the RBCs obtained from a sample of the patient's blood are separated and washed to remove antibodies not coating the cells. The cells are then reacted with polyspecific reagent antibodies (animal anti-IgG and anti-complement). Agglutination of RBC cells indicates presence of antibody (IgG) or complement components (C3d, C3b, C4b, or C4d) on the surface of the patient's red blood cells.

Differentiation between the IgG and complement components on the RBC surface is possible by using monospecific antibodies that will specifically react with an antigen showing the same specificity. For example, anti-IgG molecules (reagent antibodies) will bind specifically with the IgG molecules (serving as antigens) that have attached to the red blood cells.

Indirect Antiglobulin Test

general concept. Indirect antiglobulin test differs from the direct antiglobulin test in that it is a *two-stage process* (Figure 12-6), requiring an *in vitro* sensitization of the red blood

Box 12-2

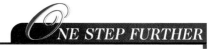

Hemolytic Disease of the Newborn

Hemolytic disease of the newborn (HDN) results from destruction of fetal red blood cells (RBCs) because of sensitization of these cells by maternal antibodies (IgG class). These antibodies are produced against fetal RBC antigens (inherited from the father) that are not present on the mother's cells. The severity of the disease varies, ranging from subclinical symptoms to intrauterine death of the fetus.

The disease is classified according to the specificity of the maternal antibodies produced, most frequent of which are the anti-A and anti-B (ABO HDN) and the anti-D (Rh HDN). Combination of anti-D and other Rh antibodies (other HDN) are also included in this classification.

Mechanism of Disease

The production of maternal antibodies occurs after the mother's exposure to the infant's incompatible RBC antigens at childbirth (i.e., fetal-maternal hemorrhage), during which fetal RBCs enter maternal blood circulation and are recognized by the mother's immune system as "foreign." Thus production of maternal antibodies against fetal antigens (not present on the mother's RBCs) follows each incompatible pregnancy, so that the first child is usually not affected. Subsequent pregnancies, however, produce a greater and greater risk of HDN in the fetus.

Sensitization (coating) of the fetal RBCs with maternal IgG antibodies occurs in vivo because of the antibodies' ability to cross the placenta and react with the fetal RBC surface antigens. The antibody-coated fetal red blood cells are then lysed and the released hemoglobin is catabolized. The resulting indirect (unconjugated) bilirubin crosses the placenta to the mother's circulation and is removed by mother's liver. In the newborn, however, because removal of the excess unconjugated bilirubin by the mother is no longer available, the bilirubin circulates in the newborn's blood and may be deposited in a variety of tissues, giving rise to such symptoms as generalized edema, jaundice, and anemia.

Immunologic Testing

Prenatal evaluation of the mother includes screening for antibodies. When an antibody of class IgG (able to cross the placenta) is detected in the mother's serum, antibody titration (quantification) may be performed periodically as a means of fetal monitoring.

Neonatal studies performed when HDN is suspected:

- *Indirect antiglobulin test* is performed on the mother's blood. If the test is positive (i.e., antibodies are present in mother's serum), a panel of RBC with known antigen specificity is used to identify the detected antibodies.
- *Direct antiglobulin test (DAT)* is performed on cord blood for presence (sensitization) of maternal antibodies on the newborn's RBCs. When the DAT is positive, the antibodies should be identified by first removing (eluting) the antibodies from the surface of the RBCs and then testing them with a panel of reagent RBCs containing antigens of known specificity.

It is important to note that the *only* blood group antibodies that are present in the cord blood are the mother's IgG class antibodies that have crossed the placenta.

Preventive Measures

The incidence of hemolytic disease of the newborn (Rh HDN) has been substantially lowered as a result of prenatal laboratory testing of Rh_o (D) negative women for the presence of clinically significant antibodies.

When anti-D antibodies are detected in the mother's serum, human IgG (anti-D), also referred to as *Rh immune globulin,* is administered during the 28th week of each pregnancy (antepartum) and again within 72 hours of delivery of a Rh_o (D) positive infant (postpartum) as well as at the time of any spontaneous abortion.

The administered anti-D globulin attaches to the D antigen sites on the fetal RBCs entering the maternal circulation, thus preventing recognition of these foreign Rh_o (D) antigen by mother's immune system and formation of anti-D immunoglobulins.

cells (reagent cells) with the circulating "free" antibodies in the patient's blood before addition of anti-human globulin (anti-IgG).

The procedure is used to detect serum antibodies, referred to in blood banking as "unexpected" antibodies, showing specificity for a particular RBC antigen.

procedure. In the *first stage* of the indirect antiglobulin procedure (sensitization), the patient's serum is allowed to react in vitro (at 37° C temperature) with red blood cells containing various known antigen specificities (panel of red blood cells).

This first stage of the reaction simulates events occurring in vivo, during which specific antibodies present in the patient's plasma attach to antigens on the RBC surface showing corresponding specificity (see Figure 12-2). This stage of the agglutination reaction is referred to as *sensitization* see Figure 12-6.

In the *second stage* of the test (hemagglutination), the antibody-coated RBCs are washed to remove unbound antibodies, and an anti-human globulin (anti-IgG) is added to promote lattice formation by binding with the antibodies on the RBC surface (sensitized cells) to produce a visible *hemagglutination reaction* (see Figure 12-6). The end-point of the reaction is interpreted as previously described (see Figure 12-3).

comments. The following clinical applications and technical considerations are important.

1. *Clinical application*
   - The indirect Coombs' test is used mainly in blood banking during compatibility testing before blood transfusion. The purpose of this test is to detect the presence of unexpected antibodies (free or circulating) in a patient's serum that may be of clinical significance, particularly in pregnancy.
   - The procedure may also be used to type certain red blood cell antigens, such as Kell antigen, which show an ability to stimulate production of specific antibodies (anti-Kell) that may cause hemolytic disease of the newborn (see One Step Further Box 12-2).

2. *Technical considerations:*
   - Improper washing or centrifugation of cells may result in a false reaction.
   - In antigen excess, prozone phenomenon may be observed (false negative).
   - Use of outdated or improperly stored reagents must be avoided.
   - Quality control is important for proper interpretation of test results.
   - Rouleaux formation (appears as stack of coins) may be mistaken for agglutination but can be differentiated microscopically.

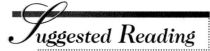

Suggested Reading

Henry JB, editor: *Clinical diagnosis and management by laboratory methods,* ed 19, Philadelphia, 1996, WB Saunders.

Review Questions

MECHANISM OF AGGLUTINATION

1. A visible direct agglutination (antigen-antibody reaction) occurs when the specific antigen has all the following characteristics, *except:*
   a. contains multiple epitopes
   b. is a soluble antigen
   c. occurs naturally on red blood cell surface
   d. is a particulate antigen

2. Agglutination reactions may be used for detecting:
   a. soluble antigens
   b. circulating antibodies in plasma
   c. naturally occurring antigens
   d. all of the above

3. An antigen-antibody reaction occurs in two steps. Select the process (step) during which binding occurs between an antigen on the surface of a particle and its specific antibody:
   a. lattice formation   b. agglutination
   c. sensitization   d. cross-linking

4. Lattice formation during an agglutination (antigen-antibody) reaction can be optimized by all of the following enhancement techniques, *except:*
   a. maintaining appropriate pH
   b. reducing ionic strength of the suspending medium
   c. increasing contact between the antigen and antibody
   d. increasing particle surface charge

5. All of the following factors affect agglutination reactions, *except:*
   a. zeta potential
   b. size of epitopes
   c. class of antibodies
   d. antigen and antibody concentration

6. A negative surface charge on a carrier particle, such as a red blood cell or an inert particle, is known as:
   a. electromagnetic potential
   b. zeta potential
   c. LISS
   d. all of the above

METHODS

7–11. Indicate whether the following statements refer to a direct or an indirect agglutination procedure:

   a. direct agglutination
   b. indirect (passive) agglutination

   ____ detects naturally occurring antigens (particulate antigens)
   ____ requires antigen-coated particles as reagent antigen
   ____ detects antibodies to group A streptococcus antigens
   ____ identifies ABO blood group antigens on red blood cells
   ____ uses antiserum (reagent antibody) to detect unknown antigen

12. A false negative agglutination reaction may be caused by:
   a. prozone phenomenon
   b. antibody excess
   c. inappropriate ratio of antigen to antibody
   d. all of the above

13. In reverse passive agglutination procedure, all of the following statements are true, *except:*
   a. antigen attaches to carrier particle
   b. antibody is attached to the carrier particle
   c. commercially prepared reagent antibodies are used
   d. red blood cells can be used as carrier particles

14. Monoclonal reagent antibodies reduce the possibility of all of the following, *except:*
    a. false positive reactions
    b. cross-reactivity between antigens
    c. heightened agglutination reaction
    d. false negative reactions

15. A procedure that is based on competition between reagent antigen and unknown antigen in a patient's serum for the same antigen-combining sites on a reagent antibody is known as:
    a. reverse-passive agglutination
    b. agglutination inhibition
    c. antibody-mediated agglutination
    d. indirect agglutination

16. An agglutination reaction in which red blood cells (reagent antigens) are reacted with unknown antibodies in serum is known as:
    a. hemagglutination reaction
    b. indirect agglutination reaction
    c. antibody-mediated agglutination
    d. none of the above

17. Which one of the following statements is *not true* when a visible agglutination is seen in an agglutination-inhibition test:
    a. indicates negative reaction
    b. indicates positive reaction
    c. indicates absence of suspected antigen in patient's sample
    d. indicates absence of soluble antigen in a patient sample

18. False negative agglutination inhibition can be avoided by:
    a. using correct amount of reagent antigen
    b. using correct concentration of antibody
    c. controlling the ratio of reagent antigen to antibody
    d. all of the above

19. A commonly used agglutination test for detecting unexpected antibodies ("incomplete antibodies") uses an anti-human globulin for all of the following reasons, *except:*
    a. reducing space between red blood cells
    b. facilitating formation of lattices
    c. bridging space between antibody-coated red blood cells
    d. promoting agglutination

20–25. Indicate next to stated application whether the statement refers to direct or indirect antiglobulin Coombs' test:

    a. direct antiglobulin test
    b. indirect antiglobulin test

    ____ detection of autoantibodies
    ____ investigation of hemolytic disease of the newborn (HDN)
    ____ detection and identification of RBC antibodies in serum
    ____ typing of RBC antigens
    ____ blood compatibility testing (crossmatching)
    ____ investigation of hemolytic transfusion reaction

CHAPTER 13

Labeled Immunoassays

CHAPTER OUTLINE

PRINCIPLES OF LABELED IMMUNOASSAYS

TYPES OF LABELS

TYPES OF PROTOCOLS IN LABELED IMMUNOASSAYS

ONE STEP FURTHER BOX 13-1: HASHIMOTO'S THYROIDITIS

METHODS

RADIOLABELED IMMUNOASSAYS

ENZYME IMMUNOASSAYS (EIA)

CHEMILUMINESCENCE IMMUNOASSAYS

IMMUNOFLUORESCENCE ASSAYS (IFA)

ONE STEP FURTHER BOX 13-2: SYSTEMIC LUPUS ERYTHEMATOSUS

ONE STEP FURTHER BOX 13-3: BULLOUS SKIN DISEASES

Upon completion of Chapter 13, the student will be prepared to:

PRINCIPLES OF LABELED ASSAYS

- Define the following terms: *analyte, ligand, reactant, solid phase,* and *reagent antibody.*
- State the main difference between a heterogeneous and homogeneous immunoassay.
- Name the type of signal or property that is produced by radioisotopes, enzymes, and fluorescent and chemiluminescent labels that can be detected by an appropriate measuring device.
- Explain the reason for the greater sensitivity of a non-competitive rather than a competitive binding assay.
- Explain the difference in protocol for a competitive and a non-competitive binding assay.
- State the purpose of a separation step (wash) in a competitive binding assay.

METHODS

- Discuss the method used in immunoradiometric assay (IRMA), radioallergosorbent assay (RAST), and radioimmunosorbent assay, indicating the type of label used, labeled reactant (antigen or antibody), type of solid phase, labeled detection device, and type of format (competitive or non-competitive).
- List the three most frequently used enzyme immunoassays.
- Name steps and reactants in a non-competitive "sandwich" technique.
- Indicate the type of detection device (instrument) used in a chemiluminescence immunoassay for measuring concentration of an analyte in the patient's sample.
- Explain the difference between direct and indirect immunofluorescence immunoassays in terms of protocol and clinical application.

adsorption - Attachment of one substance or molecule to the surface of another.

analyte - Any substance or molecule (antigen, antibody, or other molecule) that can be detected or measured in various biologic fluids or tissues using a labeled immunoassay.

binder molecules - Protein molecules, most often antibody molecules, that are attached to a solid phase for binding an analyte (ligand or antigen).

competitive binding - Labeled and unlabeled ligand molecules (antigens) compete for a limited number of antigen-specific binding sites on a reagent antibody (binder or receptor molecules) in a labeled immunoassay.

extrapolate - To derive a concentration of an analyte (unknown substance or molecules) from a standard or calibration curve that has been constructed using values obtained from standards (known analyte).

immunoassay - Method that uses an antigen-antibody reaction to detect and/or quantify antigens, antibodies, and other molecules.

label - Molecule or an atom, also known as a *signal, tag,* or a *marker,* which is attached to a reagent antigen, antibody, or other molecule, capable of producing a detectable signal.

labeled reagent antigen or antibody - Labeled molecules that are serologically indistinguishable from the analyte in the patient's sample (i.e., the label does not alter the reactivity of the labeled molecule). The term also refers to antigen or antibody molecules adsorbed onto a solid phase (solid support or phase antigen or antibody).

ligand - Also referred to as a *reactant;* it is usually a labeled or unlabeled molecule (antigen or antibody) reacting in an immunoassay.

reactant - Refers to a labeled (reagent antigen or antibody) or an unlabeled molecule (analyte or ligand to be measured) taking part in an antigen-antibody reaction.

separation step - "Wash" component that separates an unlabeled from a labeled reagent or antigen-antibody complex.

solid phase - Solid support (beads or plastic tubes) that is used for immobilization of binder molecules (antigen or antibody) during a reaction and separation process.

substrate - Material acted on by a specific enzyme.

----•----

The underlying principle in all labeled immunoassays is the detection of an antigen-antibody reaction.

Labeled immunoassays have become increasingly popular for the detection and/or quantification of such *analytes* as bacterial and viral antigens, allergens and allergen-specific antibodies, antibodies in various infectious diseases such as AIDS and hepatitis, hormones, drugs, and tumor markers. However, *most labeled immunoassays are used for the detection and/or quantification of various antigens.*

PRINCIPLES OF LABELED IMMUNOASSAYS

Most labeled immunoassays consist of the following basic components:
1. Reactants, including:
   - Labeled reagent antigen or antibody (commercially prepared ligand)
   - Analyte of interest (in patient's sample)
   - Ligand (antigen or antibody attached to solid phase [support])
2. Appropriate standards
3. Incubation step
4. Separation step (bound from free labeled reagent)
5. Detection of labeled antigen-antibody complexes by an appropriate measuring device

High specificity and sensitivity of the labeled immunoassays make these assays the methods of choice in detecting very low quantities of analytes, which previously could not be detected by then available precipitation and agglutination methods.

In the discussion that follows, these terms will be used as indicated in order to maintain consistency and clarity:
- *Reagent:* Any commercially prepared labeled antigen or antibody molecule, anti-human globulin (anti-antibody), or solid phase–bound antigen or antibody molecule.
- *Ligand:* Any molecule (labeled or unlabeled) that can combine with its complementary molecule to form an antigen-antibody complex.
- *Analyte:* A ligand (antigen, antibody, or other molecule) being analyzed in the patient's sample.
- *Reactant:* Any reacting molecule in a particular assay.

It is important to recall that any two reacting molecules can bind to form an antigen-antibody complex only when both molecules (reagent and analyte) have the same specificity or complementarity (see Chapter 5).

TYPES OF LABELS

A prototype of the *labeled immunoassay,* developed in the late 1950s, employed a *radioactive label for tagging a specific antibody (anti-insulin)* in an assay that was used to detect and quantify human insulin. This radiolabeled immunoassay was appropriately designated as a *radioimmunoassay (RIA).*

Subsequently, labeled immunoassays (Table 13-1) were developed that used a variety of labels referred to as *indicators, markers,* or *tags.* When tagged to a reagent antigen or reagent antibody molecule, the selected label (e.g., radioisotope, enzyme, or fluorescent and chemiluminescent molecule) must be able to show some property (signal) that can be measured by a detection device (see Table 13-1).

Commercially produced *monoclonal antibodies* (see Use of Monoclonal Antibodies, Chapter 10), used as reagent antibodies in labeled immunoassays, show the following characteristics:
- High specificity for a particular antigen (specific epitope)
- Low cross-reactivity with other epitopes (antigenic determinants)
- Ease of labeling with a substance that produces a signal

Table 13-1 MAJOR LABELED IMMUNOASSAYS

Assay	Label*	Solid Phase	Detection Device
RIA	Radionuclides (^{125}I, ^{57}Co, ^{3}H)	Tubes or glass beads	γ-scintillation counter
EIA	Alkaline phosphatase, horseradish peroxidase, β-galactosidase	Tubes, polystyrene beads, or microtiter plates	Spectrophotometer
ChemLum	Luminol, acridinium esters, dioxetane phosphate	Magnetic particles, microtiter plates or gels	Luminometer
IFA	Fluorescein (FITC), rhodamine (TMR)	Tissue/cell preparations (slides, microbeads, dipsticks)	Fluorescent microscope, fluorometer

* Also known as *tag, marker,* or a *signal*

RIA, radioimmunoassay; *EIA,* enzyme immunoassay; *ChemLum,* chemiluminescence; *IFA,* immunofluorescent assay; *I,* iodine; *Co,* cobalt; *H,* hydrogen; *FITC,* fluorescein isothiocyanate; *TMR,* tetramethylrhodamine isothiocyanate.

- High affinity (strength) for the specific epitope (antigenic determinant)
- Stability in their reactivity (molecule is not altered by labeling or during projected shelf-life)

Radioisotopic Labels
Radioactive elements have nuclei that decay spontaneously with the emission of energy (β and γ radiation) and can be measured by scintillation counters. This characteristic makes them suitable for use as labels in certain immunoassays.

Although several radioisotopes have been used as labels in radioimmunoassays, including ^{3}H and ^{57}Co, the radioisotopic label of choice is the gamma-emitting ^{125}I.

Enzyme Labels
Enzymes are protein molecules that catalyze (i.e., initiate or augment) a biochemical reaction by reacting with an appropriate substrate to form a breakdown or reaction product that can be measured by a spectrophotometer (see Table 13-1).

The most often selected enzymes for labels in enzyme immunoassays are *horseradish peroxidase* and *alkaline phosphatase.* Their popularity is the result of the following characteristics:

- Enzymes are not naturally occurring molecules in the patient's sample (e.g., biologic fluid or tissue)
- Enzymes have high specific activity; the specific activity is not altered by attachment to an antigen or antibody

- Enzymes show stability during performance of an assay

In general, enzyme labels are inexpensive, readily available (Table 13-2), have a long shelf-life (stability), can be adapted to automation, and cause changes that are measurable by a spectrophotometer.

Fluorochrome Labels
Several fluorochrome labels, also known as *fluorophores,* are currently available for use in the clinical laboratory. These are fluorescein isothiocyanate (FITC), rhodamine derivatives, phosphorescent labels, phycobiliproteins, and umbelliferone, among others. The most widely used fluorescent labels in detecting and quantifying drugs, hormones, proteins, and peptides in biologic fluids are fluorescein and phycoerythrin:

- *Fluorescein isothiocyanate (FITC)* is a chemical form of fluorescein that can covalently bind to protein. This fluorochrome, which emits a green color, is used to label both the reagent antibodies (antiserum) and the reagent analytes.
- *Phycobiliproteins,* such as the phycoerythrin label, may be used with fluorescein to obtain multicolor images by fluorescence microscopy, flow cytometry, immunoassays, and DNA sequencing. Phycoerythrin emits a red color.

Both fluorochromes have a characteristic absorption and emission spectrum (wavelength or light color). When these organic compounds are treated with an appropriate light, the elec-

Table 13-2 ENZYME LABELS	
Enzyme	Source
Horseradish peroxidase	Horseradish
Glucose oxidase	Aspergillus niger
Glucose-6-phosphate dehydrogenase	Leuconostoc mesenteroides
β-galactosidase	Escherichia coli
Alkaline phosphatase	Calf intestine

trons within the molecule become excited and move to a higher energy level from which they return back to a ground state, releasing energy in form of a photon (wavelength).

Fluorochromes that show the following characteristics may be used as labels in fluoroimmunoassays:

- Must not interfere with the antigen-antibody reaction
- Maintain their stability
- Have the ability to absorb excitation light
- Be able to emit appropriate wavelength (fluorescent light)

Chemiluminescence Labels

The fact that certain compounds will produce light (chemiluminescence) when oxidized makes them adaptable for use as labels or markers in several assays that are based on a similar reaction to EIA and RIA.

Major Groups of Chemiluminescence Labels
Five major groups of chemiluminescence labels are available for assays. These are: luminols, acridinium esters, oxalate derivatives, ruthenium complex, and dioxitane derivatives. However, the most widely used labels are the acridinium esters and luminols:

- *Acridinium esters:* Acridinium esters are capable of producing light by first reacting with an alkaline H_2O_2 (oxidizer) to form high-energy intermediates that then decompose to an excited fragment, which emits an intense blue flash of light (flash-type of chemiluminescence), detectable by a luminometer (detection device).
- *Luminol derivatives:* In the presence of an oxidizer (H_2O_2) and a catalyst (metal ion), luminol is oxidized to an excited-state intermediate, which on returning to its ground-state emits a blue light (chemi-

luminescence) that remains visible for minutes to hours and is detectable by a luminometer.

These chemiluminescent molecules may be used as *direct labels* by attachment (coupling or conjugation) to the reagent antibody, reagent antigen, or a DNA probe in nucleic acid hybridization assays (discussed in Chapter 15). When used as *indirect labels,* the chemiluminescence molecules serve as substrates for enzymes, such as *alkaline phosphatase, horseradish peroxidase,* and *β-galactosidase* in enzyme immunoassays, referred to as *indirect chemiluminescence immunoassays.*

Both applications of chemiluminescence labels are now used in the clinical laboratory, in commercially prepared kits, and in automated immunoassays.

TYPES OF PROTOCOLS IN LABELED IMMUNOASSAYS

Currently, two types of labeled immunoassay protocols are used in the clinical laboratory. These protocols are named according to the type of binding (*competitive* or *noncompetitive*) that occurs between a labeled molecule (generally a reagent antibody), an analyte (unlabeled antigen or ligand), and a solid phase reagent, resulting in a production of a solid phase–bound antigen-antibody complex.

In addition to the competitive and noncompetitive protocols in labeled immunoassays, a variation in these protocols is also available, known as *heterogeneous* and *homogeneous reactions* (described following).

Competitive Binding

The *competitive binding methods* are sometimes referred to as *direct* or *limited reagent methods* because the labeled and unlabeled ligand molecules (e.g., *antigen*) compete for a *limited* number of specific antigen-binding sites on the binder or receptor molecules (e.g., *high affinity reagent antibody [Ab] adsorbed on a solid phase [SP]*).

In these competitive binding reactions (Figure 13-1), the commercially prepared labeled antigen is present in an excessive constant amount so that all antigen-binding sites on the antibody molecule become occupied. If the antigen being analyzed is present in the pa-

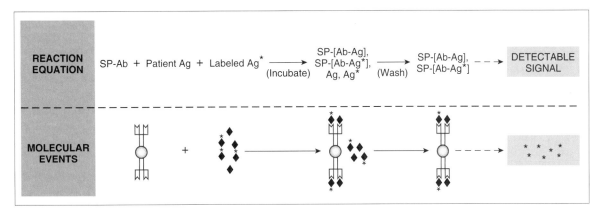

FIGURE **13-1** **Competitive Binding Reaction.**   An antigen *(Ag)* in a patient's sample (analyte) and a labeled antigen (reagent in excess amount), showing the same specificity, are allowed to compete (during incubation) for the same binding sites on an antibody *(Ab)* attached to a solid support phase (SP) to form a labeled and unlabeled antigen-antibody complex (SP-[Ab-Ag]). The labeled complex (SP-[Ab-Ag*]) emits a detectable signal that is measured with a detection device. The amount of signal is inversely proportional to the concentration of the analyte. *, detectable signal on a labeled molecule.

tient sample, it will compete with the labeled antigen for the same binding sites, thus reducing the amount of labeled antigen bound to the solid phase.

Upon separation of the *free* from the *antibody-bound labeled antigen,* the amount of label present in the bound fraction is detected by an appropriate measuring device and is indirectly proportional to the concentration of the analyte in the patient's sample.

In assays that involve analysis of an *antibody* (analyte in the patient's specimen, One Step Further Box 13-1), the labeled reagent antibody and the unlabeled antibody react competitively with an *antigen adsorbed onto the solid phase (SP-Ag).* This procedure used for detection of an antibody (analyte) is the same as in the detection of an antigen (analyte) previously described.

Reaction
When a labeled reagent antigen and an antigen (analyte) in a patient's sample are allowed to react in the reaction medium, they will compete for the *same* limited number of specific antigen-binding sites on the commercially prepared reagent antibody molecule adsorbed to a solid phase (SP-Ab).

In this initial phase of the reaction (incubation period), during which the reaction reaches

an equilibrium (see Chapter 10), the formed antigen-antibody complexes remain attached to the solid phase (SP-[Ab-Ag]). A washing step that follows the first phase is a simple way of separating the free (unbound) antigen from the bound antigen (bound to the antibody on the solid phase).

It is important to note that both the labeled and unlabeled antigens are indistinguishable from each other by serologic means and have the same reactivity or complementarity (specificity) as the reagent antibody.

The reagent antibodies (commercially prepared), also known as *receptor* or *binder molecules,* are attached by physical adsorption to a *solid phase (SP),* such as microtiter plates, plastic tubes, or sepharose beads (see Table 13-1).

Separation Step
Most of the currently available assays use a *solid phase* for both the reaction (described previously) and the separation processes *(wash)* to separate bound from free reactants.

Following the separation, either the free or bound ligand (analyte bound to solid support) can be measured by an appropriate label-detection device (see Figure 13-1). Concentration of the analyte in the patient sample may be extrapolated from a standard curve, which

Box 13-1

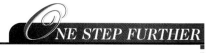

Hashimoto's Thyroiditis

Mechanism of Disease

Hashimoto's thyroiditis, an autoimmune thyroid disorder (see Chapter 7), is the most common form of thyroiditis and occurs most frequently in women. It is characterized by inflammation of the thyroid gland, which slowly progresses to a deficiency in thyroid activity (hypothyroidism), and the presence of autoantibodies (anti-thyroid antibodies) directed against several thyroid-specific antigens. The most important of these autoantibodies are anti-thyroglobulin and anti-thyroid peroxidase (TPO).

Anti-thyroglobulin autoantibodies (anti-Tg), also referred to as *thyroglobulin antibodies,* are directed against precursors of the thyroid hormones (thyroglobulin), which are found within the follicles of the thyroid gland.

Anti-thyroid peroxidase autoantibodies (anti-TPO), previously known as *anti-microsomal antibodies,* are directed against thyroid peroxidase (TPO) antigen (microsomal antigen) located within the microsomal fraction of the thyroid epithelial cells.

Anti-Tg and anti-TPO autoantibodies may also be detected in individuals with other thyroid disorders, such as hyperthyroidism and thyroid tumors. These autoantibodies may also be seen in other types of disorders, such as pernicious anemia and lupus erythematosus, and in certain healthy individuals.

Immunologic Testing

Laboratory testing for both types of circulating autoantibodies (i.e., anti-Tg and anti-TPO [in serum]) is suggested to establish diagnosis of Hashimoto's thyroiditis.

Initially, the only available test for detecting these antibodies was immunofluorescence. Currently, however, agglutination or enzyme-linked immunosorbent assay (ELISA) can also be used for this purpose.

DETECTION OF ANTI-THYROGLOBULIN (ANTI-TG)

Autoantibodies directed against thyroglobulin can be measured by a variety of methods, which include indirect immunofluorescence (IIF), enzyme-linked immunosorbent assay (ELISA), and passive hemagglutination. The most common and highly sensitive procedure for detecting anti-Tg is the passive hemagglutination method, which uses commercially prepared thyroglobulin-coated erythrocytes as the reagent antigen (see Reverse Passive Agglutination, Chapter 12).

A positive anti-Tg reaction (presence of anti-Tg) is considered a "serologic marker" for differentiating hypothyroidism from Hashimoto's thyroiditis.

DETECTION OF ANTI-THYROID PEROXIDASE (ANTI-TPO)

The most frequently used procedure for detecting anti-TPO is indirect immunofluorescence microscopy (IIF) (see later this chapter), which uses tissue sections of monkey thyroid gland as an antigen. Commercially prepared ELISA kits, containing purified microsomes or recombinant TPO, may also be used to detect TPO antibodies.

---

is constructed using standards of known concentration (refer to any clinical chemistry book).

Non-Competitive Binding

Non-competitive immunoassays or indirect method is a two-step reaction process that can be used to measure either an antigen or an antibody, using a "sandwich" technique or a typical non-competitive reaction, respectively (see following).

Non-Competitive Reaction

In a typical non-competitive reaction for the detection or quantification of an *antibody,* during the first step of the reaction (Stage I), the reagent antigen is adsorbed onto a solid phase (SP) and the analyte (antibody in patient's sample) is added and incubated to allow the analyte to react with the SP-bound antigen (commercially prepared).

After washing, the second step (Stage II), involves adding a labeled reagent antibody (anti-human globulin), in excess, to the SP-[Ag-Ab] and incubating it to allow the labeled antibody to react with the Fc portion of the patient's antibody that has bound to the SP-bound antigen during the first phase of the reaction (Figure 13-2). An appropriate detection device (see Table 13-1) can measure the "signal" emitting from the resulting labeled complex (SP[Ag-Ab-Ab]).

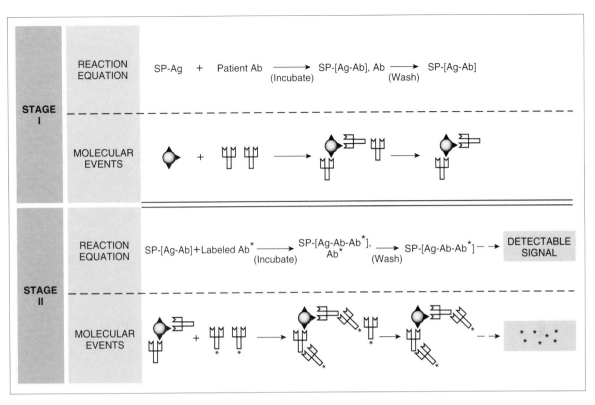

FIGURE **13-2** **Non-Competitive Binding or Indirect Method.** Typical two-step reaction during which a commercially prepared reagent antigen (Ag) attached to a solid phase (SP-Ag) is allowed to bind with an antibody (Ab) in the patient's sample (analyte), forming an antigen-antibody on the solid phase (SP-[Ag-Ab]). Addition of another commercially prepared labeled antibody (Ab*) (anti-human immunoglobulin) directed against Fc portion of the analyte results in the formation of an antigen-antibody-antibody* complex that emits a detectable signal (*).

It is important to note that when the antibody (immunoglobulin) is absent from the patient's sample, the second antibody (anti-human immunoglobulin) remains unbound and is removed by the second wash.

Thus, after the second wash, the detectable signal is generated by the bound antigen-antibody-antibody complex (see Figure 13-2). The amount of the signal, measured by an appropriate detection device, is proportional to the concentration of the analyte (antibody) present in the patient's sample.

These assays are more sensitive than the direct (competitive) assays because the unknown analyte (ligand in a sample) is allowed to participate fully and without competition in the antigen-antibody reaction. However, the procedure involves more steps and handling (i.e., it has two incubations and two wash steps).

"Sandwich" Technique

In this *variation* of the non-competitive binding technique, the *antigen* (ligand) is the analyte of interest in the patient's sample.

The antigen is first allowed to interact and bind with a reagent antibody that has been attached to a solid phase support (SP), forming a SP-[Ab-Ag] complex. After washing, a second labeled reagent antibody, when added to the reaction (in excess amount), reacts with a different site on the same ligand (antigen with more than two epitopes), and becomes "sandwiched" between the two reagent antibodies, thus forming an antibody-antigen-antibody complex SP-[Ab-Ag-Ab] that is detectable (after second wash) by an appropriate detection device (Figure 13-3).

This "sandwich" technique is extremely sensitive, detecting as little as one molecule of the analyte being tested.

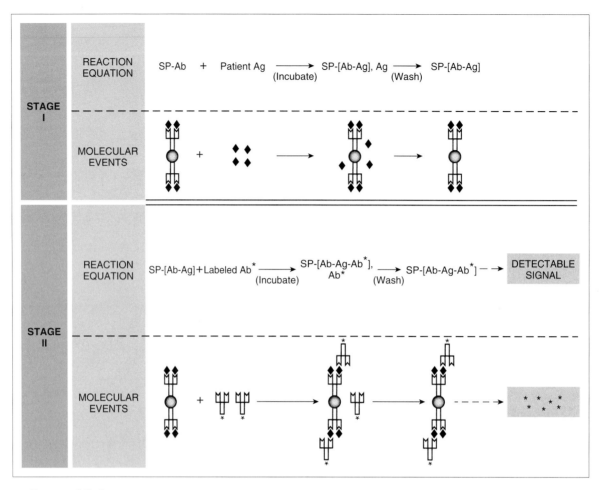

FIGURE **13-3** "Sandwich" Reaction. Variation of non-competitive binding technique, consisting of a reaction (binding) between the antigen (analyte) in the patient's sample and an antibody on the solid phase (SP-Ab). In the second stage, addition of a labeled antibody (Ab*), reacting with a different epitope on the same antigen, results in formation of fluorescent antibody-antigen-antibody complex. After removing labeled non-bound antibody (Ab*), the detectable signal (*) emitted from SP-[Ab-Ag-Ab*] can be measured.

One-Step Assay

The one-step protocol is a newer variation of the classic non-competitive binding assay, consisting of one reaction and one wash step. The simultaneously occurring reaction between an antibody on a solid phase (SP), an antigen in the patient's sample (the analyte), and a *labeled* reagent antibody (directed against a different epitope on the analyte) results in formation of an antibody-antigen-antibody complex (Figure 13-4).

By including a wash that removes any free labeled antibody present, the signal emitted from the remaining complex reflects the amount of the analyte present in the patient's sample because the signal is proportional to the concentration of the analyte.

Homogeneous and Heterogeneous Reactions

The fundamental difference between the homogeneous and heterogeneous reaction is the inclusion or absence of a separation step before detection of the signal from a labeled product.

Homogeneous Reaction

In this type of labeled immunoassay, the antigen-antibody reaction does not require a

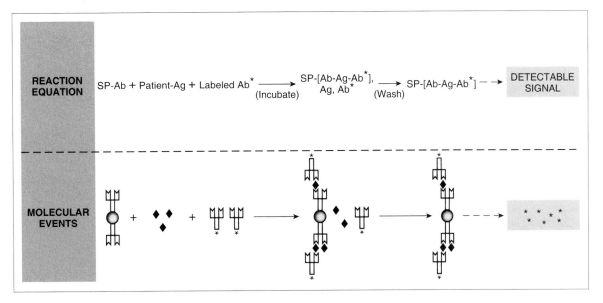

FIGURE **13-4** **One-Step Technique.** Variation of a non-competitive binding assay that allows simultaneous reaction between an antigen (Ag) in a patient's sample and a labeled antibody (Ab*) and the solid phase–bound antibody (SP-Ab). Each of the two types of antibodies shows specificity for a different epitope on the same antigen in the patient's sample. *, detectable signal.

separation step (wash) to separate the free from bound ligand (see discussion of enzyme immunoassay).

Heterogeneous Reaction

These types of labeled immunoassays require a physical separation (washing) of the free from bound ligand, which can be accomplished by including a wash (separation step).

ETHODS

RADIOLABELED IMMUNOASSAYS

Competitive Radioimmunoassay (RIA)

A classic labeled immunoassay protocol that uses the concept of competitive binding (discussed previously) allows a ligand in the patient's sample and a radiolabeled ligand (added in excess) to compete for a limited number of antigen-binding sites on a reagent antibody adsorbed onto a solid phase. As these binding sites become occupied by both the unlabeled and labeled ligands (antigens), the resulting antigen-antibody complex can be detected by a scintillation counter (see Figure 13-1). The concentration of the antigen in the patient's

sample is inversely proportional to the amount of detected radioactivity.

The type of radioactive label used affects the choice of a detection devise for measuring the emitted radiation in counts per minute (CPM). For example, ^{125}I signal (γ-rays) is measured using a solid crystal gamma counter, whereas α- and β-rays are detectable with a liquid scintillation counter.

Non-Competitive Immunoradiometric Assay (IRMA)

In this non-competitive radioimmunoassay, known as *immunoradiometric assay (IRMA)*, the basic protocol is the widely accepted "sandwich" technique (see Figure 13-3), which requires use of an excess reagent antibody, now made readily available by monoclonal antibody technology (see One Step Further Box 14-1).

The reagent antibody (radiolabeled) and the analyte (antigen present in the patient's sample) are added to a solid phase antibody (commercially prepared) and allowed to interact, producing antigen-antibody complexes.

After separating free reagent antibody from solid phase–bound antigen-antibody complexes by washing, the bound complexes are measured and the amount of radioactivity detected is directly proportional to the concentration of the antigen present in the patient's sample.

Radioallergosorbent Assay (RAST)

This radioimmunoassay, also known as an *allergen profile, allergy screen,* or *allergen-specific IgE antibody quantification,* is performed on patients with severe allergic reactions to skin tests or when testing infants to establish existence of allergy (e.g., sensitivity to food or pollen) (discussed in Chapter 7).

The protocol used in this assay is the same as in the classic radioimmunoassay (i.e., competitive reaction between a labeled reagent and an analyte [in patient's sample] for the same binding sites on a molecule adsorbed onto a solid phase) (see Figure 13-1).

However, the RAST procedure involves binding of a reagent antigen (allergen) to a cellulose disk (solid phase) in larger amounts so that more sites on the antigen (epitopes) are available for binding with the IgE present in small concentration in the patient sample and the competing radiolabeled reagent IgE molecules. The resulting radiolabeled antigen-antibody complex formed on the solid phase (cellulose disk) is detectable by an appropriate measuring device and is inversely proportional to the concentration of the IgE in the patient's sample.

Radioimmunosorbent Assay (RIST)

RIST assay uses the concept of competitive binding (previously described) to quantify IgE, an analyte present in the patient's serum.

The assay is performed by mixing a predetermined (fixed) amount of labeled reagent IgE (serving as antigen) with the unlabeled analyte (IgE in patient's sample). Both the labeled and unlabeled molecules are allowed to compete for the binding sites on reagent antibody (anti-IgE) adsorbed onto a plate (solid phase). The amount of labeled IgE that binds with the stationary anti-IgE, forming an antigen-antibody complex (anti-IgE-IgE), is inversely proportional to the amount of IgE present in the sample. Therefore, the less detectable is the signal (radioactive decay), the greater is the amount of IgE present in the sample (see Figure 13-1).

ENZYME IMMUNOASSAYS (EIA)

Enzyme immunoassays (EIA) were developed as an alternative to radioimmunoassays (RIA), which require special handling and disposal of radioactive waste to prevent contamination with radioactivity.

Initially, enzyme immunoassays were based on the same concept as competitive binding used in RIA (i.e., the enzyme-labeled ligand competing with the unlabeled ligand in patient's sample for the same [limited number] of binding sites on a solid phase–bound antibody).

In competitive binding, labeled and unlabeled antigen-antibody complexes are formed, which can be detected by the amount of enzyme (label) activity that occurs in the presence of an appropriate substrate.

Currently, a variety of enzyme immunoassays are available, which include both the competitive and non-competitive binding protocols as well as the heterogeneous and homogeneous reactions (discussed earlier and following). The most frequently and extensively used enzyme immunoassays among the variety of available techniques are the enzyme-linked immunosorbent assay (ELISA), enzyme immunoassay (EIA), and the enzyme multiplied immunoassay techniques (EMIT).

Homogeneous Enzyme Immunoassay

Homogeneous reaction refers to any antigen-antibody reaction that *does not require a separation step (wash).*

Reaction

Labeled antigen (linked with enzyme) is allowed to compete with the analyte (antigen in patient's sample) for a limited number of antigen-binding sites on an antibody that has been adsorbed on a solid phase.

Upon binding to form an antigen-antibody complex, the antigen-bound enzyme experiences a steric hindrance or some conformational change, which causes a decrease in its activity.

Therefore, with an increase in binding, there is a decrease in the enzyme activity. This decrease is detected by the amount of color change that occurs in the presence of an appropriate substrate and is inversely proportional to the concentration of the analyte, as measured by a spectrophotometer.

In this protocol, separation of the labeled from unlabeled antigen is not required because it is a reduction of the enzyme activity (i.e., a decrease in a colored product) that is measured by a spectrophotometer.

Application

The procedure is simple, rapid, and is adaptable to automation for detecting very small molecules (analytes in serum or urine), such as drugs and hormones, that are not detectable by other assays.

Heterogeneous Enzyme Immunoassay

Heterogeneous enzyme immunoassay reactions (described following) are similar to radioimmunoassays in their sensitivity and need for physical separation (washing) of free from bound ligand.

However, non-specific protein binding and cross-reactivity may pose a problem, which may be addressed with careful control of the test conditions and technique.

Competitive Enzyme Immunoassays

enzyme-linked immunosorbent assay (ELISA). In this *prototype of competitive enzyme immunoassays* (see Figure 13-1), the enzyme-labeled ligand (antigen) competes with the unlabeled analyte (antigen in the patient's sample) for a limited number of antigen-specific binding sites on an antibody molecule (adsorbed onto a solid phase).

The protocol requires a wash step to remove any unbound reagent antigen (labeled ligand).

After washing and addition of an appropriate substrate, the enzyme activity is measured by detecting a color change with a spectrophotometer. The enzyme activity is inversely proportional to the concentration of the analyte (antigen) present in the patient's sample. Thus, the higher the concentration of the analyte, the lesser is the binding of the labeled ligand and the production of a detectable activity (color change).

Non-Competitive Immunoassays

"sandwich" enzyme immunoassay. In the typical "sandwich" technique, the analyte (antigen in the patient's sample) is allowed to react with the solid phase–bound antibody (Sp-Ab) to form an antigen-antibody complex (SP-[Ab-Ag]). After washing, an enzyme-labeled reagent (second antibody) is added in excess and is allowed to react with the antibody-bound antigen, forming a "sandwich" antibody-antigen-antibody complex (SP-[Ab-Ag-Ab]. After a second wash and addition of an appropriate substrate, a colored product is produced, which is detected by a spectrophotometer (see Figure 13-3).

indirect enzyme immunoassay. Although this procedure uses a "sandwich" protocol and is sometimes referred to as the "sandwich" enzyme-linked immunoassay (ELISA) (previously described, see Figure 13-3), *the function of the analyte and ligand molecules are reversed in this procedure.* That is, the antigen is attached onto the solid phase (SP-Ag), while the antibody (analyte in the patient's sample) is the molecule that binds with the (Sp-Ag), producing an antigen-antibody complex (SP-[Ag-Ab]).

A second enzyme-labeled antibody (anti-human globulin or anti-antibody), with specificity for the analyte (antibody in the sample) when added, binds with the analyte to produce an antigen-antibody-antibody complex (SP-[Ag-Ab-Ab]). After washing and addition of an appropriate substrate, a colored product is produced that is detected by a spectrophotometer (see Figure 13-3). The concentration of the analyte (i.e., antibody) is directly proportional to the color produced (color intensity).

enzyme-multiplied immunoassay technique (EMIT). A variation of the ELISA ("sandwich" technique), sometimes also referred to as a *capture assay,* is employed for detection of very small concentrations of an antigen with multiple epitopes.

The assay may also be used to quantify specific immunoglobulins (e.g., IgM in an acute infection or IgE in an allergic response), which function as antigens in this protocol, while the anti-human immunoglobulin (e.g., anti-IgM or anti-IgE, respectively) is the antibody that is directed against the immunoglobulin (analyte in the patient's sample).

CHEMILUMINESCENCE IMMUNOASSAYS

Chemiluminescence detection technology, the newest of the label detection, has a diverse range of applications in the clinical laboratory, most important of which is the use of chemiluminescent labels in various immunoassays and nucleic acid assays, such as DNA probe assays and Southern blotting (see Chapter 15).

Although chemiluminescence immunoassays typically are categorized as *competitive* and *non-competitive binding assays* (see following discussion), as in all labeled immunoassays, these immunoassays may use either a protocol that does not require separation of bound from unbound ligand *(homogeneous)* or a protocol requiring a separation step *(heterogeneous)*, as previously described.

In both competitive and non-competitive immunoassays, chemiluminescent molecules (label) are tagged to a reagent antigen or antibody and detected as emitted light energy when an antigen-antibody reaction occurs. This light energy is emitted during oxidation of the chemiluminescent label (chemical reaction that produces energy), during an antigen-antibody reaction.

When a chemiluminescent label such as acridinium esters are used in these immunoassays, upon oxidation, they emit energy that is visible as a *flash of light.* In order to capture the flash of light (signal), however, the chemical reaction producing the energy must occur directly in front of the light detection device in a luminometer, where the reagents can be introduced into the assay tube.

In methods that use oxidation of luminol label as the source of emitted energy, the energy may be visible as a prolonged emission (*glow of light*), which lasts for minutes to hours. This type of label is useful in blotting applications (described in Chapter 15).

Non-Competitive Chemiluminescence Immunoassays

In the non-competitive or "sandwich" chemiluminescence assay, a ligand (either a reagent antigen or reagent antibody molecule, depending on the analyte of interest) is tagged with a label, such as acridinium ester.

When the analyte to be determined in the patient's sample (usually an antigen) is allowed to bind with the reagent antibody adsorbed to a solid phase (i.e., magnetic microparticles), the antigen-antibody complex that forms remains attached to the solid phase (SP). On addition of the labeled reagent antibody, a SP-antibody-antigen-antibody complex forms (SP-[Ab-Ag-Ab]) (see Figure 13-3). This complex ("sandwich") can be detected (after washing) by adding a mixture of sodium hydroxide and hydrogen peroxide to generate a flash of light (signal) that can be measured by a luminometer.

Competitive Chemiluminescence Immunoassays

As previously discussed in a competitive binding reaction, the analyte (antigen) in the patient's sample and the labeled reagent antigen (ligand tagged with a chemiluminescent label such as acridinium ester) are allowed to *compete* for antigen-binding sites on the reagent antibody adsorbed onto a solid phase (magnetic particles). The resulting antigen-antibody complexes (containing labeled and unlabeled antigens) remaining attached onto the solid phase (SP) must be washed to separate the bound from unbound (free) labeled antibody (see Figure 13-1).

After the wash step, a mixture of sodium hydroxide and hydrogen peroxide, when added to the SP-[Ag-Ab] complex directly in front of a photodetector, produces a flash of light that can be detected by a luminometer.

For this type of immunoassay, kits containing commercially prepared reagents for use in this assay are currently available for quantifying such analyte (antigen) as cancer antigen (CA 27.29), a circulating tumor marker that can be used to monitor therapy and the course of the disease.

Other Chemiluminescence Assays
Indirect Chemiluminescence Enzyme Immunoassays

Chemiluminescent substances are also capable of functioning as substrates, a characteristic that makes them acceptable for use in enzyme reactions and applicable to indirect chemiluminescence enzyme immunoassays.

Automated (Direct) Chemiluminescence Assay

Chemiluminescence has also been adapted to the automated chemiluminescence detection system, currently used for detecting and quantifying prostate specific antigen (PSA) in the serum of males with prostatic cancer.

Immunoblotting (IB)
For a discussion of protein and nucleic acid blotting procedures, see Chapter 15.

IMMUNOFLUORESCENCE ASSAYS (IFA)

Contrary to the previous belief that the body is unable to produce antibodies against "itself," a more recent understanding of the mechanism involved in an immune response to endogenous substances (e.g., autoimmune response to thyroglobulin, see One Step Further Box 13-1), has opened new opportunities for diagnosing autoimmune diseases.

Diseases such as systemic lupus erythematosus (SLE) (One Step Further Box 13-2) and Hashimoto's thyroiditis (see One Step Further Box 13-1) can now be diagnosed by presence of characteristic autoantibodies that are referred to as specific "markers" for a particular disease (Table 13-3).

Detection of these specific autoantibodies ("markers") and various other molecules of interest (e.g., proteins, hormones, and drugs) has been made possible and received a wide acceptance within the clinical laboratories by the recent advances in the development of *immunofluorescence assays.*

These immunoassays use fluorochrome labels (previously described) and a newer type of instrumentation. The fluorochrome label, which is used as a signal or a fluorescent probe, emits a fluorescent light at a wavelength of lower energy level than the excitation wavelength.

Thus immunofluorescence is the emitted light (wavelength or color) that is observed when energy is released from a fluorochrome on excitation by an incident light (wavelength providing excitation energy). For example, fluorescein isothiocyanate (FITC) has a characteristic absorption or excitation wavelength of 490 nm and an emission spectrum (517 nm) that is visible as a characteristic green color.

There are two types of immunofluorescence immunoassays: the *indirect immunofluorescence assays (IIF)* that have the capability of detecting circulating autoantibodies in serum and the *direct immunofluorescence assays (DIF)* that are used to detect deposited autoantibodies in skin or tissues (tissue biopsy) (see Chapter 7, Figure 7-3). DIF can also be used to detect bacterial and cell antigens in suspensions.

Both types of immunofluorescence techniques (i.e., direct and indirect assays), use commercially prepared fluorescein-labeled monospecific antibodies with high known specificity and sensitivity (see Chapter 14).

Direct Immunofluorescence Techniques
In direct immunofluorescence procedures, fluorochrome-labeled antibodies (reagent antibodies) are added directly to a cell suspension or tissue section to form a labeled antigen-antibody complex (Figure 13-5). The complex is detectable by fluorescence microscopy.

Direct immunofluorescence techniques (DIF) can be used to identify:
- Viral, parasitic, or fungal antigens
- Immune complexes (antigen-antibody complexes)
- Lymphocyte surface markers
- Immunoglobulins (IgG, IgA and IgM) and complement components in cells and tissues

In addition, DIF techniques are particularly useful to dermatologists in establishing differential diagnosis of various autoimmune skin diseases, such as bullous pemphigoid (One Step Further Box 13-3).

Method
When fluorochrome-labeled monospecific antibodies (commercially prepared antisera) of high specificity and sensitivity are added directly to tissue or live cell suspension containing cell surface markers or immunoglobulins, respectively and are allowed to interact, labeled antigen-antibody complexes will form at the site of complex formation (see Figure 13-5).

After removal of any unbound labeled antibody by washing, the tissue or cell preparations are viewed against a dark background in a fluorescence microscope (modified standard light microscope). A bright light (fluorescence) is observed at the site where fluorescent antigen-antibody complexes have formed. The

Box 13-2

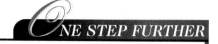

Systemic Lupus Erythematosus

Mechanism of Disease

Systemic lupus erythematosus (SLE) is a systemic rheumatic disease of unknown origin, classified as an autoimmune disease (non-organ specific hyperactivity of the immune system). The disease is characterized by presence of *polyclonal* (of multiple specificity) *autoantibodies* (see Table 13-3) that include antibodies to native DNA (anti-nDNA), known as *double-stranded DNA (dsDNA),* and antibodies to Smith antigen (anti-Sm), both usually specific for SLE and of the IgG or IgM class.

Although it has not yet been established whether viral stimulation or the patient's own DNA is responsible for the production of anti-DNA antibodies, studies indicate that formation of autoantibodies is partly genetically determined.

For example, patients with certain HLA genes are more likely to produce autoantibodies (i.e., HLA-DR2 produce anti-dsDNA, HLA-DR3 produce anti-SS-A (Ro) and anti-SS-B (La), HLA-DR4 and HLA5 produce anti-Sm and anti-RNP) (see Table 13-3).

SLE disease affects many organs, with tissue injury being mediated by circulating antigen-antibody complexes that are deposited within the affected tissue (see Immune Complex–Mediated Hypersensitivity, Chapter 7). These immune complexes form when an antibody to DNA (anti-DNA) is produced in the SLE patient and binds with the DNA antigen.

For example, in the secondary form of glomerulonephritis (see Chapter 7), associated with 50% or more of all SLE patients, the tissue damage is initiated on deposition of immune complexes in the kidney glomeruli, observed as a immunofluorescence granular pattern (IgG, IgA, IgM, and C3 complexes).

Clinical findings include arthritis of various joints, skin rash (e.g., butterfly pattern on face), renal involvement (nephritis), and less frequently an involvement of the lungs, heart, nervous system, eyes, and gastrointestinal system. Small vessel vasculitis, however, is more common.

Immunologic Testing

SERUM TESTING

Most SLE patients have elevated levels of α (acute phase reactant) and γ globulins (increased production of polyclonal IgG of various epitope specificity) and occasionally a decrease in albumin and serum complement levels. The reduction in complement occurs because of increased use in active SLE disease (formation of immune complexes) and/or reduced synthesis of complement. Although infrequently determined, the C5-C9 (membrane attack complex, see Chapter 4) is increased during hemolytic episodes.

IMMUNOLOGIC FINDINGS

SLE is characterized by the following immunologic findings:
- High titer of autoantibodies, including antinuclear antibodies (ANA) and antibodies against double-stranded DNA (anti-dsDNA) and against Smith antigen (anti-Sm)
- Low serum complement levels (C3 and C4)
- Deposits of immune complexes along the (kidney) glomerular basement membrane and dermal-epidermal (skin) junction

Additional immunologic findings include presence of cytotoxic antibodies (specific for T cell surface antigens) in many of the patients with SLE. These antibodies (in presence of complement) are capable of destroying T lymphocytes and binding on their cell surface (see Opsonization, Chapter 4).

CONFIRMATORY TESTS FOR SLE

The diagnosis of SLE can be facilitated by performing indirect immunofluorescence (IIF) procedure, radioimmunoassay (RIA), or enzyme immunoassay (EIA).

The main distinguishing features (hallmark) of active SLE are reduced serum complement levels and presence of antibodies to double-stranded DNA (dsDNA).

Table **13-3**	AUTOANTIBODIES IN SYSTEMIC LUPUS ERYTHEMATOSUS SLE	
Antibody	Substrate	Pattern*/Reaction
Anti-ANA	HEp-2 cells	Diffuse, homogeneous
Anti-dsDNA	*Crithidia luciliae*	Positive kinetoplast
Anti-Sm	ENA	Positive
Anti-RNP	ENA	Positive

*Observed by indirect immunofluorescence (IIF).
ANA, antinuclear antibodies; *HEp,* human epithelial cells; *dsDNA,* double-stranded deoxyribonucleic acid; *Sm,* Smith; *ENA,* extractable nuclear antigen; *RNP,* ribonucleoprotein.

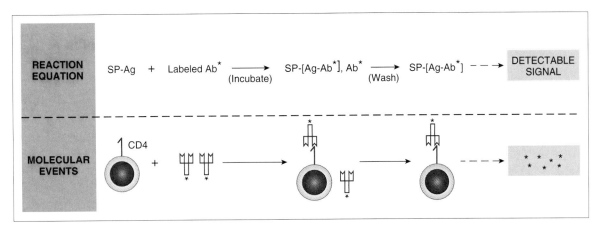

FIGURE **13-5** **Direct Immunofluorescence.** Example of a method used for the detection of helper T cells (CD4+ lymphocytes). Shown are events occurring during direct application of fluorochrome-labeled antibody (Ab*), with specificity for a CD4 marker (serving as antigen), to a suspension of lymphocytes. The fluorescent SP-[Ag-Ab]* complex formed on the surface of the CD4+ T cell is measured by detecting the emitted fluorescence. *, detectable signal on a labeled molecule.

color of the light depends on the type of fluorochrome used for tagging the reagent antibodies. For example, fluorescein isothyiocynate (FITC) emits a green color (see Chapter 7, Figure 7-3), whereas phycobiliprotein emits a red color.

Labeled antigen-antibody complexes may also be detected at cell surfaces by flow cytometry (see Immunophenotyping, Chapter 14).

Indirect Immunofluorescence Techniques

The *indirect immunofluorescence assay (IIF)* is basically a modification of the antiglobulin reaction (Coombs', discussed in Chapter 12) or a double antibody test (see Figure 13-2).

IIF assays may be used for detection of various serum antibodies with specificity for tissues, such as bullous pemphigoid and pemphigus antibodies in skin disease (see One Step Further Box 13-3), and for detection of autoantibodies (Table 13-3) directed against native DNA antigens (nDNA), nuclear antigens (ANA), mitochondrial antigens (AMA), smooth muscle antigens (ASMA), and parietal cell antigens (APCA).

Anti-glomerular basement membrane (anti-GBM) antibodies in renal disease (see Chapter 7) have also been detected by this method, although recently, anti-GBM antibodies are more commonly detected by immunoblotting (see Chapter 15) and/or ELISA.

More recently, indirect immunofluorescence assays have been used to identify anti-neutrophil cytoplasmic antibody (ANCA), as an important adjunct to histologic studies in the diagnosis of patients with Wegener's granulomatosis (see Evaluation of Neutrophil Function, Chapter 14).

Method

serum sample. In a non-competitive indirect immunofluorescence (IIF) procedure used to detect free antibody (ligand) in the patient's sample, the ligand is reacted with a tissue antigen (e.g., HEp 2 cells fixed to a slide, serving as a solid phase [SP] antigen) to form an antigen-antibody complex (SP-[Ag-Ab]).

After washing, a second antibody (labeled anti-human immunoglobulin) is added and allowed to bind with the (SP-[Ag-Ab]), forming a fluorescent antigen-antibody-antibody complex (SP-[Ag-Ab-Ab]), which is then measured in a fluorometer.

The concentration of the antibody in the patient's sample is extrapolated from a constructed standard curve and reported in ml/dL.

tissue sections. In detecting autoantibodies in tissue sections, the labeled reagent antibody is placed directly over the tissue and allowed to bind with the previously formed antigen-

Box 13-3

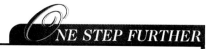

Bullous Skin Diseases

Mechanism of Bullous Pemphigoid Disease

Bullous skin diseases, which are characterized by blistering of skin and the presence of autoantibodies (specific disease markers) that bind to various skin structures, have now been linked to autoimmunity (see Chapter 7). The concept of autoimmunity has altered both the classification and the clinical diagnosis and management of the various blistering skin diseases, such as bullous pemphigoid disease.

The primary stimulus for the production of autoantibodies in bullous pemphigoid disease is not known. However, the initiation of the disease occurs as the circulating IgG binds to the bullous pemphigoid antigen (a basic glycoprotein named after the disease) in the lamina lucida at the dermal-epidermal junction, forming an antigen-antibody complex (see Chapter 7, Figure 7-3).

These complexes (formed at the dermal-epidermal junction) activate complement, resulting in an inflammatory response (see Chapter 1), that causes separation of the epidermis from the dermis.

It is interesting to note that this self-limiting disease can be transferred to animals by injecting the patient's antibodies.

Immunologic Testing

DIRECT IMMUNOFLUORESCENCE ASSAYS

In these assays, performed on the patient's skin (biopsy), a characteristic linear deposition of autoantibodies (IgG) is found at the skin dermal-epidermal junction in many patients (50% to 90%) with bullous pemphigoid. Linear deposits of complement component (C3) are also seen at this junction in almost all bullous pemphigoid patients, occasionally even in the absence of the immunoglobulin deposition. These deposits (e.g., IgG) can be identified by adding labeled antibody (e.g., reagent anti-IgG) with specificity for the IgG autoantibody and viewing them with a fluorescence microscope for presence of specific fluorescence (see Figure 7-3, A).

INDIRECT IMMUNOFLUORESCENCE ASSAYS

These assays are used to identify circulating IgG in the patient's sample, by allowing the IgG to bind in vitro to a target tissue (e.g., monkey esophagus) at the dermal-epidermal junction. After addition of a reagent antibody (labeled anti-IgG), the tissue is examined for presence of fluorescent antigen-antibody complexes (see IIF, text see Figure 7-3, B).

Differential diagnosis of blistering diseases is based mainly on immunofluorescence and histopathology and less on clinical features.

antibody complex, forming a fluorescent complex.

Evaluation of fluorescence in the tissue, using fluorescence microscopy, includes such observations as:

- Distribution or pattern of deposits (e.g., granular or linear)
- Extent of staining (e.g., focal or diffuse)
- Type of reactants (e.g., IgG)
- Location of the deposits (e.g., IgG along basement membrane)

Photographs are taken of tissues as a permanent record of microscopic findings by IIF.

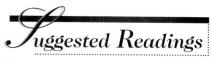

Suggested Readings

Henry JB, et al, editors: *Clinical diagnosis and management by laboratory methods,* ed 19, Philadelphia, 1996, WB Saunders.

Rose NR, et al, editors: *Manual of clinical laboratory immunology,* ed 5, Washington, DC, 1997, American Society for Microbiology.

Review Questions

PRINCIPLES OF LABELED IMMUNOASSAYS

1–5. Match the following terms with the *best* related statements:

_____ analyte
_____ ligand
_____ reactant
_____ solid phase
_____ substrate

a. labeled or unlabeled molecule (antigen or antibody)
b. antigen, antibody, or other molecules of interest detectable in tissues or biologic fluids
c. immobilizes antigen or antibody molecules
d. reagent or analyte participating in antigen-antibody reaction
e. material acted on by an enzyme

6. All of the following substances or elements can be used as a "signal" or label in a variety of immunoassays, *except:*
   a. radioisotopes
   b. fluorochromes
   c. enzymes
   d. substrates

7. Enzymes such as horseradish peroxidase are used as labels in immunoassays because of all of the following characteristics, *except:*
   a. stability during performance of an assay
   b. high specific activity
   c. emission of high energy photons
   d. absence from tissues and blood

8–11. Indicate a detectable signal for each of the listed labels:

_____ alkaline phosphatase
_____ acridinium esters
_____ phycoerithrin
_____ fluorescein isothiocy- anate

a. green color wavelength
b. colored product
c. blue flash of light (chemi- luminescence)
d. red color fluorescence

12. Select the labels that can be applied to automated immunoassays:
   a. chemiluminescent molecules
   b. enzymes
   c. fluorochromes
   d. radioisotopes

13. In competitive binding assays, all of the following statements are true, *except:*
   a. the labeled and unlabeled antigen can be serologically distinguished from each other
   b. labeled and unlabeled antigen compete for a limited number of antigen-binding sites on antibody
   c. labeled antigen is present in excess
   d. labeled and unlabeled antigen compete for the same binding sites

14. Select the method that is *not* used to separate free reactant (antigen) from the bound antigen in a competitive immunoassay:
   a. washing
   b. binding with free antibody
   c. binding with antibody adsorbed to solid phase
   d. binding with antibody adsorbed to sepharose beads

15. Labeled immunoassays consist of all of the following components, *except:*
   a. labeled antigen or antibody
   b. separation step
   c. label-detection device
   d. unlabeled analyte (in sample)

16. Select the statements that relate to a noncompetitive immunoassay:
   a. detects antigen or antibody in sample
   b. uses a "sandwich" protocol
   c. uses labeled reagent antibody with specificity for human immunoglobulin
   d. all of the above

17. The main difference between a heterogeneous and homogeneous protocol is:
   a. inclusion or absence of a separation step
   b. type of label used

c. inclusion or absence of an anti-human immunoglobulin

d. type of solid phase (support) used

METHODS

18–24. Match name of labeled immunoassay with its appropriate acronym:

```
____ ELISA      a. Radioimmuno-
____ EMIT          sorbent assay
____ IRMA       b. Radioimmunoassay
____ RIST       c. Immunoradiometric
____ RAST          assay
____ IIF        d. Indirect immuno-
____ RIA           fluorescence
                e. Radioallergosorbent
                   assay
                f. Enzyme-linked
                   immunosorbent
                   assay
                g. Enzyme-multiplied
                   immunoassay
```

25. Select an enzyme immunoassay that requires a separation of free from bound enzyme–labeled ligand:
a. ELISA
b. "sandwich" enzyme immunoassay
c. EMIT
d. All of the above

26. All of the following statements differentiate enzyme-linked immunosorbent assay from the "sandwich" type immunoassay, *except:*
a. need for separation (wash step)
b. competition for specific antibody between enzyme-labeled ligand and unlabeled analyte
c. addition of a second antibody (anti-human immunoglobulin)
d. two-step reaction process

27. Select an enzyme immunoassay protocol from those listed following in which a reduction of enzyme activity is measured as a colored product, thus not requiring a separation step:
a. heterogeneous
b. homogeneous
c. competitive binding
d. non-competitive binding

28. All statements that follow are applicable to a chemiluminescence reaction, *except:*
a. magnetic microparticles are used as a solid phase
b. wash is not required for separating bound from unbound (free) labeled antibody
c. non-competitive and competitive binding protocols are available
d. luminometer is used to measure chemiluminescence

29. Chemiluminescence is emitted during oxidation of the label in a chemiluminescence immunoassay and is detectable as:
a. a flash of light
b. a glow of light
c. light energy
d. all of the above

30. Fluorochrome labels can be used in direct immunofluorescence assays to detect:
a. immune complexes
b. various microorganisms
c. lymphocyte surface markers
d. all of the above

31–37. Match the two types of immunofluorescence assays with their descriptive statements:

a. direct immunofluorescence
b. indirect immunofluorescence

____ protocol is similar to antiglobulin (Coomb's) test
____ useful in diagnosing autoimmune skin diseases
____ protocol includes addition of labeled antibodies to the tissues or cells
____ detects specific (free) autoantibodies
____ uses fluorometer for detection of fluorescein-labeled antigen-antibody complex
____ detects anti-neutrophil cytoplasmic antibody (ANCA)
____ fluorescence produced during the reaction is detectable by immunofluorescence microscope

38. All of the following statements are *true* for the production of a characteristic emission

wavelength by fluorescein isothiocyanate (FITC), *except:*

a. excitation by an incident light
b. characteristic absorption of light
c. oxidation of fluorescein molecules
d. excitation energy

39. Select the statement(s) that apply to the type of observation made when evaluating fluorescence in tissues by fluorescence microscopy:

a. location of fluorescent deposit
b. extent of staining
c. distribution or pattern of deposits
d. all of the above

Special Techniques

Learning Objectives

Upon completion of Chapter 14, the student will be prepared to:

FLOW CYTOMETRY

- State two characteristics of the somatic cell hybridization that make this procedure particularly valuable for production of reagent monoclonal antibodies.
- List the major components of the flow cytometer.
- Define forward light scatter (FALS) and side scatter (90 degrees) in terms of the cell properties measured.
- Describe the benefit of using more than one fluorochrome for labeling monoclonal antibodies for flow cytometric analysis.
- State two ways in which flow cytometric data can be shown in terms of frequency distribution.
- List clinical applications of immunophenotyping by flow cytometry.
- Name two types of flow cytometric methods most commonly used for tumor cell analysis.
- Explain how measurement of tumor cell DNA content in DNA cell cycle analysis can serve as measurement of tumor cell growth and aggressiveness.
- Describe how the T cell flow cytometric histogram is used in interpreting compatibility or incompatibility between donor and recipient T lymphocytes.

COMPLEMENT ASSAYS

- Describe the hemolytic assay used to evaluate all complement components of the classical pathway.
- Name the two most frequently used immunoassays for quantifying complement levels.
- State the reason for correct preparation and storage of serum sample for complement analysis.
- Describe the two reaction steps in the complement fixation procedure.
- Explain the main difference in interpretation of the positive and negative end points in tubes set up as serial dilutions in the complement fixation test vs. the anti-streptolysin O (ASO) titration procedure.
- Explain the principle of hemolysis inhibition procedure.

FUNCTIONAL ASSAYS

- List the names of five cell separation techniques, indicating the most frequently used technique.
- Define the following terms: *allogeneic cells, HLA, two-way MLR, immunocompetent responders, stimulator cells.*
- Describe the cellular events that occur during mixed lymphocyte response.

HISTOCOMPATIBILITY TESTING

- Describe phenotyping procedure for class I HLA, which uses microcytotoxicity.
- Explain two ways by which the microcytotoxicity test for class I HLA differs from class II HLA.
- Explain the main difference in testing for HLA antibodies and HLA phenotyping in terms of patient specimen, type of reagent, procedure used, interpretation of test results.

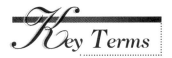

Key Terms

alloantigens - Molecules (antigens) expressed on cells of a genetically dissimilar individual (e.g., donor), which are recognized by the immune system (host) as foreign.

allogeneic - Genetically dissimilar (non-identical) members of the same species (e.g., cells from another individual with different HLA antigens).

cell lysis - Disruption of cell membrane by complement or cytotoxic T cells, resulting in cell destruction by release of cell content. Presence of "ghost" cells (cell outlines) and stain uptake by dead cells indicates cell lysis.

CH$_{50}$ - Refers to the functional assay of complement activity detected by hemolysis (50%) of reagent cells, sensitized with specific antibodies. The assay tests the sequential activation of all complement components in the classical pathway.

cluster of differentiation (CD) - Antigenic markers expressed on leukocytes, used to characterize various leukocyte populations by such tissue immunophenotyping procedures as flow cytometry and serologic tissue typing (microcytotoxicity), using antigen (CD)-specific monoclonal antibodies.

complement fixation - Refers to complement use in an antigen-antibody reaction, during which the complement becomes activated and forms complement components (fractions) that cause cell lysis.

cytotoxicity - Effector mechanism of cell-mediated immune response, in which cytotoxic T cells direct their cytotoxic effect toward cells bearing foreign (e.g., incompatible HLA) antigens, causing target cell lysis.

DNA aneuploidy - Refers to cells that are not diploid and which contain abnormal DNA content; serves as a reliable indicator of neoplasia (tumor).

DNA cell cycle - Refers to phases in cell replication (i.e., G_0/G_1, S, G_2/M phases) that can be analyzed by measuring DNA content at each phase to assess cell growth and cancer aggressiveness.

DNA ploidy - Term *diploid* is used to indicate presence of two copies of each chromosome (except ova and sperm) in normal cells. Ploidy analysis can be done by flow cytometry to predict effectiveness of chemotherapy and outcome of certain malignancies.

histocompatibility antigens - Terminology used in transplantation immunology to describe class I MHC molecules expressed on surface of all nucleated cells, also known as *human leukocyte antigens (HLA)*.

human leukocyte antigens (HLA) - Human leukocyte antigens are also known as *histocompatibility antigens* and *MHC antigens*. The term is often used in transplantation and denotes identification of MHC by tissue typing procedures.

immunophenotyping - Procedure that allows classification of cells based on the antigen or marker expressed on their cell surface. It can provide information that identifies a specific cell lineage and the cell's maturation stage.

in vitro - Used to designate reactions or procedures performed in a laboratory.

major histocompatibility complex (MHC) - Refers to a region on the human chromosome that codes for MHC molecules (antigens) expressed on certain cells. MHC molecules show unique specificity in each individual.

microcytotoxicity - In vitro procedure used for tissue typing or detection of antibodies to HLA. The procedure is based on lysis of target cells (in the presence of complement) that express antigens on their cell surfaces of the same specificity as the reagent antibodies.

mixed lymphocyte reaction - One-way or two-way MLR is performed as a culture of two allogeneic cell populations, expressing dissimilar HLA on their cell surface. The procedure is used to evaluate the ability of one or both of these cell populations to respond to the dissimilar HLA by proliferating.

monoclonal antibody - Homogeneous antibody that originates from a single clone of B lymphocytes (single cell line) with specificity for a single epitope (antigenic determinant).

target cell - Cell displaying foreign antigens that are responsible for evoking an immune response. For example, in a cell-mediated response, cytotoxicity is directed against the target cell (causing cell lysis).

Flow Cytometry

Flow cytometry has been accepted as a versatile and useful tool for both research and clinical diagnostic immunology. Applications in clinical immunology include identification of cell surface antigen (markers), post-transplantation monitoring, and assessing progress of many malignant diseases (briefly described following).

Availability of monoclonal antibodies with almost unlimited antigen specificities and quantities produced by hybridoma and newer technologies (One Step Further Box 14-1) makes the flow cytometry procedure a particularly attractive tool for such clinical applications as:

- *Phenotyping*
- *Cell sorting*
- *DNA analysis*
- *Miscellaneous studies*

Box 14-1

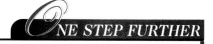

Production of Monoclonal Antibodies

The blood of any individual who has been immunized through actual infection or vaccination contains a variety of antibodies produced in response to the stimulating antigens. Although each antibody is produced by a single clone of B cells that has a unique structure and specificity for the antigen that stimulated its production, there is a basic structural similarity that is observed among all antibodies.

This similarity in structure allowed early researchers to isolate mixtures of antibodies (heterogenous or polyclonal antibodies) from the blood of immunized individuals and to propose a general antibody structure (see Chapter 5, Figure 5-7).

However, the heterogeneity (diversity) of these polyclonal antibodies (derived from more than one clone of B cells), prevented detailed analysis of the antibody structure.

The complete amino acid sequence of an individual antibody molecule was subsequently identified when the method of producing a single antibody with a single specificity for a particular antigenic determinant became available. These antibodies (originating from a single B cell clone) are known as *homogenous* or *monoclonal antibodies*.

Somatic Cell Hybridization (Hybridoma Technology)

With the development of somatic cell hybridization (cell fusion) technology by Kohler and Mildstein (1975), production of large quantities of monoclonal antibodies (mAbs) became possible. Originating from a single B cell clone, the monoclonal antibodies (homogenous antibodies) produced by this hybridoma technology showed single specificity for an antigenic determinant (epitope).

Thus production of monoclonal antibodies by somatic cell hybridization expanded the field of immunology and impacted on research in other disciplines as well as the area of clinical diagnosis and therapy.

PROCEDURE

Somatic cell hybridization is based on the fact that members of each B lymphocyte clone (originating from a single cell) express the same variable (V) region throughout their life, thus maintaining the same specificity for a particular antigen (one antigenic determinant).

The procedure involves fusion (in vitro) of mouse enzyme–deficient myeloma cells (immortalized cells, not able to synthesize antibodies) with B lymphocytes (able to produce antibodies) obtained from a mouse that has been immunized with a particular antigen. The resulting hybridomas (B cells + myeloma cells) are cultured (grown) in microtiter plates in media that is able to select hybridoma cells from other cells (i.e., unfused B cells that do not survive and myeloma cells that are not able to proliferate).

Thus the myeloma cells (hybrid cells) that are able to grow in this selective medium (hypoxanthine, aminopterin, thymidine [HAT]) produce antigen-specific monoclonal antibodies that can be identified by enzyme-linked immunosorbent assay (ELISA). These hybrid cells are then cloned in culture media or in ascitic tumors in mice (injected with the hybridoma) to expand the quantity of specific monoclonal antibodies.

Although the procedure is labor intensive and an inefficient process, the monoclonal antibodies thus produced can be frozen (cryopreserved) for long periods of time for future use.

Two characteristics of the somatic cell hybridization make this procedure particularly valuable:
- Production of specific monoclonal antibodies directed against a known and predetermined antigenic determinant (epitope)
- Use of monoclonal antibodies to identify unknown antigens in a mixture, based on their specificity for only one antigenic determinant (epitope)

Recombinant DNA Method

This method was originally proposed by Huse and colleagues (1989) for construction of the murine Fab gene library (using mouse splenic tissue as a source of Ig genes) and *E. coli* bacteriophage vector system. The human monoclonal antibody library, which was subsequently developed, uses a similar method. However, the source of B cells (Ig genes) are blood lymphocytes or bone marrow.

PROCEDURE

Construction of a gene library begins with isolation of messenger RNA (mRNA) from lymphoid tissue of a donor who has been immunized with a selected antigen; the mRNA is then converted into double-

Continued

Box 14-1—cont'd

ONE STEP FURTHER

stranded DNA (dsDNA) using reverse transcriptase and DNA polymerase. The thus produced mixture of conserved Ig V_H and V_L chain gene fragments is subjected to polymerase chain reaction (PCR), which amplifies these gene fragments (see Chapter 15).

The mixture of the amplified V_H and V_L Ig gene fragments is cloned into a plasmid vector, which will be expressed in *E. coli* bacteriophage as bacterio-

phage fusion protein (Fab gene fragments fused with bacteriophage surface coat protein).

Each recombinant bacteriophage contains a different combination of heavy and light chain variable region genes, which express antibodies with different specificities. This random gene rearrangement (V_H and V_L chain gene "shuffling" in the bacteriophage), has the potential for generating as many as 10^{8-10} different gene combinations.

Table 14-1	**SELECTED PHENOTYPIC CELL SURFACE MARKERS**
CD Marker*	Cell Population
CD3,5,7	All T lymphocytes
CD4	Helper T lymphocyte
CD8	Cytotoxic/suppressor T lymphocyte
CD19,20,22	B lymphocytes
CD10	Immature B lymphocytes
CD16,56	Natural killer (NK) cells
CD13,14,33	Monocytes/granulocytes
CD45	All leukocytes
CD41,61	Platelets (thrombocytes)
CD34	Progenitor (stem) cells

*Cluster of differentiation marker.

With the ongoing development and improvement in software, hardware, and reagents, new applications of flow cytometry in clinical immunology and other disciplines are constantly emerging.

REAGENT MONOCLONAL ANTIBODIES

Specific monoclonal antibodies, those originating from a single cell line, are completely homogeneous and selective in their reactivity. This is because each antibody is synthesized by a single clone of B lymphocytes with a specificity for a single epitope.

Thus reagent monoclonal antibodies show no cross-reactivity with other cells and can serve as a reliable indicator for the presence of specific cell receptors or markers that identify a particular cell type (Table 14-1). For example, a fluorochrome-labeled monoclonal antibody (anti-CD4) specific for CD4 receptor on the surface of a helper T cell will target only helper

T cells, forming detectable fluorescent antigen-antibody complexes (see also Direct Immunofluorescence Techniques, Chapter 13).

FLOW CYTOMETRIC METHODS

The components of a flow cytometer include a light source with focusing optics, a flow system, signal detectors and converters, and a computer system for data collection, processing, and storage.

By combining light scatter and labeled monoclonal antibodies, a flow cytometer can measure the properties of a single cell as it moves in a fluid medium (flow system based on hydrodynamic focusing) past a stationary set of signal detectors.

As the cell passes through a laser beam (light source) and disrupts the beam, there are two events that occur (Figure 14-1).

Light Scatter
The two types of light scatter are:
- *Forward light scatter (FALS):* Light scattering at a forward angle provides information on the cell size.
- *Light scatter at a 90 degree angle to the laser beam:* This event provides information on the granularity or nuclear structure of the cells.

Detection of Fluorescence
The cell sample is first reacted with fluorochrome-labeled monoclonal antibodies to form labeled antigen-antibody complexes on the cell surface. As the cells pass through the laser beam, the fluorochrome absorbs energy from the laser light and emits light at a different (longer) wavelength but one of lower energy

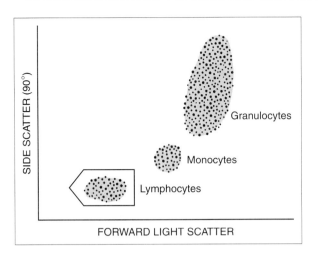

FIGURE **14-1** **Dot Plot Histogram.** Shown are light-scattering characteristics of leukocytes obtained by flow cytometry. The forward light scatter depicts size of the cells, while cell granularity is shown by side scatter of light. Note position of lymphocytes, reflecting their smaller size and reduced granularity compared to monocytes and granulocytes. A **gate** surrounding the lymphocytes indicates that this cell population has been selected for analysis.

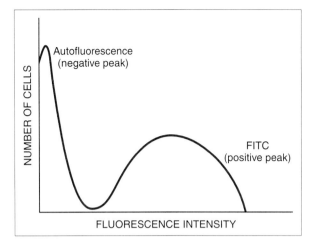

FIGURE **14-2** **Single Parameter Histogram.** A diagrammatic representation of a histogram showing autofluorescence (negative peak) and fluorescein isothiocyanate (FITC) positive cells (positive peak), as measured at 530 nm wavelength.

level. The amount of energy emitted is proportional to the amount of fluorochrome present on the cell surface or within the cell.

It is now possible to use two or more different color fluorochromes for labeling antibodies, such as fluorescein isothiocyanate (FITC), phycoerythrin (PE), and propidium iodide (PI), thus allowing for a simultaneous detection of each immunofluorescence of an individual cell (Figure 14-2). The number of wavelengths emitted represents the number of different fluorochromes present in the sample.

However, in order that the scattered light and the emitted wavelengths are in a format that can be of diagnostic value, they must be converted to digital signals for computer-enhanced data analysis by analog-to-digital converters (ADCs).

Data Collection and Processing

There are two ways of collecting digital data, both of which produce frequency distribution.

Histogram Method

In this method, data measured in single parameters is shown in frequency distributions. The histogram method stores frequency distribu-

tion of operator-selected variables, known as "raw data," that cannot be reprocessed.

List Mode Method (Dot Plot)

This method stores data from each cell for all pre-selected variables, making it possible to generate frequency distributions on more than one cell population in the sample without reprocessing the sample.

A two-variable histogram, showing a typical light scatter pattern of a normal sample, is presented in Figure 14-1 with a cell population of interest selected by an electronic "gating."

CLINICAL APPLICATION

Flow cytometry has gained acceptance in clinical laboratory practice as a diagnostic and prognostic tool in determining a variety of benign and malignant diseases, in tissue/organ transplantation, in determining immunodeficiency disorders, and in other applications.

Measuring large numbers of cells, identifying (phenotyping) and sorting cells according to specific cell surface markers, and analyzing DNA are some of the most frequent uses of flow cytometric analysis.

Cell Sorting

Flow cytometry with cell sorting capability can separate cells by size or an antibody marker. Its clinical application is to separate various populations of cells.

In the cell sorting procedure, the patient's cells are allowed to react with fluorochrome-labeled monoclonal antibodies showing specificity for the various cell surface markers. Binding that occurs between the surface marker (antigen) and the labeled monoclonal antibody with the same specificity produces labeled antigen-antibody complexes on the surface of the particular cell.

The labeled cells are then separated (sorted) according to the fluorescent signal (wavelength) that is emitted.

Immunophenotyping

This most frequently used flow cytometric procedure allows classification of cells based on the antigen or marker expressed on their cell surface (see Table 14-1). Thus immunophenotyping can provide information that identifies a specific cell lineage and the cell's maturation stage.

In immunophenotyping, when cells expressing a specific marker are exposed to fluorochrome-labeled monoclonal antibodies (mAbs), such as fluorescein isothiocyanate (FITC) or phycoerythrin (PE), with the corresponding antigen specificity, fluorescent antigen-antibody complex will form on the surface of these cells. The fluorescence (wavelength) emitted by the fluorochrome label is detected by the flow cytometer.

A two-color immunofluorescence (i.e., two different fluorochromes that absorb light at a similar wavelength and emit light at two different wavelengths [orange and green]) is also useful and has been frequently applied to enumeration of CD3+/CD4+ cells in patients infected with HIV (see Figure 14-2).

Clinical application of immunophenotyping includes pre-transplantation evaluation (see Chapter 6), monitoring of immunotherapy and immune reconstitution and chemotherapy in immunodeficiency diseases, establishing prognosis in HIV-positive patients, and diagnosing congenital immunodeficiency disease.

HLA Phenotyping

Individual class I major histocompatibility complex (MHC), also known as *human leukocyte antigen* (HLA-A, HLA-B, and HLA-C antigens) and *class II MHC molecules* (HLA-DR and HLA-DQ), have been defined by serologic testing using reagent monoclonal antibodies (produced against distinct class I HLA and class II HLA) (see Testing for Histocompatibility in Transplantation [tissue typing], Chapter 8).

In flow cytometric HLA phenotyping, specific fluorochrome-labeled monoclonal antibodies for each HLA specificity are used and allowed to react with the class I and II HLA. The procedure for identifying the HLA specificity (phenotype) is performed as described previously in the discussion on immunophenotyping.

Tumor Cell Phenotyping

Immunophenotyping of tumor cells by flow cytometry is performed according to the protocol described previously. However, as in HLA typing, the monoclonal antibodies used are fluorochrome labeled and antigen specific.

For example, leukemia-associated antigens such as terminal deoxynucleotidyl transferase (TdT) (a cytoplasmic marker) and common acute lymphoblastic leukemia antigen (CALLA) (a cell surface marker, now officially designated as CD10) are used mainly as markers of hematopoietic cancers (Table 14-2).

Diagnosis and Prognosis of Malignancy

Although many flow cytometric methods have been developed for use in tumor cell analysis, two types of analysis (i.e., DNA content analysis and cell-surface antigen analysis [immunophenotyping]) are most commonly used.

Thus, by identifying cell surface markers by immunophenotyping (see Table 14-2) and quantifying DNA content of the individual cells (described following), it is now possible to identify cells in such hematologic malignancies as acute lymphoblastic leukemia (ALL), lymphoma, non-lymphocytic leukemia, and chronic lymphocytic leukemia (CLL).

DNA analysis can be used to support morphologic evaluation (microscopic) of stained cells or tissue, thus serving as a diagnostic and prognostic tool in the management of many cancers, such as breast, colon, etc.

DNA Content Analysis

DNA ploidy. Normal cells that contain two copies of each chromosome are diploid, and all

Table 14-2	PHENOTYPES IN SELECTED HEMATOLOGIC MALIGNANCIES	
Malignancy	Phenotype	Comments
All (T cell)	CD3+, CD7+, CD5−	Loss of any normal T cell marker (e.g., CD5) Tdt+, usually children
ALL (B cell)	CD10/22+, CD19+	Tdt+, usually in children
CLL (B cell)	CD 5/19+, CD20+, CD22+	Weak expression of monoclonal L chain (κ or λ), usually in adults
Lymphoma	CD19+, CD20+, CD22+	Monoclonal κ- or λ-L chain sIg+ (sIgG or sIgM)

*Electrophoretically separated.

ALL, acute lymphoblastic leukemia; *CLL,* chronic lymphocytic leukemia; *sIg,* surface immunoglobulin; *CD,* cluster of differentiation, *CD10/22+,* co-expression; *CD5/19+,* co-expression; *L,* light chain; *Tdt,* terminal deoxynucleotidyl transferase.

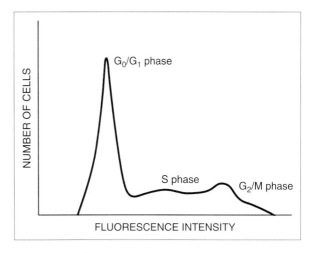

FIGURE **14-3** DNA Cell Cycle Histogram. Histogram represents fluorescence intensity in cell replication analysis. The quantity of S phase fraction (SPF) shown on the histogram correlates with the proliferative activity of tumor cells and their aggressiveness. For example, a good correlation is seen between an observed SPF and the survival of a patient with breast carcinoma. *G,* growth (cell cycle over 24 hours); G_0/G_1 *phase,* pre-DNA synthesis phase; *S phase,* DNA synthesis; G_2/M *phase,* post-DNA synthesis.

cells (excepting ova and sperm) that are not diploid are considered aneuploid and can serve as a reliable indicator of neoplasia.

Ploidy analysis can be used (as a research procedure) during chemotherapy to monitor the effectiveness of treatment in eliminating the aneuploid clone and in predicting the outcome of certain malignancies.

Analysis of tumor ploidy is performed by flow cytometry, which determines the total amount of nuclear DNA in individual tumor cells. The DNA index (DI), used to determine ploidy of a tumor is a calculated ratio of DNA fluorescence of tumor cells to fluorescence of normal cells (Figure 14-3), when control and tumor cells are analyzed simultaneously.

The DNA Index (DI) of a diploid tumor is 1, and DI more or less than 1 indicates an aneuploid tumor, which is typically a sign of poor prognosis in carcinoma of the ovary, bladder, colorectum, and in melanoma.

DNA-specific fluorescence-emitting dye, such as propidium iodide, is used as a label that binds to the nuclei of the tumor cells.

The amount of DNA of each cell is measured by the intensity of DNA-specific fluorescence, emitted as the cells pass through a laser beam of a flow cytometer, and is directly proportional to the amount of DNA present in the cell.

DNA cell cycle analysis. It is also possible to measure DNA content at various cell cycle phases during cell replication (i.e., G_0/G_1, S, G_2/M phases [see Figure 14-3]) to assess cell growth and cancer aggressiveness.

The analysis is performed by staining the nuclei of cells with various DNA stains and measuring the DNA content of the cell in a flow cytometer. The amount of the DNA of the cell is proportional to the amount of DNA that has been synthesized by the cell and is directly proportional to the aggressiveness of the tumor.

Thus, the more DNA that has been synthesized, the more aggressive is the cancer, and cells going through the S phase show DNA synthesis that is directly proportional to their aggressiveness.

Other Applications
Leukocyte Cross-Matching (Histocompatibility Testing)
This highly sensitive automated cross-matching method (100 times more sensitive than macroscopic serologic procedures) for detecting HLA antibodies is typically performed in situations such as (1) previous graft rejections, (2) living related donors (after negative T cell and positive B cell serologic cross-match), and (3) patients on a waiting list for donors (cadavers).

procedure. In this procedure, separation of T and B lymphocytes is accomplished electronically by tagging B cells with a fluoresceinated goat anti-human reagent (FITC-IgG antiserum). Separate peaks for T and B cells will be observed on a histogram (tracing of fluorescence).

Briefly, fluorescent anti-human antibody is added to donor lymphocytes that have been incubated with patient serum. The labeled reagent antibodies bind to surface immunoglobulins (sIg) of donor B cells. The goat anti-human antiserum (FITC-labeled) also binds to T cells, which express a donor HLA patient HLA-specific antibody complex that is bound to their surface. This HLH/Ab complex forms when the HLA antibodies are adsorbed (bound) to donor T cells from patient serum during incubation.

test interpretation. B cells are identified by their fluorescence peak on a histogram. Donor T cells, showing fluorescence because of the presence of donor HLA/patient HLA antibodies/goat anti-human (FITC-labeled) complex on their surface, produce a separate characteristic peak, which is compared with the histogram tracing of a positive control serum and a negative (normal) control serum tracing (i.e., normal T cell peak).

T cell histogram, that is comparable to the positive control serum, is indicative of the presence of antibodies (patient's serum) against class I antigens (donor T cells) This cross-match result is considered positive, indicating existence of incompatibility between the donor and the patient.

COMPLEMENT ASSAYS

Complement analysis may serve as an important tool for detection of complement deficiency that may be associated with such conditions as infectious, autoimmune, or inflammatory diseases.

The role that the complement system plays in the defense of the body against foreign antigens by antibody-mediated cell lysis (blood cells, bacteria, and enveloped viruses) has been discussed in Chapter 4.

In vivo cell lysis or damage can be initiated by either antigen-antibody complexes (classical pathway) or by C3b (alternative pathway) activation of complement. Both activation pathways ultimately form a membrane attack complex (MAC) that causes disruption of the cell membrane and cell lysis (see Chapter 4 and Figure 4-3).

Thus, performing an in vitro study for total hemolytic activity of complement, known as the CH_{50} and AH_{50} functional assays (described following), can serve as a screening test for complement abnormalities.

For quantifying individual complement components such as C3, C4, and factor B, the most frequently used assays are nephelometry and ELISA.

ASSAYS FOR COMPLEMENT ABNORMALITIES

It is important to remember that complement components are protein in nature and as such are heat labile. Thus, when stored above $-70°$ C, complement will readily undergo a breakdown and lose its activity. Therefore collection and storage of serum samples for analysis of complement by immunoassays (e.g., rate nephelometry and ELISA) and functional assays (e.g., total hemolytic assay) requires immediate separation of serum from clotted blood and storage at $-70°$ C or lower to preserve its maximal activity integrity.

There are two types of tests that can be used to evaluate complement:
- *Hemolytic complement activity assays*
- *Immunoassays*

Complement Activity Assay (Hemolytic Titration)
The hemolytic activity assay can be used as a screening test for congenital deficiency of complement components that affect the total hemolytic activity of serum (entire complement sequence, which is required to produce cell lysis).

There are two functional assays, known as CH_{50} and AH_{50} assays, that reflect the sequential activation of all of the components of the classical and alternative pathways, respectively, so that when any one of the components is missing, the resulting value for both assays will be 0 U/mL.

CH_{50} Hemolytic Assay

Total hemolytic activity (i.e., the entire complement activation sequence [C1 to C9] required for production of lysis of antibody-coated cells [antibody-mediated hemolysis]) is quantified by determining the dilution of serum (complement) needed to lyse 50% of sheep red blood cells (SRBC) that have been sensitized with rabbit anti-sheep antiserum (antibody or hemolysin):

(SRBC + Hemolysin) → Sensitized SRBC

Sensitized SRBC + Serum Complement→
Hemolysis of SRBC

The amount of hemolysis (total complement activity) produced in each dilution of this assay (prepared as a serial dilution) is detected by a spectrophotometric measurement of absorbance (concentration) of hemoglobin released from the lysed SRBC.

A standard curve (using controls) is constructed by plotting the amount of absorbance (hemoglobin released from SRBC) against an increasing amount of fresh guinea pig serum added (source of complement) in order to standardize the system.

Reciprocal of the serum dilution is expressed as the CH_{50} test result (CH_{50} units/mL of serum).

A microtiter version of the CH_{50} is also available and so are commercially prepared reagents for CH_{50} assay.

AH_{50} Hemolytic Assay

This functional assay is performed to evaluate alternative pathway–dependent lysis, using unsensitized rabbit red blood cells (RRBC) and human serum complement (patient's serum).

A serial dilution of the patient's serum (containing complement) is prepared and incubated with the RRBC. The reaction occurs as follows:

Serum Complement + RRBC → Hemolysis of RRBC

The amount of hemoglobin released from the hemolyzed RRBC is detected by the spectrophotometric reading of optical density (OD) and extrapolated from a previously constructed standard curve.

Immunoassays for Complement Components

The availability of commercially prepared antibodies directed against major complement components and complement inhibitors make determination of each of the complement components and control proteins possible by such immunoassays as nephelometry and enzyme-linked immunosorbent assay (ELISA) (discussed in Chapter 13).

However, results of immunoassays provide only a molecular concentration (quantity) of a particular complement component in serum. Thus any information regarding the quality or functional integrity of the complement molecule is obtained by functional studies (discussed previously).

Newer methods, such as an automated system, are currently being considered as a possible replacement for these functional studies (i.e., CH_{50} and AH_{50}).

Interpretation of Test Results

A direct correlation has been observed between reduced C3 level detected by immunoassays and reduction in CH_{50} total hemolytic activity (described previously).

The significance of reduction in complement activity and the reduction or increase in complement level are discussed following.

Reduced Complement Levels

Reduced levels have been attributed to one or more of the following mechanisms: (1) complement consumption during an in vivo formation of antigen-antibody complexes (immune complexes), (2) reduced synthesis of complement, (3) increased catabolism of complement, and (4) presence of an inhibitor.

Reduction in Serum Complement Activity

Reduction in complement activity has been observed in a variety of diseases, such as lymphoma, allograft rejection, infective hepatitis with arthritis, severe combined immunodeficiency, systemic lupus erythematosus with glomerulonephritis, and immune complex disease.

Although complement deficiencies are uncommon (1 in 10,000), the patient with the deficiency may have a life-threatening situation.

Increased Levels of Complement

Although increased complement levels have been observed in a variety of diseases (e.g., gout, diabetes, thyroiditis, acute rheumatic fever, and rheumatoid arthritis), the significance of these observations has not been established. However, it has been suggested that the increase in the complement level is the result of its overproduction.

COMPLEMENT-DEPENDENT TECHNIQUES

Cytotoxicity Tests

These complement-dependent techniques (using complement as a reagent) are discussed under functional studies (see following).

Complement Fixation Tests

The classic complement fixation test uses complement as a reagent. Because complement fixation occurs after the binding of antigen and its specific antibody, complement can serve as the indicator of the presence of a specific antigen or antibody in the test sample.

Procedure

The complement fixation test consists of a two-step in vitro reaction (Figure 14-4).

Before testing, complement present in the patient's serum must be inactivated by heating to 56° C for 30 minutes.

- *Stage 1 (test system):* Involves interaction between a known antigen and an antibody (analyte) in the patient's serum in the presence of complement. Various dilutions of serum are dispensed into tubes, according to a standard titration procedure, to which an antigen of known specificity and a predetermined amount of guinea pig complement is added. The interaction between the test components during incubation results in formation of antigen-antibody complexes and consumption of complement.
- *Stage 2 (indicator system):* Measures remaining complement in the test mixture by employing the hemolytic assay as follows: sheep red blood cells and he-

molysin are added to the test system. After additional incubation and centrifugation, the tubes are visually evaluated for hemolysis.

Interpretation of Test Results

positive results. These results are reported as the highest tube dilution showing no hemolysis. The lack of hemolysis indicates that the specific antibody is present and that the complement has been consumed during stage I and is not available to produce cell lysis during stage II of the reaction (positive result).

negative results. These results show the presence of hemolysis and an absence of the particular antibody tested. The hemolysis occurs because complement has not been confirmed in stage I and is available in stage II to produce hemolysis (negative result). The amount of complement fixed (consumed) during this reaction is proportional to the amount of antibody present in the test serum.

Hemolytic Assays

The use of complement as a reagent has been discussed under the assay for complement hemolytic activity (see previously), in which sheep red blood cells (SRBC), sensitized with rabbit antibody directed against the SRBC, have been exposed to complement.

The quantity of hemolysis of SRBC (hemoglobin release) produced by added guinea pig complement is determined by spectrophotometry.

Hemolysis Inhibition Assays (ASO)

Detection of an antibody response to streptococcal exotoxins produced by group A streptococci, involves the most important anti-toxin antibodies such as anti-streptolysin O, anti-DNase B, anti-NADase, and antihyaluronidase used to diagnose and document acute rheumatic fever or post-streptococcal glomerulonephritis (both being a sequelae of streptococcal infection), particularly in situations where the organism may no longer be present.

Previously the most frequently used procedure for detecting streptococcal antibodies was the *anti-streptolysin O (ASO) titer.* These streptococcal lysins or antibodies (specific for the streptolysin O antigen) are capable of destroying (lysing) erythrocytes and leukocytes.

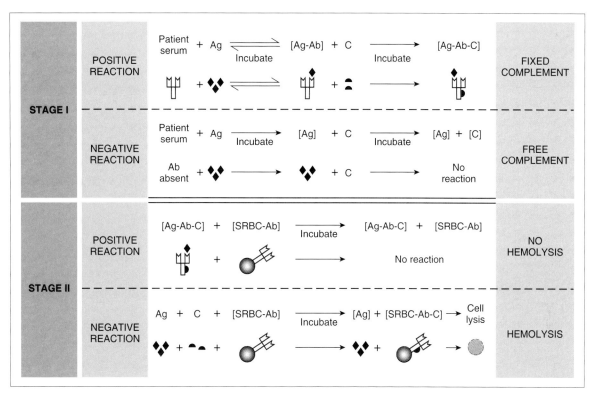

FIGURE **14-4** Complement Fixation Test. This test consists of two steps. **Stage I** (test system) reaction that removes reagent complement from the medium, when antigen-specific antibodies are present in the patient's serum. This is accomplished by formation of an antigen-antibody-complement complex (positive test). **Stage II** (indicator system). Because reaction in Stage I is not detectable, an indicator system (SRBC-Ab) is added to the procedure, to show absence of hemolysis of SRBCs when complement is absent (bound in Stage I). Hemolysis indicates a negative result when specific antibodies are absent and free complement is available and is activated to produce cell lysis. *Ag*, antigen; *C*, complement; *Ab*, antibody; *SRBCs*, sheep red blood cells.

The ASO titer results are used in diagnosis of post-streptococcal infections (i.e., glomerulonephritis and rheumatic fever).

Procedure

The procedure is a hemolysis inhibition technique and is based on the ability of the anti-streptococcal antibodies (anti-streptolysin O) to inhibit or neutralize the hemolytic activity of streptolysin O (oxygen-labile, hemolytic streptococcal exotoxin) produced by group A streptococci during their multiplication. Human red blood cells (RBCs) are used in the procedure to serve as an indicator of cell lysis (hemolysis).

This hemolysis inhibition technique involves preparation of serial dilution of patient's serum in tubes, addition of commercially pre-pared streptolysin O, and incubation of the mixture. After addition of RBCs and further incubation of the mixture, the tubes are centrifuged and visually evaluated for hemolysis (Figure 14-5). Controls must be included in the procedure.

Hemolysis of RBCs is inhibited (no hemolysis will be seen) when patient's serum contains anti-streptolysin O (specific antibodies to streptolysin O). As the dilution of serum increases, the concentration of antibodies in serum decreases. Therefore the reciprocal of the highest serum dilution showing no hemolysis is considered as the ASO titer.

Interpretation of Test Results

Serum antibody titer (ASO titer) is reported as the reciprocal of the highest serum dilution

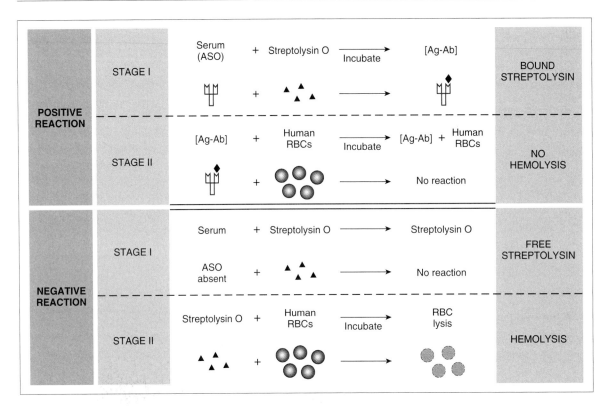

FIGURE **14-5** **Anti-Streptolysin O (ASO) Test.** An example of a two-stage hemolysis inhibition technique, in which the reagent streptolysin O is prevented from lysing human red blood cells (RBC) in Stage I by having been bound to specific antibodies (ASO), present in the patient's serum. In this procedure, hemolysis inhibition (no observable hemolysis) is a positive reaction, indicating presence of ASO antibodies in the patient's serum. *Ag,* antigen; *Ab,* antibody; *(Ag-Ab),* antigen-antibody complex; *ASO,* anti-streptolysin O; *RBCs,* red blood cells (erythrocytes).

showing no hemolysis (see Figure 14-5). However, a single titer is not diagnostically significant, requiring a repeat of the procedure in 2 weeks. A four-fold rise in the titer (two tubes) is considered of clinical significance.

A negative result, however, does not rule out the presence of glomerulonephritis or acute rheumatic fever because individuals may respond differently to streptococcal antigens, thus requiring laboratory and clinical findings for final diagnosis.

FUNCTIONAL ASSAYS

Lymphocytes are a preferred cell population for conducting functional studies for immune competence and histocompatibility testing.

CELL SEPARATION TECHNIQUES

Any one of the cell separation techniques, briefly described following, can be used for isolation of mononuclear leukocytes (lymphocytes, monocytes) from circulating blood. The selection of technique depends on the assay to be performed.

Density Gradient Separation

Density gradient separation of mononuclear cells is based on the fact that neutrophils and erythrocytes are denser than the mononuclear cells. Therefore, by employing a solution of greater density than the mononuclear blood cell population (but one of lesser density than erythrocytes and neutrophils), mononuclear cells can be separated from other blood cells.

The procedure consists of layering anti-coagulated venous whole blood, over a Ficoll-Hypaque or Histopaque (Sigma) solution dispensed into a centrifuge tube. After centrifugation, a layer of mononuclear cells that forms at the interface between the plasma and the Ficoll solution can be removed (aspirated and washed in buffered saline solution), thus separating lymphocytes and other mononuclear cells from cells that pass through the Ficoll solution and settle at the bottom of the tube.

This cell isolation technique is suitable for use in such procedures as cell-mediated cytotoxicity and tissue typing (discussed following).

Magnetic Separation

Separation of cell populations can be performed with commercially prepared magnetic beads (plastic with magnetic core), coated (sensitized) with monoclonal antibodies (mAb) with specificity for a selected cell surface marker (e.g., CD19 marker for B lymphocytes).

The procedure consists of mixing the immunomagnetic (mAb-coated) beads with cells in the patient's sample. Cells that are recognized by the specific antibody coating the beads will be bound and then removed by exposure to a magnetic field.

Because of the specificity of the mAb-coated magnetic beads, the cell population isolated by this method is highly purified. The procedure is also faster than the traditional density gradient methods.

Panning (Plating)

This procedure is used to separate cell subpopulations from the total cell population.

A plastic plate is coated with an antibody of selected antigen specificity, and the test cells are applied to the plate. Cells having the same antigen specificity as the antibodies on the plate will bind to the antibodies and the free cells (antigen negative) can be washed off.

Nylon Wool Column (Straw Method)

The "straw method" is based on the principle that B lymphocytes adhere to nylon wool (packed in a straw) during an incubation period, while the T lymphocytes are flushed out with the media.

However, although the procedure is simple and easy to perform, it is time-consuming, and the B cell population is not completely pure because of contamination with T cells.

The method is an inexpensive way of separating large quantities of T and B lymphocyte populations.

Cell Sorting (Flow Cytometry)

This method of separating cells uses a very sophisticated instrument (fluorescence-activated cell sorter) that combines the analytic capability of flow cytometry and its ability to sort cells according to their specific surface marker.

The advantage of this method is that various lymphocyte populations, such as T and B cells, can now be separated (sorted). However, the use of cell separating by flow cytometry is mainly used in research although it is now slowly gaining popularity in a clinical laboratory setting.

In this procedure, the lymphocytes are allowed to react with fluorochrome-labeled monoclonal antibodies with specificity for the selected cell surface marker. The binding that occurs between the surface marker (antigen) and the labeled monoclonal antibody with the same specificity produces labeled antigen-antibody complexes on the surface of the lymphocyte.

Thus labeled lymphocytes are then processed in the cell sorter according to the manufacturer's instructions and separated (sorted) according to the fluorescent signal (wavelength) that is emitted. The separated cells can then be collected in tubes or directly placed into a microtiter plate.

The cells sorted by flow cytometry remain viable and sterile throughout the process and can be used for cell analysis as well as functional assays (cell cultures) (discussed following).

CELL CULTURES

Lymphocyte cultures can be used for evaluating immune competence or functional capacity of T and B lymphocytes by using various stimuli (e.g., mitogen, antigen, or human leukocyte antigen [HLA]) on allogeneic cells (stimulator cells from another individual with different HLA antigens) to activate lymphocytes and trigger their proliferation.

Cell Culture Technique

A lymphocyte culture is usually set up in triplicate in a microtiter plate. A predetermined concentration of stimulating antigen or mitogen and separated patient's lymphocytes (suspended in an appropriate medium) are added to the wells. The cell culture is then incubated to allow the cells to respond to the antigenic stimulus. A normal cell culture control, consisting of patient's cells without the stimulus, is also prepared and processed simultaneously.

Before harvesting the cells, a labeled DNA precursor (^{3}H-thymidine) is added to the cell culture mixture for incorporation into new DNA molecules, synthesized during additional incubation time.

After incubation, the cells are collected by a cell-harvesting device and the amount of radioactivity emitted from the cells (^{3}H-thymidine incorporated into newly synthesized DNA) is measured as counts per minute (cpm) in a liquid scintillation counter.

The patient's actual response to the stimulus is determined by subtracting cpm of radioactivity obtained from the normal cell culture control (i.e., patient's cell culture without antigenic stimulus) from cpm obtained from the patient's cell culture with antigenic stimulus, thus measuring the amount of newly (de novo) synthesized DNA. The amount of newly synthesized DNA is indicative of the patient's immune competence (i.e., lymphocyte responsiveness to an antigenic stimulation).

Lymphocyte Activation and Proliferation

As the resting peripheral blood lymphocytes are stimulated (activated) by an antigen or a non-specific mitogen (plant lectins or other substances added to the cell culture mixture [see previously]), the lymphocytes enter a process known as *transformation* or *blastogenesis* as evidenced by such cell cycle events as synthesis of protein, RNA, and DNA that lead to cell division (mitosis) and proliferation of the activated cells.

The degree of new (de novo) DNA synthesis is determined by the cpm emitted from ^{3}H-thymidine (measured by scintillation counter) that has been incorporated into the DNA during its synthesis in a cell culture.

Thus DNA synthesis serves as a marker for lymphocyte activation and proliferation and the ability of T and B lymphocytes to respond to an antigen or mitogen stimulation (e.g., *Candida* antigen or phytohemagglutinin [PHA], respectively). The assay measures the functional capacity (immune competence) of the T and B lymphocytes.

Antigen Stimulation

Stimulation of lymphocytes by antigens is limited to only those lymphocytes that are specifically sensitized to the particular stimulating antigen. Therefore the total DNA synthesis is low under standard cell culture conditions and requires a longer culture time for maximal response.

Normal individuals show a good correlation between the in vitro antigen stimulation technique and the skin tests for an allergic response (delayed-type hypersensitivity [DTH], see Chapter 7) by the same antigen.

Mitogen Stimulation

Unlike the antigenic stimulators, stimulation of lymphocytes by mitogens is non-specific (i.e., not requiring previous cell sensitization) (Figure 14-6). This allows for stimulation of large number of lymphocytes.

Mixed Lymphocyte Reaction (MLR)

Immune response to genetically incompatible tissue HLA antigens can be produced and evaluated by setting up a cell culture (described previously).

When two allogeneic cell populations (cells from two different individuals), containing dissimilar HLA (class I and class II major histocompatibility complex antigens [MHC]) on their cell surface, are used in a cell culture, the procedure is known as a *mixed lymphocyte culture (MLC)*, or a *mixed leukocyte reaction (MLR)*, used interchangeably. As the two allogeneic cell populations are allowed to interact and recognize the dissimilar (foreign) HLA on their cell surfaces, the events that follow are cell activation and proliferation (described previously).

The MLR can be set up as either a "one-way" or "two-way" protocol, see Chapter 4 and Figure 6-4.

"one-way" protocol. In a one-way MLR, the patient's lymphocytes are exposed to a foreign histocompatibility antigen (HLA) located on

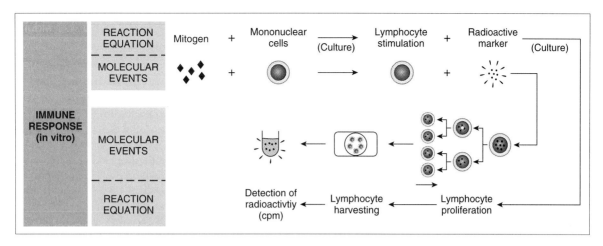

FIGURE **14-6** **Lymphocyte Stimulation by Mitogens.** Shown is response of patient's mononuclear cells to stimulation with a mitogen (plant lectin serving as an antigen) that does not require specific recognition by patient's lymphocytes. This in vitro technique is used to evaluate patient's immune response in microtiter plates. The amount of cell proliferation is measured by incorporation of a radioactive marker, such as ^{3}H thymidine, into newly synthesized DNA and detecting the emitted radioactivity in counts per minute (cpm). The amount of radioactivity is directly proportional to the efficiency or integrity of the immune response.

the surface of unrelated (allogeneic) lymphocytes. These cells, serving as stimulator cells, are treated with mytomycin C or irradiated to prevent them from responding and synthesizing DNA, but without making them non-viable.

The one-way MLR procedure is performed using the antigen stimulation technique procedure (see previously).

The immunocompetent-responding lymphocytes (patient's cells), when activated by the allogeneic HLA, will synthesize new DNA and proliferate, incorporating labeled thymidine (^{3}H-thymidine) into the newly synthesized DNA.

Therefore the total response (synthesis of DNA) originates from the patient's lymphocytes (responder cells).

The amount of the new (de novo) DNA synthesis, as detected by the amount of radioactivity emitted from the responders (patient's cells) in a scintillation counter, is a measure of the degree of lymphocyte responsiveness, which is a measure of the patient's T cell function.

"two-way" protocol. When both cell populations are immunocompetent (able to proliferate) and are mutually stimulating and responding because of differences in their MHC antigens, either of the two populations can serve as an inducer (stimulator) of the immune response and the other as a responder to the non-self HLA stimulus. The reaction is known as a two-way MLR.

Thus the amount of DNA synthesis produced during the two-way MLR represents a total response of both sets of cells and can be used to predict the success of a graft or cell-mediated rejection of graft by the host's immune system in a transplantation procedure.

CYTOTOXICITY ASSAYS

Lymphocyte-mediated cytotoxicity consists of three stages, which include (1) conjugate formation (i.e., direct membrane-to-membrane contact between the cytolytic cell [cytotoxic lymphocyte] and the target cell to form a conjugate), (2) triggering of various membrane and cellular metabolic events, and (3) pore formation in the target cell membrane by lymphocyte secretions (e.g., perforin) and/or non-secretory events, resulting in release of cytoplasmic granules (see Chapter 7). These events can be produced in vitro in a cytotoxicity assay that can be used to evaluate cytotoxic T lymphocyte function. A commonly used technique is described following.

Chromium (^{51}Cr) Release Assay

This commonly used in vitro lymphocyte-mediated cytotoxicity assay is used as an indicator of the efficiency of cytotoxic T lymphocytes (CTL) in lysing such target cells as tumor cells, allogeneic tissue cells, or virally infected cells.

Radioactive chromium (^{51}Cr) is used in this assay as a marker of target cell lysis because of its ability to bind intracellular proteins of target cells (other potential radioactive labels include ^{3}H-proline and ^{3}H-thymidine). Thus, when target cell lysis occurs, the chromium-labeled proteins are released from the labeled target cells and the amount of chromium released is proportional to the quantity of lysed cells.

The target cell lysis by CTLs occurs without the participation of antibodies or complement (see Chapter 1 and Figure 1-13).

Procedure

Briefly, lymphocytes are incubated with chromium (^{51}Cr)-labeled target cell population. After centrifugation of the incubated cell mixture, ^{51}Cr-containing supernatant fluid is removed and quantified by detecting emitted gamma rays on a gamma scintillation counter (Figure 14-7).

The amount of ^{51}Cr released from lysed cells is indicative of the CTL function.

EVALUATION OF NEUTROPHIL FUNCTION

As previously described in Chapter 1, polymorphonuclear neutrophils (PMNs, present in the bloodstream and extravascular spaces) play a central role in host defense against infection.

In assessing the function of these PMNs, other components of the immune response, such as immunoglobulins (antibodies), complement, and chemotactic factors, must also be considered. Disorders that are associated with PMN function may be the result of a qualitative or quantitative abnormality of the PMN.

For example, in a *qualitative disorder,* although the total number of neutrophils is either normal or highly increased, their antimicrobial function is not effective. This is seen in chronic granulomatous disease (see Chapter 7), in which the normal or increased number of PMNs cannot destroy certain intracellular microorganisms because of a deficiency in any one of the stages or activities that occur during phagocytosis.

Methods

Nitroblue Tetrazolium Dye Reduction Test (NBT Test)

Neutrophils have the ability to reduce NBT dye on ingestion of certain particles (e.g., latex) after respiratory burst (H_2O_2 generation). Failure to generate hydrogen peroxide (H_2O_2) and to reduce NBT dye is of diagnostic value in determining overall reduction of phagocytic function of neutrophils (see Immunodeficiency, Chapter 7).

Flow Cytometry

In many laboratories, flow cytometry (discussed previously) has replaced the NBT test for detection of chronic granulomatous disease.

Chemiluminescence

Neutrophils emit a small amount of energy (chemiluminescence) during the respiratory burst, which can be amplified by adding luminol in the presence of ingestible latex particles. The photons of light emitted can be measured in a luminator (see Chapter 13).

The test measures the overall phagocytic activity of neutrophils.

Anti-Neutrophil Cytoplasmic Autoantibodies (ANCA)

Detection of ANCA is performed primarily to evaluate patients who have or are suspected of having primary small vessel vasculitis not associated with connective tissue or chronic inflammatory conditions.

These vasculitis-associated autoantibodies are directed against two main enzymes (antigens): proteinase 3 (PR3) and myeloperoxidase (MPO).

procedure. Indirect immunofluorescence technique (IIF) (described in Chapter 13) for detection of anti-nuclear antibodies can be adopted for detecting two fluorescence-staining patterns of ANCA (i.e., cytoplasmic [cANCA] and perinuclear [pANCA]). The IIF technique is performed on ethanol-fixed leukocytes.

Negative serum control and positive cANCA and pANCA controls are processed together

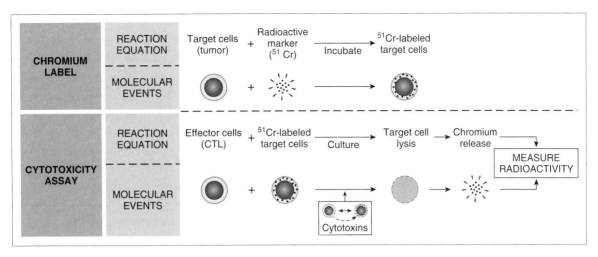

FIGURE **14-7** **Cytotoxicity Assay.** This chromium release assay is used for determining efficiency of cytotoxic T lymphocytes (CTLs).   The cytotoxic activity of the CTL (CD8+ effector cells) is detected by incorporating a radioactive chromium marker (^{51}Cr) into target cells (abnormal or infected cells). Radioactivity is measured when target cells are lysed by cytotoxins released by CTLs.

with the patient's serum. A positive cANCA in the patient's serum is further tested by enzyme-linked immunosorbent assay (ELISA), as described in Chapter 13.

HISTOCOMPATIBILITY TESTING

PHENOTYPING

Tissue Typing Procedures

Tissue typing (phenotyping), also known as *serologic tissue typing* or *human leukocyte antigen (HLA) typing procedure,* is used for the detection of various cell surface markers that include the human leukocyte antigens (HLA) present on the cell surface of a potential donor's and recipient's mononuclear cells.

Class I major histocompatibility complex (MHC) molecules consist of HLA-A, HLA-B, and HLA-C antigens, whereas the class II MHC molecules are IILA-DR, DQ, and DP antigens (see Chapter 6).

Both classes of MHC antigens (molecules) can be individually identified with a panel of selected alloantibodies (HLA typing sera) that are highly specific for the particular HLA, using the following procedures.

Microcytotoxicity Test for Class I HLA

The microcytotoxicity procedure (see Chapter 6, Figure 6-8) is an in vitro tissue typing method used for typing of isolated blood mononuclear cells (lymphocytes).

In histocompatibility testing, the tissue typing procedure is performed on the donor and recipient blood mononuclear cells as a component of donor and recipient (patient) pre-transplantation testing, discussed in Chapter 6.

procedure. The microcytotoxicity procedure is based on the antibody-mediated (complement-dependent) lysis of target cells that carry antigens (class I and class II MHC) of the same specificity as the reagent HLA antibody (see Chapter 6, Figure 6-8).

Isolated blood mononuclear cells (see cell separation, discussed previously) are reacted with a reagent panel of antisera (HLA antibodies of known specificities). Complement is added to the test system and becomes activated when binding occurs between reagent antibody and the corresponding HLA on the cells being tested. The activated complement initiates a cytotoxic destruction or lysis of the target cells (see Chapter 4, Figure 4-3, and Chapter 6, Figure 6-8).

The cytotoxic effect (target cell lysis) can be observed microscopically as a cell uptake of a dye, such as eosin or trypan blue.

test interpretation. The test is considered positive for a specific cell marker (HLA) when at least 50% of the mononuclear cells have been destroyed, as shown by the dye uptake (eosin or trypan blue).

Microcytotoxicity Test for Class II HLA

Tissue typing procedure for class II HLA (HLA-DR/DQ typing) is similar to class I HLA typing, differing only by:

- The specificity of antisera (HLA-DR, HLA-DQ antigen specific).
- Monoclonal cell preparation for testing. B lymphocytes (expressing class II HLA) are enriched by separating T cells from B cells to ensure that an adequate number is available for typing (see separation techniques, previously discussed). (Resting T lymphocytes [lacking class II HLA antigens] comprise approximately 80% of peripheral blood lymphocytes).

Microcytotoxicity Tests for HLA Antibodies

The standard microcytotoxicity procedure (see previous discussion and Chapter 6, Figure 6-8) may be applied to detection and cross-match of the following antibodies.

HLA Cytotoxic Antibodies

The donor or recipient serum (source of HLA antibodies) is tested against a panel of known type T and B lymphocytes to detect and identify antibodies according to their HLA specificity.

HLA Autoantibodies (Autologous Cross-Match)

The recipient serum (source of antibodies) and cells (source of antigens) are tested against each other to detect the presence of antibodies directed against self-antigens, known as *autoantibodies*. It is important to distinguish autoantibodies (non-specific anti-lymphocyte antibodies), from specific antibodies (alloantibodies) directed against the donor antigens (see discussion following).

Donor-Specific Alloantibodies (Major Cross-Match)

Patient serum is tested against the potential donor cells to detect the presence of any antibodies in the patient serum that may react with HLA (class I or class II MHC molecules) located on the cells of the potential donor.

CROSS-MATCHING

Mixed Lymphocyte Reaction (MLR) Cross-Match

Donor and recipient lymphocytes are combined in tissue culture medium and cultured according to the two-way mixed lymphocyte reaction (MLR) previously described and presented in Chapter 6, Figure 6-4.

The strength of the MLR is proportional to the extent of the differences in HLA identities (expressed on the donor and recipient lymphocytes). Thus the MLR is useful in selecting a donor (organ or tissues) that is least stimulatory to the patient's immune system (i.e., shows the lowest response in the mixed lymphocyte culture) and therefore is most compatible (see also Chapter 6).

Flow Cytometric Cross-Match

In this procedure (described earlier), donor T cells, showing fluorescence because of the presence of donor HLA antigen/patient HLA antibodies/goat anti-human (FITC-labeled) complex on their surface, are detected as a separate characteristic peak on a histogram (see Figure 14-2), which is compared with histogram tracing of a positive control serum.

The cross-match is considered positive or incompatible (i.e., incompatibility between donor and patient exists) when the T cell histogram indicates presence of HLA antibodies in the patient serum with specificity for Class I HLA on donor T cells as evidenced by a positive peak (see Chapter 6).

When HLA antibodies are absent, normal T cell peak is seen (see Figure 14-2).

Lymphocytotoxicity

Chromium-Release Assay

This commonly used in vitro lymphocyte-mediated cytotoxicity assay (see Figure 14-7) can be used as an indicator of the degree of compatibility (or incompatibility) between allogeneic cells (donor and recipient cells) in pretransplantation testing (see Chapter 6).

The procedure (see previously described cytotoxicity assays and Figure 14-7) involves lysis of allogeneic tissue cells (target cells) by cytotoxic T lymphocytes (CTL) with release of radioactive chromium (^{51}Cr) that serves as an end-point and a marker of target cell lysis.

The amount of chromium released is proportional to the quantity of lysed cells and is indicative of the degree of incompatibility that exists between the two allogeneic cell populations.

Suggested Readings

Giklas PC: Complement tests. In Rose NR, et al, editors: *Manual of clinical laboratory immunology,* ed 5, Washington, DC, 1997, American Society for Microbiology.

McCoy JR, et al: Basic principles in clinical flow cytometry. In Karen D, editor: *Flow cytometry in clinical diagnosis,* Chicago, 1989, ASCP Press.

Wiik A: Antinuclear cytoplasmic antibodies. In Rose NR, et al, editors: *Manual of clinical laboratory immunology,* ed 5, Washington, DC, 1997, American Society for Microbiology.

Review Questions

Flow Cytometry

1. Reagent antibodies used in flow cytometry can be characterized by all of the following statements, *except:*
   a. are known as monoclonal antibodies
   b. originate from a single clone of B cells
   c. show specificity for one epitope
   d. are heterogeneous

2. Select two procedures that are currently used for production of monoclonal antibodies:
   a. molecular cloning
   b. somatic cell hybridization
   c. recombinant DNA method
   d. DNA synthesis

3. The most frequently used fluorochromes for labeling monoclonal antibodies in flow cytometry are all those listed following, *except:*
   a. acridinium esters (AE)
   b. propidium iodide (PI)
   c. phycoerythrin (PE)
   d. fluorescein isothiocyanate (FITC)

4. In flow cytometry, selection of a cell population of interest in a sample is performed by electronic "gating" of:
   a. light scatter pattern
   b. histogram frequency distribution
   c. digital data
   d. all of the above

5. Cell sorting by flow cytometry requires the capability of separating cells according to their:
   a. size and cell density
   b. size and fluorescent signal
   c. cell density and cell surface antigen
   d. cell surface marker and cell density

6. Clinical application of immunophenotyping includes all of the following, *except:*
   a. detecting HLA incompatibility
   b. phenotyping leukemia-associated antigens
   c. enumeration of lymphocyte subpopulations
   d. establishing prognosis for HIV-positive patients

7. Analysis of tumor ploidy can provide information regarding which of the following statements:
   a. determine amount of nuclear DNA in individual tumor cell
   b. predict outcome of certain carcinomas
   c. determine effectiveness of chemotherapy in eliminating aneuploid clone
   d. all of the above

8. Select the cell cycle phase in which DNA synthesis is directly proportional to cancer aggressiveness:
   a. G_0/G_1 phase
   b. S phase
   c. G_2/M phase
   d. none of the above

9. Leukocyte cross-matching is performed by flow cytometry for detecting HLA antibodies in which of the situations listed:
   a. previous graft rejection
   b. living related donors
   c. patients on a waiting list for donors
   d. all of the above

Complement Assays

10. For quantifying individual components, such as C3, C4, and Factor B, two of the most frequently used assays are:
    a. nephelometric analysis
    b. enzyme-linked immunosorbent assay
    c. complement fixation test
    d. hemolytic complement activity assay

11. Spectrophotometric measurement of hemolysis produced from sensitized sheep
red blood cells after exposure to patient's
serum can provide information regarding:
a. total quantity of serum complement
b. total hemolytic activity of complement
c. complement activation
d. all of the above

12-17. Match the following statements with the
appropriate hemolytic assay:

   a. CH_{50}
   b. AH_{50}

   ____ evaluates alternative pathway–
   dependent lysis
   ____ uses unsensitized rabbit red
   blood cells
   ____ microtiter version is available
   ____ patient serum is a source of
   complement
   ____ uses sensitized sheep red blood
   cells
   ____ uses complement as a reagent

18. Reduced complement levels may be caused
by all of the following mechanisms, *except:*
a. complement consumption during in
vivo formation of immune complexes
b. reduced synthesis of complement
c. decreased catabolism of complement
d. presence of an inhibitor

19. Select procedures that use complement as
a reagent:
a. complement fixation test
b. hemolytic complement activity assay
c. hemolysis inhibition assay
d. hemolytic assays

20. Serum antibody titer (ASO titer) is reported as the reciprocal of highest serum
dilution showing:
a. hemolysis
b. no hemolysis
c. agglutination
d. all of the above

21. A rise in antibody titer (ASO procedure) is
considered clinically significant when the
rise is:
a. two-fold
b. four-fold
c. two tubes above normal
d. all of the above

FUNCTIONAL ASSAYS

22. Select the technique(s) used for separating
mononuclear cells from other blood cells:
a. flow cytometry
b. density gradient
c. straw method
d. all of the above

23. Resting peripheral lymphocytes can be
induced to proliferate by:
a. plant lectins
b. *Candida* antigen
c. phytohemagglutinin
d. all of the above

24. DNA synthesis can serve as a marker for:
a. lymphocyte ability to respond to antigen
b. lymphocyte proliferation
c. functional capacity of T and B lymphocytes
d. all of the above

25. In vitro antigen stimulation technique
shows good correlation with:
a. skin tests
b. delayed-type hypersensitivity (DTH)
c. in vivo stimulation with the same
antigen
d. all of the above

26. Newly (de novo) synthesized DNA during
blastogenesis that leads to cell division
(mitosis) during a cell culture technique is
measured by:
a. luminometer
b. scintillation counter
c. nephelometer
d. spectrophotometer

27. When two allogeneic cell populations are cultured to evaluate an immune response to dissimilar (genetically incompatible) human leukocyte antigens (HLA), the procedure is known as:
    a. histocompatibility culture
    b. mixed lymphocyte reaction
    c. antigen stimulation procedure
    d. in vitro immune response

28. Chromium release assay can be used to evaluate:
    a. in vitro cytotoxicity
    b. cytotoxic lymphocyte (CTL) function
    c. target cell lysis
    d. all of the above

29. Polymorphonuclear leukocyte function can be evaluated by all the listed procedures, *except:*
    a. flow cytometry
    b. NBT
    c. ELISA
    d. ANCA

HISTOCOMPATIBILITY TESTING

30. In a microcytotoxicity assay, complement is added to the test system (cells + reagent antibodies) and becomes activated when binding occurs between:
    a. reagent antibody and corresponding HLA on the cells being tested
    b. reagent antibody and the target cell
    c. reagent antibody and the cytotoxic T cell
    d. none of the above

31. Select laboratory procedures that assist in evaluating the *compatibility* between donor and recipient before transplantation (pre-transplantation testing):
    a. flow cytometry
    b. lymphocytoxicity
    c. mixed lymphocyte reaction
    d. all of the above

32. Microcytotoxicity is a procedure that can be used in:
    a. HLA tissue typing
    b. HLA cytotoxic antibody detection
    c. lymphocyte compatibility testing (cross-matching)
    d. all of the above

33. In performing lymphocyte major cross-match, the following antigens or antibodies are detected:
    a. alloantigens on cells of potential donor
    b. HLA alloantibodies in host serum
    c. autoantibodies against host lymphocytes
    d. all of the above

34. A panel of T and B lymphocytes of known HLA specificity is used to detect HLA cytotoxic antibodies in:
    a. donor serum
    b. recipient serum
    c. donor and recipient serum
    d. all of the above

35. In a microcytotoxicity typing procedure, cells incubated with reagent antibodies (anti-HLA-DR2) and complement show eosin uptake, while cells incubated with anti-HLA-DR3 do not take up the stain. The HLA type of test cells is:
    a. HLA-DR2
    b. HLA-DR3
    c. HLA-DR2/DR3
    d. none of the above

36. The ability (immunocompetence) of T cells to proliferate in response to an alloantigenic stimulus may be evaluated by:
    a. microcytotoxicity
    b. mixed lymphocyte reaction
    c. flow cytometry
    d. all of the above

37. Tissue typing procedure for detection of class II HLA is similar to class I HLA typing procedure, *except for:*
    a. specificity of the typing antisera
    b. test interpretation
    c. absence of complement
    d. all of the above

Molecular Techniques

Upon completion of this chapter, the student will be prepared to:

STRUCTURE AND SYNTHESIS OF DNA

- Describe the DNA and RNA molecules by comparing their structure, chemical composition, and function.
- Explain what is meant by "semi-conservative replication" in DNA synthesis.
- Define the following terms: *gene, coding gene, mRNA, codons, template, primer, complementary molecule, nucleotide, transcription,* and *translation.*

DNA ISOLATION

- Describe the function of restriction enzymes in DNA isolation.

NUCLEIC ACID ANALYSIS

- Define the following terms: *hybridization, probe, target, amplicons,* and *amplification.*
- Explain the process of hybridization, including the components and their role in the process.
- State characteristics that are common to Dot blot, Southern blot, Northern blot, and in situ hybridization.
- Describe Southern blot hybridization.
- State the main difference between in situ hybridization and other hybridization assays.
- Explain the general principle of target amplification procedures.
- Describe the function of the following PCR components: template (target), primers, dNTPs, and DNA polymerase.
- State main differences between PCR and LCR.
- Describe a situation in which the signal amplification method can be the method of choice.
- State one application for each of the following hybridization assays: Dot blot, restriction fragment length polymorphism (RFLP), Northern blot, and in situ hybridization.
- Give an example for each of the following applications of molecular techniques to clinical diagnosis: detection of infectious agents and hemolytic disorders, diagnosis of genetic disorders, forensic medicine, and histocompatibility testing.

allele - Any alternative form of gene occupying a particular locus on a chromosome.

amplicons - DNA targets previously amplified.

amplification - Production of additional copies of a genetic sequence (nucleic acids).

base pair (bp) - Nucleotide (adenine, guanine, cytosine, thymine, or uracil) and its complementary base on the opposite strand.

blotting - Transfer or fixation of nucleic acids onto a solid matrix (nitrocellulose or nylon membrane) before hybridization.

cDNA - Complementary DNA that has been produced from mRNA by using reverse transcriptase.

clone - Genetically identical group of cells originating from a single precursor cell.

coding region - Section of the gene responsible for the genetic code (exon).

denatured DNA - Two single strands that result when hydrogen bonds are broken on a double-stranded DNA from exposure to changes in pH, temperature, or nonphysiologic concentration of salt, detergents, or organic solvents.

DNA sequencing - Method of determining the order of base pairs along a particular stretch of DNA.

dsDNA - Double-stranded DNA.

endonuclease - Enzyme that cleaves the covalent bonds between adjacent nucleotides.

exon - Coding sequence of a gene.

gene - Segment of DNA that codes for a specific product (protein).

genotype - Genetic structure of an individual, also referring to alleles present at a particular position(s) on a chromosome.

hybridization - Process by which two complementary single-stranded nucleic acid molecules (base sequences) bind (reanneal) to form a double-stranded molecule.

intron - Region of a gene that does not code for a protein.

label - Radioactive or nonradioactive tag or a marker that generates a signal, indicating the presence of the labeled molecule or probe.

mapping - Method used to determine location of a gene on a chromosome.

mRNA (messenger RNA) - Form of genetic information present in cell cytoplasm that is translated from nucleotide sequences into amino acid sequences of the protein.

nucleotide - Basic building block of nucleic acids, consisting of a nitrogenous base (purine and pyrimidine), pentose sugar (deoxyribose), and phosphoric acid.

oligonucleotide - Short sequence of nucleotides (base pairs) (can be chemically synthesized).

polymerase chain reaction (PCR) - System used to amplify a single target sequence of DNA to facilitate its detection.

primer - Short nucleic acid sequence (DNA or RNA), containing a free 3'-OH end that is able to bind with a complementary single-stranded DNA to form a dsDNA fragment.

probe - Known labeled sequence of DNA or RNA that is used in a hybridization process to detect any complementary sequence of target polynucleotides.

restriction enzyme - Bacterial endonuclease that recognizes specific short base sequences in the DNA and cleaves the DNA at or near a specific location of the recognition site (target).

stringency - Environmental condition (i.e., salt, formamide, and temperature) that affects the amount of base pair mismatches in a hybrid molecule during hybridization. High stringency requires nearly perfectly matched hybrids.

template - Single DNA strand that serves as a "blueprint" in complementary DNA replication and complementary RNA transcription processes.

transcription - Process by which a mRNA is produced from a DNA template.

translation - Process of producing a polypeptide product (protein) from mRNA.

With the discovery of the *double helical nature of the DNA molecule,* an explosion of research followed, resulting in such important discoveries as *polymerase chain reaction (PCR)* procedure for amplification of selected DNA segments (nucleic acids) and its application to a variety of molecular techniques (e.g., Southern blot and in situ hybridization). These procedures provided the basis for current understanding that a change in even a single base pair in the particular gene code can be responsible for a serious disease (e.g., sickle cell anemia).

As the general interest in molecular biology and DNA technology increases and clinicians become more aware of the potential of DNA technology for establishing diagnoses of various disease states, genetic disorders, microbial infections, and malignancies, more DNA research procedures will be considered for adoption into the clinical laboratory.

STRUCTURE AND SYNTHESIS OF DNA

Deoxyribonucleic acid (DNA) is a molecule that carries within its structure the genetic information and all the instructions (genes) for maintaining life and for the transfer of information to successive generations.

Research findings showing that genes determine the structure of proteins (i.e., "one gene, one protein concept") preceded identification of the molecular structure of a *gene as a group of adjacent nucleotides that code for (specify) each amino acid.* These findings opened new opportunities for identifying and altering the heredity of a gene.

DNA STRUCTURE

The DNA molecule is a double-stranded molecule (dsDNA) that exists in a double helix conformation (Figure 15-1). Each strand (a single-stranded DNA molecule, ssDNA) is composed of four building blocks, deoxyribonucleoside triphosphates (dTTP, dCTP, dATP, dGTP), each of which consists of a sugar molecule, a triphosphate group, and one of four possible bases: thymine (T), cytosine (C), adenine (A), or guanine (G).

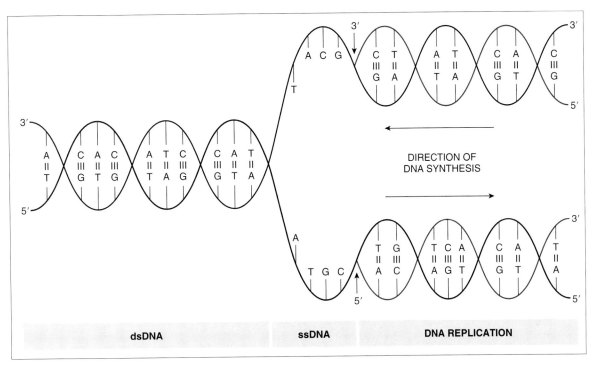

FIGURE **15-1**   **DNA Molecule.**   Diagrammatic representation of a double-stranded (ds) DNA molecule forming a helix. This DNA structure consists of complementary base pairs, held together by double
and triple hydrogen bonds (e.g., T=A, C≡G). Shown also is a portion of DNA consisting of two single
strands (ssDNA) with disrupted hydrogen bonds, which result when dsDNA helical structure becomes
denatured before DNA synthesis and replication. The DNA replication occurs in a 5′ to 3′ direction,
producing two dsDNA molecules that consist of "parent" and newly synthesized "daughter" strands.

The backbone of the ssDNA is a sugar molecule (deoxyribose), connected by phosphate
groups. Attached to the first carbon of each
sugar molecule is one of the four possible bases
(T, C, A, or G).

The dsDNA is a stable molecule, which can
be denatured or unwound into two single
strands (ssDNA) by disrupting base pair bonds
or hydrogen bonds by a change in pH or by
extreme heat or formamide, respectively (see
Figure 15-1).

In vivo, *DNA molecules* consist of highly
compacted units, known as *chromosomes.* A
chromosome is a genetically specific DNA molecule, to which many proteins are attached.
These DNA-associated proteins maintain the
structure of the chromosome and are involved
in regulating gene expression.

Each human cell nucleus contains 23 pairs
of chromosomes of unique base-pair sequence
and characteristic length, which can be made
visible by special dyes (Figure 15-2). *These 46
chromosomes constitute the human genome.*

RNA molecule differs from DNA in several
ways, which include structure, chemical composition, and function. RNA exists only as a
single-stranded molecule and is less stable and
therefore readily degraded by RNA-specific
enzymes, known as *RNAses.* It contains a
unique base (uracil [U]), which is chemically
similar to thymine (T) in that it is a specific
base pair to adenine (A).

DNA Synthesis

Most protein synthesis occurs in the cytoplasm. Because the DNA molecule is located
within the nucleus, the information of DNA
(nucleotide sequence) for protein (and new
DNA) synthesis must be communicated to the

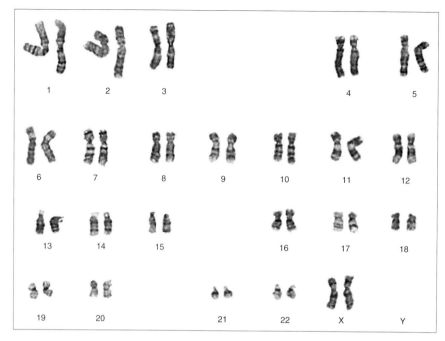

FIGURE **15-2** **Human Genome.** *Normal karyotype,* showing 23 pairs of chromosomes (with visible banding), which constitute the human genome.

cytoplasm by an intermediate molecule known as *ribonucleic acid (RNA).*

Three different RNA molecules are involved in protein synthesis: ribosomal RNA (rRNA), transfer RNA (tRNA), and messenger RNA (mRNA).

DNA Replication

DNA synthesis is known as a semi-conservative replication, in which each "parent" strand of the double-stranded DNA (dsDNA) serves as a template to direct the synthesis of a new ("daughter") strand. The replication is exact (see Figure 15-1).

Before replication, unwinding of the helix and separation of the DNA strands takes place. This allows a short RNA sequence, complementary to the single-strand DNA sequence, to be synthesized by RNA polymerase to serve as a *primer.*

DNA polymerase proceeds with the DNA synthesis according to the template, linking deoxyribonucleotides in the 5′ to 3′ position (see Figure 15-1) to produce two dsDNA molecules. The two dsDNA molecules consist of the original DNA (parent) and the new DNA (daughter) molecules with the same base pair sequence,

thus *conserving* the original DNA strand (semi-conservative replication).

Transcription

Protein synthesis is initiated by activation of a particular *gene,* which is that region of the DNA molecule that specifies (codes for) the amino acid sequence of a protein.

Thus *one gene contains the amino acid sequence (exon) that codes for one protein.*

These coding sequences *(exons)* of the gene compose only a part of the human genome. The remaining DNA sequences are non-coding *(introns* or "junk DNA"), which may have some functional tasks not yet fully defined.

As the gene is activated, a copy of the gene (code) is made in the form of a messenger RNA (mRNA) in the cell nucleus by a process known as *transcription* and is carried to the cytoplasm where the protein synthesis occurs.

The mRNA is synthesized from a single strand of the DNA. The complementary DNA strand is not used in this process.

When damage occurs to the DNA in vivo (e.g., temperature or UV), the damaged nucleotides are replaced with new ones, using the intact strand as a template. This process reduces the number of alterations that could lead to a mutation (discussed following).

Translation

The mRNA carries units of three bases (triplets) known as *codons,* each of which specifies the order of amino acids of a protein to be synthesized.

Twenty different amino acids are used in protein synthesis, but only four nucleotides (adenine, guanine, thymine, and cytosine arranged in triplets and in 64 different combinations) code for the 20 amino acids that can be synthesized.

DNA Synthesis

DNA synthesis occurs in a 5′ to 3′ direction (see Figure 15-1) and requires the following components.

Template

Template is a single DNA strand that serves as a "blueprint" for producing:
- *Complementary DNA molecules during DNA replication*
- *Complementary RNA molecules in the transcription process*

The transfer RNA (tRNA) molecules are also known as a templates during protein synthesis from mRNA in the *translation* process (i.e., the nucleic acids [mRNA] are "translated" into amino acids [protein]). In this process, the information flows from DNA to RNA to protein:

$$\text{DNA} \rightarrow \text{RNA} \rightarrow \text{PROTEIN}$$
$$\text{(Transcription)} \quad \text{(Translation)} \quad \text{(Synthesis)}$$

DNA Polymerase

This enzyme can synthesize DNA only in the 5′ to 3′ direction, so that one new DNA strand can be continuously synthesized as the dsDNA opens for replication. The other new DNA strand can be synthesized in only short segments in the 3′ to 5′ direction, which are then joined by a DNA ligase.

Primer

The primer consists of a short RNA sequence that is used to synthesize DNA in the 3′ to 5′ direction and is complementary to the DNA sequence on a single strand to be replicated.

Nucleotide Triphosphates (ATP, TTP, CTP, GTP)

Nucleotides are the building blocks of nucleic acids. Each nucleotide contains a phosphate group, a sugar (deoxyribose in DNA and ribose in RNA), and either purine (adenine or guanine) or pyrimidine (cytosine or thymine in DNA and cytosine or uracil in RNA). When many nucleotides are linked together, they are known as *polynucleotides.*

DNA ISOLATION

DNA EXTRACTION

Classic Procedure

The classic procedure for DNA isolation from cells consists of four steps:
- *Release of DNA from cells:* A detergent is added to cells to solubilize the cell membrane by producing a hole in the membrane, thus releasing the cell contents. Subsequent addition of the enzyme protease results in digestion of the released cellular and nuclear proteins, resulting in the release of DNA.
- *Extraction of DNA: Organic extraction (phenol-chloroform extraction) of DNA* is accomplished by an addition of organic solutions (phenol-chloroform) to the solubilized cells, producing two phases: upper aqueous phase containing the extracted DNA and a lower organic phase with protein and lipid molecules. *Non-organic extraction* can be performed, when non-organic reagents are chosen, by adding protein precipitating agent to the previously solubilized cells. The proteins will precipitate out of the solution and form a pellet at the bottom of a tube. The extracted DNA will remain in the supernatant.
- *DNA precipitation:* The extracted DNA strands (molecules) are precipitated out of solution with sodium or ammonium acetate and cold absolute ethanol ($-20°$ C) and centrifuged. The formed DNA pellet at bottom of the tube is removed with absolute ethanol and washed with 70% ethanol.

- *DNA solubilization:* Washed DNA is resuspended in water or buffer.

RNA Extraction

Extraction of RNA from cells is performed in three steps, when RNA is to be isolated:

- Lysing cells to remove the RNA by guanidine thiocyanate agent
- Precipitation of the released RNA by isopropanol and ethanol
- Resuspension of the RNA-containing pellet in diluent

DNA DIGESTION

Restriction Enzymes

Bacterial restriction enzymes are endonucleases (restriction endonucleases) that have the ability to recognize short DNA base pair sequences and to cleave (digest) the phosphodiester bonds (covalent bonds) between adjacent nucleotides at a specific recognition site located on a DNA molecule. Thus the digested DNA molecule consists of 4 to 8 recognition sequences.

The restriction enzymes originate from certain bacteria, which normally produce these enzymes as a means of protection against phagocytosis by bacteriophages (phagocytes). These bacterial enzymes are named according to the bacteria from which they are derived.

For example, the restriction enzyme Eco RI (Eco, *Escherichia coli;* R, RY13 strain; and I, first nuclease to be isolated) is isolated from *Escherichia coli,* while the restriction enzyme Hind III is isolated from *Haemophilus influenzae* (Hin, *Haemophilus influenzae;* d, Rd strain; and III, third isolated nuclease).

NUCLEIC ACID ANALYSIS

Nucleic acid analysis is performed to characterize DNA and RNA molecules through methods that include electrophoretic separation of the molecules, hybridization and amplification assays, and other methods such as restriction fragment length polymorphism (RFLP).

Many procedures currently available combine these assays to produce a new protocol, such as Southern blotting.

The discussion that follows is intended to provide basic concepts of DNA molecular techniques, which have been applied to direct detection of infectious agents, identification of certain hemolytic and genetic disorders, forensic analysis, and histocompatibility testing.

ELECTROPHORETIC SEPARATION OF DNA

Gel electrophoresis can separate the restriction enzyme–digested DNA according to the size (molecular weight or length) of the nucleotide sequences, a property that is used to characterize the size of a nucleic acid fragment. The electrophoresis format is analogous to that used in separating proteins.

Briefly, the DNA sample is mixed with gel-loading buffer (made heavy with sucrose or Ficoll for loading) and with gel-loading dye (a visual marker for molecules being separated) before being placed into wells, submerged under buffer in agarose gel ("submarine gel").

DNA molecular weight standard, producing bands of known size that are referred to as "DNA or RNA ladders" is placed in adjacent wells and electrophoresed together with the sample (Figure 15-3). The distance of migration of an unknown sample is compared with the standard to determine the size of the base pair of the sample.

The electrophoresed gels are stained with ethidium bromide and the integrity of the DNA sample evaluated under UV light.

After electrophoretic separation, the DNA is transferred from the agarose gel to a nylon membrane by vacuum or capillary transfer method and then baked at 80° C.

HYBRIDIZATION ASSAYS

The hybridization reaction is highly specific and can be used for determining nucleic acid content of an unknown sample by allowing fragments of known nucleic acid composition *(probe)* to locate the matching (complementary) sequences in the unknown sample, under conditions appropriate for complementary base pairing.

Base pairing can occur between the complementary strands of DNA-DNA, DNA-RNA, or RNA-RNA duplex structure.

As previously discussed, DNA is a stable double-stranded structure, made up of two strands of DNA that are held together by many

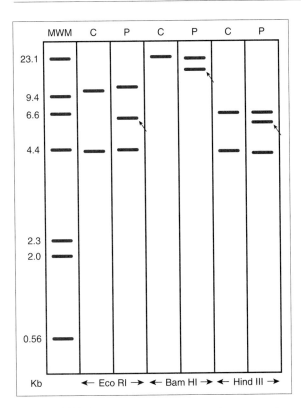

FIGURE **15-3** **Southern Blot Hybridization.** A diagrammatic representation of a membrane (gel) that has been "probed" with Jβ$_I$/β$_{II}$ probe (see text). In lane 1 is depicted a molecular weight marker (MWM) that is used as a reference. Note *arrows* in lanes 3, 5, and 7, pointing to abnormal blots (β chain gene) (i.e., rearrangement of T cell receptors). *Eco RI, Bam HI,* and *Hind III* are enzymes used for digesting DNA (see text). *C,* control (placental DNA) digested with each enzyme; *P,* patient's DNA digested with each enzyme.

hydrogen bonds between complementary base pairs (see Figure 15-1). *The binding between the strands is reversible and base-sequence specific.*

Thus, if the DNA is denatured to produce two separate single strands (ssDNA), the strands can be *annealed* (re-formed) to produce a double-stranded DNA (dsDNA) by the process known as *annealing.*

When one of the DNA strands is labeled with a signal-emitting tag, the labeled DNA is referred to as the *probe* and the process of annealing is known as *hybridization.*

As the labeled probe hybridizes with the sample DNA (nucleic acids), hybridization

products (hybrids) are formed, representing the hybridized DNA sequence of interest, which is detectable by the signal emitted from the label.

Hybridization Components

All hybridization assays contain the following common basic components.

Probe

A *probe* is a short sequence of DNA or RNA molecule, consisting of 15 to 45 base pairs (oligonucleotides). It can be tagged with such labels as radioisotopes (e.g., ^{32}P, ^{35}S, or ^{125}I), enzymes (e.g., alkaline phosphatase or peroxidase) or biotin (e.g., avidin-enzyme or avidin-fluorochrome) and used to detect a target nucleic acid sequence of interest.

For example, in HLA phenotyping procedure, sequence-specific nucleotide probes (unique for each HLA antigen specificity) are prepared by using small segments of single-stranded DNA and amplifying the selected DNA segment containing the gene of interest, using PCR technique (discussed following).

Target Nucleic Acids

A *target* is either a DNA- or RNA-selected nucleic acid sequence or fragment to be identified.

Reaction Conditions

Environmental conditions such as *stringency* of the hybridization solutions affect the base pairing reaction.

For example, a *low stringency* (high salt concentration, low temperature, and low denaturant) will allow base pair mismatching. However, as the stringency of the solution increases, fewer mismatches are tolerated in a hybrid duplex, so that at *high stringency* (low salt, high temperatures, and high denaturant) a mismatched base pairing is not allowed to occur and even a single mismatched base pair is capable of disrupting the duplex.

Methods of Detection

Depending on the type of label used for tagging the particular probe, the following methods are available for detection of signal from the labeled hybrids (hybridization products):

- *Scintillation counting or autoradiography for radioisotopic labels*
- *Autoradiography for chemiluminescent labels*
- *Colorimetric or fluorescent methods for enzyme/substrate labels*

Hybridization Methods

Conceptually, all hybridization assays are similar in that they require a nucleic acid fragment of known sequence (labeled DNA probe) that locates the matching (complementary) nucleic acid sequences in an unknown sample.

Presence of appropriate reaction conditions for complementary base pairing is essential as is the detection device for detecting hybridization product *(probe-sample hybrids)*.

Southern Blot Hybridization

This elegant hybridization technique, known as *Southern blot,* combines electrophoretic separation of DNA fragments by size with a hybridization procedure, which reveals the location of the sample DNA fragments (see Figure 15-3).

procedure. Briefly, Southern blotting technique consists of extraction of the DNA to be tested from cells of the peripheral blood test sample although DNA can be isolated from a variety of samples. The isolated DNA is then digested into fragments (gene segments) with selected restriction endonucleases (previously discussed). The endonucleases cleave the DNA molecule between base pairs at specific recognition sites. These restriction enzymes differ from each other by the base pairs they recognize and by the size and number of DNA fragments that are produced during the digestion, which vary according to the enzyme used.

Following digestion, the DNA fragments are then electrophoretically separated through agarose gel by size. The gel is then stained with a dye that fluoresces under UV light, thus pinpointing the location of the DNA fragments.

In preparation for the next step (i.e., hybridization), the gel is then exposed to acid and base solutions, which break the hydrogen bonds between the base pairs, thus producing the DNA as a single-stranded molecule.

The gel is then soaked in a neutralizing solution, blotted (transfer of DNA) onto a membrane by capillary action or by vacuum transfer, and baked to increase binding between the DNA and the membrane. This is followed by incubation of membrane in a hybridization solution that contains the specific *probe* (biotin-labeled DNA), which has also been denatured to allow binding with complementary *target* DNA fragments.

After hybridization, the membrane is washed and the probe is prepared for detection by incubating with an enzyme/substrate label (e.g., streptavidin/alkaline phosphatase). The site (band) where the probe has hybridized to the DNA on the membrane can be seen as a color produced by the biotin–streptavidin–alkaline phosphatase complex, thus indicating the location of the DNA fragments (see Figure 15-3).

Controls are processed simultaneously with the sample to check enzyme activity (completeness of digestion) and to provide molecular weight markers for gel electrophoresis (see Figure 15-3).

restriction fragment length polymorphism (RFLP). The RFLP is based on the fact that when a normal and a variant gene of the same gene locus (polymorphic locus) are digested with a restriction enzyme, the resulting normal restriction fragments (band pattern) will be of a different size than the pattern resulting from the abnormal gene.

This fact allows RFLP to be used in determining polymorphism of HLA alleles (One Step Further Box 15-1) *and for identification of an abnormal gene responsible for a particular genetic disease. In the latter, classic RFLP analysis can demonstrate presence of a mutation.*

When the restriction site (genomic DNA sequence) has been changed by a mutation, the restriction enzyme is not able to cut the DNA at that particular location. Based on this fact, the RFLP is used to diagnose diseases associated with a change in genomic DNA (DNA sequences).

Differences in restriction fragment size (polymorphism) because of a deletion, point mutation, or different number of repeat copies of DNA produce abnormal gene product, causing a particular genetic disease.

RFLP procedure. Briefly, the procedure involves extracting genomic DNA (test DNA) from the patient's cells and digesting the DNA

Box 15-1

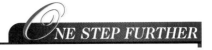

Molecular Fingerprinting

Application of molecular techniques to tissue typing mainly in forensic medicine and pre-transplantation testing has provided a more precise way of identifying human leukocyte antigens (HLA). This is based on the fact that HLA loci (nucleotide sequences), which code for individual HLA antigens, can be identified, thus establishing the polymorphism of the HLA alleles.

The following molecular techniques have been developed for detection of polymorphism of HLA alleles:

- *RFLP:* Restriction fragment length polymorphism (RFLP) uses Southern blotting technique to identify HLA loci (nucleotide sequences) that code for individual HLA antigen (see following).
- *SSP:* Sequence-specific priming (SSP) detects polymorphism generic to allele-level HLA antigens, using PCR/gel electrophoresis technique.
- *SSOP:* Sequence-specific oligonucleotide probing (SSOP) is a technique that uses PCR/hybridization of probes to PCR product to detect HLA alleles.
- *SBT:* Sequence base typing (SBT) is a procedure that uses PCR/nucleotide sequencing of PCR product to detect alleles at the exact sequence level.

Restriction Fragment Length Polymorphism (RFLP) Technique (Molecular Fingerprinting)

This tissue typing procedure is the first of the molecular methods used in HLA typing to identify nucleotide

sequences (HLA loci) that code for individual HLA antigen.

The method is particularly useful when serologic HLA typing (see Chapter 14) is unsuccessful because of lack of expression of HLA molecules, seen in such abnormalities as lymphopenia or increased cell fragility.

Procedure. Briefly, genomic DNA (patient's DNA) is extracted from the patient's cells and the DNA fragments visualized using Southern blotting technique (previously described). The process involves:

- Digestion of cellular DNA by restriction endonuclease
- Separation of digests (mixture of DNA fragments) by gel electrophoresis
- Transfer of DNA fragment gel pattern to support membrane by blotting (Southern blotting)
- Exposure of blot to individual cDNA probes (nucleotide sequences that encode individual HLA antigens), thus serving as specific markers for HLA antigen present in the DNA sample (test DNA).

Test interpretation. HLA antigens are identified by comparing patient's *band patterns* (restriction fragment length polymorphisms [RFLP]) with the band patterns of the controls that have been subjected to the same test protocol.

The band patterns (RFLP) are characteristic for each HLA specificity and are as unique for each individual as is the DNA. Thus RFLP tissue typing is sometimes referred to as *molecular fingerprinting,* because it distinguishes one individual from another.

---

with restriction endonuclease. The resulting DNA fragments are then separated by gel electrophoresis and transferred to a support membrane by blotting (Southern blotting, see preceding discussion).

The blot is then exposed to individual cDNA probes, which serve as specific markers for a particular polymorphic locus, such as the HLA antigens.

The band patterns (restriction fragment length polymorphism) that appear on the blot

are compared with band patterns produced by the controls that have been subjected to the same test conditions.

Dot Blot Hybridization

This hybridization protocol, also referred to as *Immunoblot,* involves immobilization of the sample DNA (nucleic acids) in a *solid phase* (matrix) such as a cellulose or nylon membrane. DNA immobilization facilitates simultaneous handling of samples (multiple samples on a single membrane) through the various steps of hybridization and increases standardization of the assay.

For example, in the PCR amplification procedure (see following), the amplified DNA sequence is blotted onto a nitrocellulose or nylon membrane, and the membrane is incubated in a solution containing a labeled probe. The probe is then labeled with a radioisotopic or non-isotopic label, such as an enzyme or biotin, and the signal emitted from the label is detected, as described previously.

Positive and negative controls are included and processed with the sample and are used in the interpretation of results.

interpretation of results. Detection of a signal from the label by an appropriate detection device indicates that the probe has hybridized with the target (DNA) at a particular location.

Northern Blot Hybridization

Using RNA as a target, *Northern blot* procedure is generally used to investigate gene expression. The extracted RNA is mainly ribosomal (rRNA) with 1% to 2% of mRNA content. The RNA is a single-stranded molecule, composed of shorter strands than DNA and does not require digestion before electrophoresis.

After electrophoresis, the fractionated (according to molecular weight) RNA can be transferred to nitrocellulose or nylon membranes, which covalently bind nucleic acids. The transfer from agarose gels can be either by capillary action or by vacuum transfer. Hybridization is performed with labeled DNA or RNA probes as in Southern blotting and detected by an appropriate device (e.g., spectrophotometer).

As in Southern blotting, the bands produced in Northern blotting indicate the presence and size of nucleic acids in the sample that have hybridized to the specific probe used in the assay. Lack of bands indicates absence of sequences complementary to the probe.

DNA Chip Technology

Although currently this novel version of solid-support hybridization technique is used only in research to identify alterations in genes, it is believed that chip technology has a potential to replace standard methods of genotyping and to overall improve the existing gel-based methods

of genetic tests now used to detect genetic defects producing such diseases as cystic fibrosis or hereditary breast cancer or to more rapidly identify infectious agents.

In this technique, biochips, also known as *biologic chips* or *microarrays* (smaller than a postage stamp), serve as a solid support for a variety of combinations of relatively short oligonucleotides (pieces of genetic sequences used as probes). These oligonucleotide pieces are attached to the biochip surface and are identical to the gene sequences that are to be evaluated for any alterations.

The chip allows thousands of biologic reactions to be performed simultaneously and has been compared to computer chips, which simultaneously perform thousands of mathematical calculations.

procedure. Briefly, DNA to be tested is obtained from patient's blood and amplified by PCR to produce multiple copies. The DNA is then copied into single-stranded RNA, which is labeled with a fluorescent dye, and fragmented into small pieces. A normal copied RNA is used as a control.

Both samples (patient and normal control) are inserted into a chip containing the selected probe, and, after *hybridization,* the chip is washed to remove any sample not bound to the probe.

evaluation of results. The samples are examined for the presence of a localized fluorescence which, when present, indicates that *the DNA matching (hybridization) has occurred between the complementary sequences.*

However, when the area of the DNA sequence to be hybridized contains a mutation, that area will not hybridize and will show less fluorescence intensity during the scan than the normally hybridized sequences.

The test is considered normal (i.e., mutations are absent) when both the patient and the control (normal samples) hybridize identically with the probe.

Fluorescent In Situ Hybridization (FISH)

In situ hybridization procedure is a highly specialized molecular technique used to probe for (or localize) DNA or RNA target and to diagnose structural or numerical chromosomal abnormalities (e.g., duplication, deletion, or translocation) (Figure 15-4).

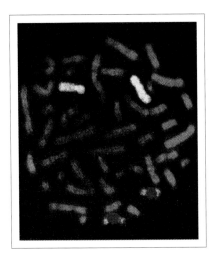

FIGURE **15-4**   **Fluorescent In Situ Hybridization (FISH Analysis).**   Shown is an abnormal karyotype of a female patient. Note the abnormal number of chromosomes (47) with the additional 47th chromosome being a derivative of chromosome 9 (stained pink color). Normal xx chromosomes are stained green. (Courtesy Monmouth Medical Center, New Jersey.)

probing for DNA. When genomic DNA is the target, the probe is able to locate specific, variant nucleic acid sequences in cells or chromosomes, thus providing a particular piece of genetic information and its location in histologic preparations (tissue, cell, or chromosome), without destroying the morphologic integrity of the structures.

When a foreign DNA is the target (usually of viral origin), a probe can be used to detect virally infected cells.

probing for RNA. In situ hybridization for messenger RNA allows identification of cells that express a specific gene. Thus probing for the presence or absence of mRNA can complement the DNA in situ hybridization procedure as well as certain immunocytochemical techniques.

procedure. In the fluorescent in situ hybridization (FISH) procedure, the solid support is a slide that holds the material to be analyzed (cells, tissues, or chromosomes) through all steps of the hybridization protocol that include:

- *Sample preparation of cells* grown in tissue cultures and harvested at metaphase, at which point their growth is arrested
- *Preparation of slides* by standard histologic methods

Table **15-1**	AMPLIFICATION TECHNIQUES	
Technique	Target AMP	Signal AMP
PCR	+	−
LCR	+	−
NASBA	+	−
bDNA	−	+

Amp, amplification; *PCR,* polymerase chain reaction; *LCR,* ligase chain reaction; *NASBA,* nucleic acid sequence–based amplification; *bDNA,* branched DNA.

- *Digesting sample* (before hybridization) by various enzymes, such as protease, DNase, or RNase
- *Hybridization of the sample* with a probe contained in a hybridization solution
- *Removal of unhybridized probe* by washing in series of graded salt washes
- *Detection of signal (fluorescence)* by a fluorescent microscope
- *Counterstaining* to facilitate microscopic visualization of morphology (see Figure 15-4)

Thus in situ hybridization is the only form of hybridization that combines morphologic analysis with genetic analysis and allows localization of genetic information.

NUCLEIC ACID AMPLIFICATION METHODS

Rapid growth in the development and application of molecular technology to the diagnosis of human disease has produced many DNA techniques, such as procedures for amplification of specific nucleic acid sequences (selected segments of DNA) to increase the concentration of target nucleic acids.

Currently, two basic amplification technologies are available for use in the clinical laboratory. These are (Table 15-1):

- *Target amplification methods*
- *Signal amplification methods*

Target Amplification Procedures

These amplification procedures generate many copies of selected nucleic acids, thus allowing the use of less sensitive detection methods (also less expensive).

DNA target amplification methods (see Table 15-1) include methods that produce new copies of original target nuclei (e.g., PCR) and those that amplify the probe (e.g., LCR).

Most common of the amplification methods are:

- Ligase chain reaction (LCR)
- Nucleic acid sequence–based amplification (NASBA)
- Transcription-mediated amplification (TMA)
- Polymerase chain reaction (PCR)

An inherent problem associated with the target amplification methods is a *contamination of the sample with amplicons* (DNA targets already amplified). Thus, to avoid any contamination with amplicons, the following precautions have been recommended:

- Designating a separate room for each activity (i.e., reagent preparation, sample processing, amplification, and detection of sample)
- Using dedicated supplies and equipment for each activity
- Using controls (negative, weakly positive, and all reagent control, except DNA template)
- Altering (digesting) amplicons

Polymerase Chain Reaction (PCR)

Since the introduction of *polymerase chain reaction (PCR)* technique in 1985, this technique has been the procedure of choice in many clinical laboratories for diagnosing such disease states as infectious diseases, genetic disorders, and cancer.

PCR is a molecular technique for exponential amplification of a selected DNA sequence (gene segment of interest) of known specificity (i.e., production of multiple copies of a DNA sequence by a twofold amplification of target genetic material with each replication cycle).

Because PCR enables production of many copies of a selected DNA sequence without resorting to cloning, it is particularly useful in quantification of DNA and inclusion in methods that require large quantities of specific nucleic acid sequences.

components of PCR. The PCR procedure involves the use of the following reactants:

- *Template (target):* Isolated genomic DNA segment or complementary DNA that serves as a template for amplification. Both strands of DNA can be used as templates. Target sequences must be carefully se-

lected because the degree of specificity of the amplification reaction depends on the specificity of the target sequences selected.
- *Primers:* Two oligonucleotide primers that are complementary to both ends of the DNA segments (3′ and 5′) to be amplified. The selected primer sequences must be compared to ensure that they will not hybridize with each other.
- *dNTPs:* Deoxynucleosidetriphosphates (i.e. dATP, dTTP, dGTP, dCTP (abbreviated as A, T, G, C) are the "building blocks" for DNA.
- *DNA polymerase:* Taq DNA polymerase, originating from the bacterium *Thermus aquaticus* (thermostable even at 94° C), is used to synthesize a specific region of DNA.

reaction. In a typical PCR, the starting material consists of a very small amount of target genomic DNA (sample material) containing the sequence to be amplified and defined by the primers used.

Two oligonucleotide primers that direct the starting point for DNA synthesis, a thermostable DNA polymerase, a defined solution of salts, and an excess amount of each of the four nucleotide triphosphates are added to the target DNA.

The PCR reaction proceeds through a series of cycles, consisting of three steps within each cycle (Figure 15-5):

- *Denaturation:* Heating of target DNA to *separate the strands. The reaction occurs as follows:* the PCR mixture, containing the previously listed reactants is heated in a thermal cycler to 94° to 96° C to denature (separate) the DNA molecules and produce single stranded DNA.
- *Annealing of primers:* After denaturation of DNA, primers are added in excess to the reaction mixture and cooled to 50° to 65° C to allow the oligonucleotide primers to anneal (bind) to the complementary sequences of the target DNA (both strands).
- *Extension of primers:* The temperature of the reaction medium is then raised to 72° C to allow the Taq polymerase to extend (synthesize) the primer (one base at a time) according to the gene sequence of the target DNA. Thus, the synthesis of a new DNA strand proceeds in the 5′ to 3′ direction as follows: DNA polymerase is allowed to bind to the 3′ end of the primer that has annealed to the DNA target (template). A complementary copy of the target

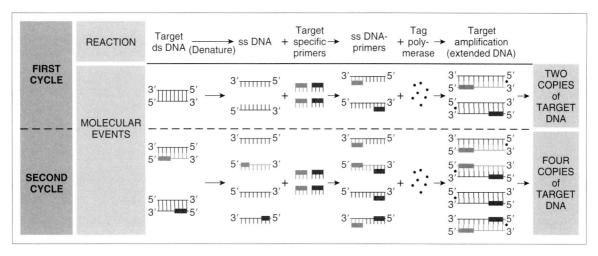

FIGURE **15-5** **Polymerase Chain Reaction (PCR)** Represented are two discrete cycles, showing exponential amplification of target sequences of DNA. As many as 25 to 40 such cycles may be required for effective amplification.

sequence is produced, using dNTPs present in the reaction mixture. Thus, by providing one DNA strand as the template, the Taq polymerase will synthesize a second strand of DNA (see Figure 15-5).

- *Exponential amplification:* As each replication cycle is repeated, both the extended primer and the original nucleic acid serve as templates for the next DNA replication cycle. The target sequence (DNA segment) is doubled with each cycle (see Figure 15-5). Thus the number of cycles that will be repeated depends on the efficiency of the reaction. Usually 25 to 40 cycles are required for amplification of 10^5-10^6 fold increase in the target (DNA segment). After that many cycles, a plateau is reached because of exhaustion of primers, inactivation or insufficient amount of enzyme, or product re-association.

detection of PCR products. Examination of amplification products to determine the specificity of the amplified gene segments can be performed by gel electrophoresis or hybridization assays.

- *Gel electrophoresis:* After amplification, the amplified target sequence (DNA sample) can be identified by electrophoretic assay (discussed in Chapter 11) and compared with DNA molecular weight standards.
- *Hybridization:* Amplified target nucleic acid sequence (DNA) can be identified by

dot blot hybridization, discussed previously.

clinical application of PER. The first application of PCR was for the diagnosis of sickle cell disease. Since then, the use of PCR has been expanded to include such diagnostic and research areas as oncology, genetics, infectious diseases (One Step Further Box 15-2), and forensic medicine (see One Step Further Box 15-1).

Ligase Chain Reaction (LCR)

Another method for cyclic (thermal) *target amplification* is the ligase chain reaction (LCR), which involves repeated cycles of denaturation and annealing, but, instead of the DNA polymerase used in the last step of the PCR, the enzyme is a thermostable DNA ligase.

Unlike the target sequence in the PCR, target sequence in the LCR must be completely known in order to prevent even a single base pair mismatch at the area of ligation, which would prevent the ligation from occurring.

The advantage of LCR over PCR is that it is able to detect *point mutations (at ligation site),* such as the mutation responsible for cystic fibrosis. Thus, LCR can be used as an adjunct to PCR or other amplification procedures because PCR can produce large number of target molecules (see Figure 15-5), and LCR can then be used to distinguish the locus of interest.

Box 15-2

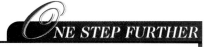
ONE STEP FURTHER

Direct Detection of Infectious Agents

All infectious agents contain a genome that is composed of either DNA or RNA molecules. Because each genome carries nucleic acid sequences that are unique and specific for the particular organism, complementary probes to these specific sequences can be designed.

A probe can selectively bind to the complementary (targeted) nucleic acids in presence of other non-targeted nucleic acids (showing different sequences).

Thus, by using a specific DNA probe, it is possible to identify the organism responsible for the current infection. This assay is analogous to immunologic assays that detect presence of an infectious organism rather than the immune response of the host to the organism (e.g., antibodies).

With the introduction of nucleic acid amplification technology such as PCR into the DNA probe assay,

amplification of any selected (targeted) nucleic acid sequence became possible. This allowed for identification of infectious organisms in certain situations, such as when:

- A clinical specimen contains a variety of pathogenic organisms, requiring separate protocol for identification
- Infectious agent cannot be cultured outside the host [e.g., Hepatitis C virus (HCV)]
- Organism can be cultured only with difficulty (e.g., *M. tuberculosis*)
- Currently available assays (e.g., ELISA) are able to detect seroconversion status but are not useful after seroconversion (appearance of antibodies in serum)
- Characterization of an organism to subspecies level is required in epidemiologic studies

Nucleic Acid Sequence-Based Amplification (NASBA)

NASBA is a novel nucleic acid amplification technology, which is used to amplify target RNA nucleic acid sequences several million-fold (10^6-10^9 amplifications) in a continuous chain reaction, employing three enzymes:

- *Reverse transcriptase (RT):* Makes complementary DNA (cDNA) copy from RNA (by reverse transcription), which serves as a template for further replication
- *Ribonuclease H (RNase H):* Degrades the RNA that has been hybridized to DNA (RNA:DNA hybrid), allowing binding of a second oligonucleotide primer and synthesis of a complete, double-stranded cDNA copy of the RNA
- *T7 RNA polymerase:* Produces multiple copies of RNA from DNA but requires a *promoter region* to begin the reaction.

amplification reaction. The RNA replication (NASBA) is similar to the DNA replication (PCR) in that it involves inclusion of nucleotide primers.

One of the primers, however, contains a promoter sequence for T7 RNA polymerase that anneals to the target. Because this primer is not

complementary to the target, it "hangs off" the end of the template. The reverse transcriptase extends the other end of the primer and the ribonuclease then degrades the RNA in the RNA:DNA hybrid. This allows the second oligonucleotide primer to bind and complete the synthesis of a double-stranded cDNA copy of the RNA.

The cDNA is used as a transcription template by the T7 RNA polymerase for production of many copies of the original target RNA.

In the NASBA procedure, inclusion of internal RNA standards into the amplification reaction (before nucleic acid isolation), allows the standards to be amplified together with the patient's viral RNA. The amplified samples are then hybridized and the patient's viral RNA and the standards' RNAs are quantified by electrochemiluminescence.

Inclusion of the internal standards makes the assay more accurate and reproducible and reduces the possibility of reporting lower viral load values because of enzyme inhibitors that may be present in the patient's sample.

The patient's viral load is calculated from the patient's and the standards' results (One Step Further Box 15-3).

Box 15-3

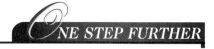

Testing for Acquired Immunodeficiency Syndrome (AIDS)

Human immunodeficiency virus-1 (HIV-1) was identified in the early 1980s as the causative agent of the acquired immunodeficiency syndrome (AIDS) pandemic. Since that time, the structure and function of HIV has been well researched, allowing development of better prevention strategies and new approaches to laboratory testing and management of the infection.

HIV is a retrovirus, consisting of two strands of ribonucleic acid (RNA) core and several enzymes, encapsulated by an outer lipid envelope containing the gp120 antigen. This antigen is of particular interest because of its involvement in binding the virus to surface CD4 receptors on the helper T lymphocyte.

The HIV genome consists of three major genes that code for various viral structural components: glycoproteins in the outer envelope (gp120 and gp41) coded by *env* gene, the core proteins (p55, p40, and p24) coded by *gag*, and the enzyme proteins that include reverse transcriptase (p66 and p51), protease (p11), and integrase (p32) coded by *pol* gene. These structural components are antigenic and can induce the host's humoral immune response to produce antigen-specific antibodies that are detectable by various immunologic laboratory methods (see discussion following).

Clinical Course of HIV Infection

PRIMARY HIV INFECTION

This phase of the infection is characterized by a burst of viremia during which the virus is detectable in peripheral mononuclear cells and plasma. The high level of viremia is rapidly reduced as HIV antibodies appear and are detectable in plasma by such immunologic techniques as ELISA (see Chapter 13).

CLINICAL LATENCY

Clinical progression of HIV infection can differ significantly among virally infected individuals. Some infections progress very rapidly, while others remain asymptomatic (latent) for 10 or more years. During this period of *clinical latency,* the viral replication occurs in lymphoid tissues with only a small amount of virus in the peripheral blood. The HIV replication and destruction by the immune system during this phase is at equilibrium.

CLINICAL AIDS

Eventually, the immune system fails to maintain the equilibrium because of continuous viral replication and reinfection of CD4+ lymphocytes. At this point, the infection progresses to *clinical AIDS.* The clinical phase of AIDS is characterized by severe depression of the immune response (immunodeficiency) because of depletion of helper T (CD4+) lymphocytes by the viral infection. The immunodeficiency results in increased susceptibility to opportunistic infections and neoplasms, such as *Pneumocystis carinii* and Kaposi's sarcoma, respectively.

Detection of HIV Infection

Until the development of molecular techniques to quantify viral RNA (viral load, see text), enumeration of CD4+ lymphocyte counts by flow cytometry (see Chapter 14) was the best marker available for monitoring HIV infection and the patient's response to therapy. Currently, however, research findings indicate that by combining results of the viral load (number of viral particles) with the CD4+ cell counts, more reliable prognosis and therapeutic assessment are possible.

There are several methods currently available for the diagnosis of an HIV infection.

ANTIBODY DETECTION

Screening for presence of HIV-1 antibodies in the patient's serum can be conducted by such immunologic methods as enzyme-linked immunosorbent assay (ELISA), discussed in Chapter 13. However, repeatedly positive ELISA results require performance of a confirmatory test, such as Western blot (briefly described following).

Western blot test. This test uses reagent HIV antigen that is electrophoretically separated into components and blotted. The patient's serum is then added to the blot and allowed to react with each of the separated HIV components (i.e., antigens p24, p31, and gp41 or gp120/160). A *labeled* anti-human globulin is then applied to the blot and allowed to bind with formed antigen-antibody complex (when antigen-specific antibodies are present in a patient's sample), thus forming a band at a characteristic location. This allows identification

Continued

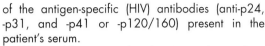 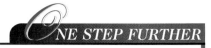

Box 15-3—cont'd

of the antigen-specific (HIV) antibodies (anti-p24, -p31, and -p41 or -p120/160) present in the patient's serum.

Western blot is considered positive when at least two out of three possible antibodies are detected in the patient's serum.

ANTIGEN DETECTION
Detection of HIV-1 antigen (mainly p24) is possible by such immunologic methods as RIA and EIA (see Chapter 13).

DETECTION OF VIRAL NUCLEIC ACIDS
Development of such molecular methods as PCR for the amplification of DNA and RNA (see text) has facilitated progress in the development of highly sensitive molecular methods for detection of HIV nucleic acids.

There are two ways that these molecular techniques can be used to study HIV:
- *Qualitative detection of virus in infected individuals:* Amplification of HIV DNA by such a method as polymerase chain reaction (PCR) (see Figure 15-5) is useful for detection of HIV-1 in infants of HIV-infected mothers before seroconversion (appearance of antibodies in serum) and when indefinite immunologic results must be resolved.
- *Quantification of HIV viral particles (viral load):* A procedure referred to as "viral load"

can be performed by such a method as NASBA (see text) to establish the quantity of HIV particles present in the patient's serum (see text). The quantity of viral particles reflects the balance between viral proliferation and destruction of the virus by the immune system (viral turnover). This viral "turnover" is very rapid in that approximately 30% of the virus is replenished each day. Thus, in order to obtain significant "viral load" values, it is important to observe changes over time or the response to therapy.

Measurement of HIV viral load (burden) levels has greatly facilitated the management of HIV infection by evaluating viral response to retroviral therapy (chemotherapy), predicting progression to AIDS and death, and predicting viral transplacental transmission from mother to fetus.

Interpretation of results. The level of plasma HIV RNA shows a good correlation with the stage of the infection, showing viremic spike after the initial infection, suppressed levels during the long latent period of the infection, and increased viremia with progression to clinical AIDS.

Evaluation of the CD4+ lymphocyte count and the HIV viral load, which typically increases as the CD4+ count decreases, provides information that best monitors the progression of an HIV infection.

clinical application of NASBA. The NASBA procedure is particularly suitable for detection of viral RNA. For example, NASBA can be adopted to quantifying HIV-1 nucleic acid (viral load) in HIV infection (see One Step Further Box 15-3).

Transcription-Mediated Amplification (TMA)
This procedure for amplification of RNA is similar to NASBA (see previous discussion) in that it also uses three enzymes:
- *Reverse transcriptase (RT):* Makes a complementary copy (cDNA strand) from RNA by reverse transcription.
- *Ribonuclease H (RNase H):* Degrades RNA that has been hybridized to DNA (RNA:DNA hybrid).

- *T7 RNA polymerase:* Unwinds DNA and makes multiple copies of RNA; the RNA amplicons (previously replicated RNA) are then used in further cycles to produce more RNA replicons.

The TMA procedure can produce as many as 106 to 109 amplifications of the original RNA target, which becomes degraded during this amplification process.

Signal Amplification Methods
Signal amplification methods have been designed to increase the signal strength by increasing the concentration of the label (fluorochromes or enzymes) attached to the target nucleic acid.

Several methods have been developed that use the signal amplification concept to detect viral nucleic acids. These include:

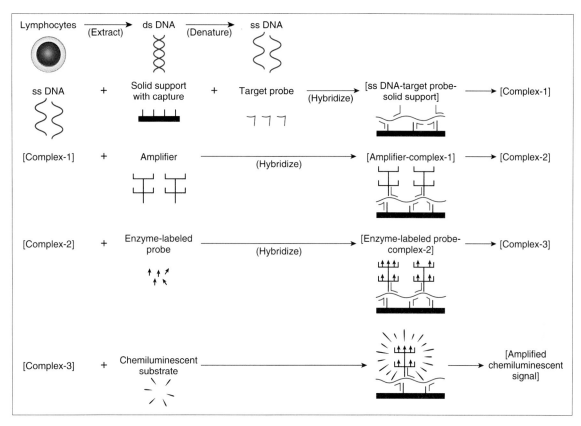

FIGURE **15-6** **Branched DNA Assay.** In this assay (see text), amplification of signal is produced by using a series of probes, an amplifier, enzyme label, and a chemiluminescent substrate on a solid support. The amount of signal detected by a luminometer is proportional to the amount of DNA present in the patient's sample (e.g., viral load). (Modified with permission from Bayer Corporation, Diagnostics Division, Tarrytown, New York.)

- *Multiple enzymes:* The simplest of these methods is one that allows attachment of multiple labels to each probe.
- *Multiple probes:* Several short probes that are complementary to different regions of the target show significant improvement in signal strength, as compared with a single probe.
- *Two-tiered probes:* This probe system consists of a primary (unlabeled) probe and a series of enzyme-labeled secondary probes.
- *Multiple probes–multiple enzymes system:* This is a most powerful system for signal amplification. It consists of primary probe, a secondary *(branched)* probe, and short enzyme-labeled tertiary probes. For example, HIV-1 Branched DNA assay (bDNA) uses a signal amplification system (Figure 15-6) that can be performed in one working area of the laboratory without product carry-over contamination.

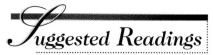

Juggested Readings

Bodner, et al: 1995 Nomenclature for factors of the HLA system, *Tiss Antigens* 46:1-18, 1995.

Cormican MG, Pfaller MA: Molecular pathology of infectious disease. In Henry JB, editor: *Clinical diagnosis and management by laboratory methods,* ed 19, Philadelphia, 1996, WB Saunders.

Dupont B: "Phototyping" for HLA: the beginning of the end of the HLA typing as we know it, *Tiss Antigens* 46:353-354, 1995.

Farkas DH: Clinical applications of molecular techniques, *Lab Med* 24(10):633-636, 1994.

Friedrich MJ: New Chip on the block: the arrival of biochip technology, *Lab Med* 30(3):181-188, 1999.

Revets H, et al: Comparative evaluation of NASBA HIV-1 RNA QT, AMPLICOR-HIV Monitor, and QUANTIPLEX HIV RNA assay: three methods for quantification of human immunodeficiency virus type 1 RNA in plasma, *J Clin Microbiol* 34(5):1058-1064, 1996.

Stoler MH: Tissue in situ hybridization. In Henry JB, editor: *Clinical diagnosis and management by laboratory methods,* ed 19, Philadelphia, 1996, WB Saunders.

Weedn VW, Swarner SL: Forensic identity testing by DNA analysis. In Henry JB, editor: *Clinical diagnosis and management by laboratory methods,* ed 19, Philadelphia, 1996, WB Saunders.

Wiedbrauk DL: Molecular methods for virus detection, *Lab Med* 23(11):737-742, 1992.

Wisecarver J: The ABCs of DNA, *Lab Med* 28(1):48-52, 1997.

Unger ER, Piper MA: Molecular diagnostics: Basic principles and techniques. In Henry JB, editor: *Clinical diagnosis and management by laboratory methods,* ed 19, Philadelphia, 1996, WB Saunders.

Review Questions

STRUCTURE AND SYNTHESIS OF DNA

1-10. Match the following terms with appropriate statements:

_____ allele
_____ clone
_____ exon
_____ denatured DNA
_____ gene
_____ nucleotide
_____ endonuclease
_____ primer
_____ probe
_____ blotting

a. transfer of nucleic acids onto solid phase
b. alternative form of gene
c. genetically identical cells from single cell
d. coding sequence of gene
e. building block of nucleic acid
f. carries genetic information
g. two single DNA strands
h. breaks covalent bonds between nucleotides
i. known labeled sequence of DNA or RNA
j. short nucleic acid sequence that can pair with single-stranded DNA

11. All the following statements apply to the DNA molecule, *except:*
a. is a stable single-stranded molecule
b. determines the structure of protein
c. exists in vivo in highly compacted units (chromosomes)
d. is composed of nucleic acid sequences

12-15. Match the following statement with the appropriate molecule:

a. DNA
b. RNA

_____ exists as a single-stranded molecule
_____ carries codons for specific amino acids in protein synthesis
_____ part of the human genome
_____ serves as a template for synthesis of new DNA strand

16. DNA replication products consist of the original "parent" DNA and a new "daughter" DNA molecules with the same base pair sequence. This type of replication uses:
a. dsDNA template
b. four nucleotide triphosphates
c. mRNA primer
d. all of the above

DNA ISOLATION

17. After release of DNA from cells, the DNA can be extracted by the following procedure(s):
a. solubilization with a detergent
b. addition of phenol-chloroform solutions
c. solubilization with sodium acetate and cold absolute alcohol
d. addition of protein precipitating agent

18. Restriction enzymes are used in the DNA isolation procedure to:
a. recognize short DNA base pair sequences
b. digest phosphodiester bonds at specific location on the DNA molecule
c. digest DNA into 4 to 8 recognition sequences
d. all of the above

NUCLEIC ACID ANALYSIS

19. bDNA assay uses the following principle:
    a. signal amplification
    b. detection of immunofluorescent signal
    c. detection of target DNA
    d. amplification of target DNA

20. Gel electrophoresis is a component of nucleic acid analysis that is used to separate digested DNA molecule according to:
    a. size of nucleotide sequences
    b. molecular weight of nucleotide sequences
    c. length of nucleotide sequences
    d. all of the above

21. The process used for re-forming of two single strands (ssDNA) into double-stranded DNA (dsDNA), when one strand is labeled, is known as:
    a. annealing
    b. hybridization
    c. base pairing
    d. target binding

22. A labeled fragment of known nucleic acid composition, used to locate its matching sequence in an unknown sample, is known as:
    a. target
    b. probe
    c. signal
    d. none of the above

23. Selected environmental condition(s) (stringency) that support base pairing of complementary nucleic acid sequences and minimal mismatches during hybridization are:
    a. low salt
    b. high temperatures
    c. high denaturant
    d. all of the above

24. Controls are included with the unknown sample in a hybridization procedure to:
    a. provide molecular weight markers for gel electrophoresis
    b. check completeness of enzyme activity
    c. determine size of the base-pairs
    d. all of the above

25. Restriction fragment length polymorphism (RFLP) is a procedure used to diagnose diseases associated with abnormal gene product (change in DNA sequences) caused by:
    a. deletions
    b. point mutations
    c. number of repeat copies of DNA
    d. all of the above

26. The Southern blot procedure consists of two procedures, which are:
    a. hybridization
    b. polymerase chain reaction
    c. gel electrophoresis
    d. in situ hybridization

27. When investigating gene expression by employing RNA as the target, the procedure used is the:
    a. Southern blot
    b. Northern blot
    c. Western blot
    d. none of the above

28. All the following procedures are used to generate large amounts of nucleic acids, *except:*
    a. ligase chain reaction (LCR)
    b. nucleic acid sequence–based amplification (NASBA)
    c. polymerase chain reaction (PCR)
    d. hybridization

29. Select a DNA amplification procedure that is based on signal amplification and is suitable for quantifying HIV-1 nucleic acid:
    a. branched DNA assay (bDNA)
    b. nucleic acid sequence–based amplification (NASBA)
    c. polymerase chain reaction (PCR)
    d. ligase chain reaction (LCR)

30. Examination of PCR products (amplified gene segments) can be performed by using:
    a. dot blot hybridization procedure
    b. gel electrophoresis
    c. signal amplification
    d. target amplification

31-38. Match the following methods with the relevant statements:

    a. PCR
    b. Southern blot hybridization
    c. RFLP
    d. in situ hybridization

    ____ uses DNA probe to detect target nucleic acid sequence
    ____ able to detect virally infected cells
    ____ signal detected by fluorescent microscopy
    ____ exponential amplification of sample DNA
    ____ combines electrophoretic separation of DNA fragments with hybridization procedure
    ____ uses restriction enzyme for digesting gene locus
    ____ can demonstrate presence of gene mutation
    ____ target amplification method

39-43. Match each molecular technique with its clinical application:

    ____ PCR
    ____ NASBA
    ____ LCR
    ____ RFLP
    ____ branched DNA (bDNA)

    a. diagnosing genetic disease, oncology, infectious diseases
    b. HLA typing by molecular method
    c. able to detect point mutations (e.g., cystic fibrosis)
    d. detection of viral load
    e. useful in detecting viral RNA

APPENDIX

ANSWERS TO REVIEW QUESTIONS

CHAPTER 1

1. b
2. a
3. a
4. d
5. a
6. b
7. c
8. c,g
9. d,e
10. a,b,f
11. b
12. d
13. c
14. a
15. a
16. b
17. a
18. a
19. b
20. b
21. a
22. b
23. d
24. c
25. c
26. a
27. c
28. a,b,d
29. d
30. a
31. d
32. c
33. c
34. b
35. b
36. c
37. c
38. a
39. b
40. a
41. b
42. d
43. c
44. b
45. d
46. a,c
47. a
48. c
49. a,b,d
50. a,b,c,d
51. a,c
52. b
53. a,b,c,d
54. a,b,c,d
55. d
56. a
57. c
58. a
59. c
60. d
61. c
62. d

CHAPTER 2

1. b
2. d
3. b
4. b
5. a
6. a
7. b
8. b
9. a
10. a
11. d
12. c
13. b
14. c
15. b
16. d
17. b
18. b
19. d
20. a
21. b
22. b
23. a
24. a
25. d
26. c
27. d
28. b
29. d
30. a
31. d

CHAPTER 3

1. d
2. d
3. a
4. b
5. d
6. d

7. e
8. c
9. b
10. e
11. b
12. c
13. a
14. b
15. a
16. c
17. d
18. b
19. cluster of differentiation
20. a,b,c
21. a
22. a,b
23. b
24. a
25. a,b
26. a,b
27. b
28. a
29. b
30. a,b
31. b
32. a
33. d
34. c
35. b
36. a
37. c
38. b
39. d
40. a
41. b

CHAPTER 4
1. c
2. b
3. d
4. d
5. c
6. b
7. d
8. b
9. c
10. a
11. b
12. b
13. b
14. c
15. a,b,c,d

CHAPTER 5
1. a,d
2. f
3. c,g
4. e,f,c
5. b
6. a
7. d
8. a
9. c
10. d
11. d
12. c
13. d
14. c
15. b
16. b
17. a
18. c
19. d
20. b
21. a
22. d
23. a,f
24. a,d
25. c,g
26. g
27. e,f
28. d
29. d
30. c
31. b
32. b
33. a
34. b
35. a,b,c,f
36. a
37. f,e
38. g
39. d
40. b
41. a
42. d

CHAPTER 6
1. d
2. b
3. b
4. d
5. c,b
6. c,d
7. a

8. c,d
9. c,e
10. a,h
11. b
12. f
13. g
14. a
15. b
16. c
17. c
18. c
19. c
20. d
21. d
22. d
23. b
24. d
25. d
26. d
27. b
28. d
29. b
30. b
31. c

CHAPTER 7

1. b
2. b
3. d
4. d
5. c
6. b
7. a,e
8. e,d
9. c
10. d
11. d
12. b
13. d
14. a
15. a
16. b
17. d
18. d
19. a
20. a
21. d
22. d
23. d
24. a
25. b

CHAPTER 8

1. b
2. d
3. b
4. b
5. b
6. a
7. b
8. b
9. c
10. b
11. a
12. c
13. b,c,d
14. d
15. d
16. b
17. d
18. d
19. d
20. b
21. a
22. c
23. c,d
24. d
25. b
26. c
27. d
28. e
29. a
30. c
31. d
32. c

CHAPTER 9

1. b
2. d
3. a
4. b
5. d
6. c
7. b
8. a
9. d
10. b
11. a
12. c
13. e
14. f
15. d
16. a,b,c,d

17. d
18. a
19. d
20. d
21. c
22. $1/10 = 0.2$ mL/x or x = 5 mL total volume; 5 mL − 0.2 mL serum = 4.8 mL saline (diluent) required
23. b
24. b
25. $0.2 \text{ mL} \times 100/2\% = 20/2 = 10 \text{ mL}$ of 2% total cell suspension
26. d
27. a
28. b
29. b
30. a
31. b

CHAPTER 10

1. c
2. a
3. b
4. c
5. a
6. a
7. b
8. b
9. a
10. b
11. c
12. d
13. d
14. a
15. c
16. c
17. d
18. c
19. b
20. c

CHAPTER 11

1. c
2. d
3. a
4. b
5. b
6. b
7. d
8. b
9. c

10. a
11. b
12. c
13. a
14. b
15. b
16. d
17. b
18. d
19. c
20. d
21. b
22. b
23. d
24. d
25. b
26. a
27. c
28. b
29. d

CHAPTER 12

1. b
2. d
3. c
4. d
5. b
6. b
7. a
8. b
9. b
10. a
11. a
12. d
13. a
14. d
15. b
16. a
17. b
18. c
19. a
20. a
21. a
22. b
23. b
24. b
25. a

CHAPTER 13

1. b
2. a

3. d
4. c
5. e
6. d
7. c
8. b
9. c
10. d
11. a
12. a
13. a
14. b
15. b
16. d
17. a
18. f
19. g
20. c
21. a
22. e
23. d
24. b
25. d
26. a
27. b
28. b
29. d
30. d
31. b
32. a
33. a
34. b
35. b
36. b
37. a
38. c
39. d

CHAPTER 14

1. d
2. b,c
3. a
4. a
5. b
6. a
7. d
8. b
9. d
10. a,b
11. b
12. a
13. a

14. a
15. b
16. b
17. a,b
18. c
19. a,c,d
20. b
21. b
22. d
23. d
24. d
25. d
26. b
27. b
28. b
29. c
30. a
31. d
32. d
33. b
34. d
35. a
36. b
37. a

CHAPTER 15

1. b
2. c
3. d
4. g
5. f
6. e
7. h
7. j
9. i
10. a
11. a
12. b
13. b
14. a
15. a
16. d
17. b,d
18. d
19. a
20. d
21. b
22. b
23. d
24. d
25. d
26. a,c

27. b
28. d
29. a
30. a,b
31. b,c,d
32. d
33. d
34. a
35. c

36. a
37. c,d
38. a
39. a
40. d,e
41. c
42. b
43. d

Index

A

Abnormal controls, quality control specimens and, 205
Abnormal immune responses; *see* Immune response, abnormal
Abortion, clonal, T lymphocytes and, 31
Absorbed light, immunoturbidimetry and, 248
Accessibility, epitopes and, 49
Accessory cells, 58, 66, 71-74
   definition of, 3, 55
Accuracy, definition of, 193
Acquired immune response, 7, 11
Acquired immunodeficiencies, 163, 164-165, 181
Acquired immunodeficiency syndrome (AIDS), 163, 164-165, 182, 183, 329-330
Acridinium esters, 274, 282
Activated B lymphocytes, 70, 98
Activation
   definition of, 3
   of specific immune response, 23-24
Active immunity, 11, 27-29
Acute cellular graft rejection, 139
Acute graft rejection, 139
Acute rubella, 262-263
Acute vascular graft rejection, 139
ADCC; *see* Antibody-dependent cell-mediated cytotoxicity
Adjuvants, 46
Adsorption, definition of, 255, 271
Affinity
   antibody, 116-117
   antigen-antibody reactions and, 219, 220, 221
   definition of, 213
Affinity constant, antigen-antibody reactions and, 221
Affinity maturation, 99
AFP; *see* Alpha-fetoprotein
Ag-Ab; *see* Antigen-antibody complexes
Agammaglobulinemia
   Bruton's, 163-164
   definition of, 149
   X-linked, 163
Agglutination, 254-289
   absence of, 263
   antibody-mediated, 264-265
   antigen-antibody reactions and, 225
   definition of, 213, 255
   direct, 225, 258-260
   factors affecting, 257-258
   indirect, 260, 261, 262-263
   mechanism of, 257-258
   methods using, 258-265, 266-267
   passive, 225, 260, 261, 262-263
   reverse passive, 225, 260-261, 264
   visible, 263

Agglutination enhancement techniques, 257
Agglutination inhibition, 225, 262-264, 265
Agglutination reaction, 256, 258-265
Agglutinins, cold, 187, 197
Aggregates, 222
   definition of, 255
   formation of, agglutination and, 257
   insoluble, 224
AH_{50} hemolytic assay, 299
AIDS; *see* Acquired immunodeficiency syndrome
Alkaline phosphatase, enzyme labels and, 273
Allele, definition of, 125, 315
Allergen, 151
   definition of, 149
Allergen profile, 280
Allergen-specific IgE antibody quantification, 280
Allergic contact dermatitis, 156
Allergic reaction, 151, 188
   definition of, 175
Allergy, immediate, 151-153
Allergy screen, 280
Allo, definition of, 3
Alloantibodies
   definition of, 125
   donor-specific, 308
Alloantigens, 42, 126
   definition of, 125, 291
   molecular basis for recognition of, 133-135
   recognition of, by helper and cytotoxic T cells, 134-135
   role of T cell receptors in, 133-134
   in vitro recognition and response to, 135-136
Allogeneic, 126
   definition of, 125, 291
Allogeneic graft, 131-132
   definition of, 125
Allograft, 126, 131-132
   definition of, 125
   recognition of, by CD8+ lymphocytes, 135
   recognition of, by CD4+ T lymphocytes, 134-135
Alloreactive, definition of, 125
Allotype, definition of, 91
Allotypic variations, 115
Alpha H chain, 106
Alpha-fetoprotein (AFP), 45
Alternative pathway, complement activation and, 83, 85
Alum precipitate, adjuvants and, 46
Aluminum hydroxide, adjuvants and, 46
AMA; *see* Anti-mitochondrial antibodies
Amplicons
   definition of, 315
   DNA target amplification and, 326
Amplification, definition of, 315
ANA; *see* Anti-nuclear antibodies

Immunoprecipitation, 224-225, 230, 231
Immunoprecipitin, 230
    definition of, 229
Immunoprecipitin curve, 216
Immunoprecipitin formation, 216, 232
Immunoproliferative disorders, 166-167, 168, 187-188
Immunoradiometric assay (IRMA), 279-280
Immunosuppression, 179
    deficiency caused by, 165
    definition of, 126, 150
    with drugs, 141
    posttransplantation, 133
    pretransplantation, 140
    in transplantation, 141-142
Immunoturbidimetry, 247-249
In vitro, definition of, 126, 292
In vitro recognition and response to alloantigens, 135-136
In vivo, definition of, 126
Inactivation of complement, 199-200
Inappropriate assembly of membrane proteins, tumor
        markers and, 44
Inappropriate immune response, 185
Incompatibility, graft rejection and, 126
Indications for immunologic testing, 176
Indicators, labeled immunoassays and, 272
Indirect agglutination, 260, 261, 262-263
Indirect antiglobulin test, 265
Indirect chemiluminescence enzyme, 282-283
Indirect enzyme immunoassay, 281
Indirect exclusion of paternity, 143
Indirect immunofluorescence assays (IIFs), 283, 285-286
Infection
    bacterial, 178
    congenital, 178
    detection of, 177-178
    extracellular, 29
    immunity induced by, 27
    intracellular, 29, 46
    past, detection of, 177-178
    primary, 177
    recent, diagnosis of, 177
    rubella, 262-263
    viral, 178, 179
Infection control, 194-195
Infectious, definition of, 4-5
Infectious agents
    direct detection of, 328
    immune response to, 176
    testing for immune response to, 176-178
Infectious waste, 197
Infectivity
    antigen classification according to site of, 46, 48
    extracellular, 29
    immunity and, 29
    intracellular, 29
Inflammation
    graft rejection and, 138
    immunologic events during, 12
    natural immune responses and, 11, 12-14
    regulation of, 14
Insoluble aggregate, 224
Insoluble multivalent antigens, 225

Insulin-dependent diabetes mellitus, 187
Interferons (IFNs), 46, 81
    definition of, 5
Interlaboratory control, 205
Interleukin, 80, 81
    definition of, 5
Interleukin-2, 138, 139
Interleukin-4, 139
Interleukin-5, 139
Interleukin-6, 14
Internal quality control, 205
Intracellular antigens, 46, 48, 67
Intracellular infection, 29, 46
Intracellular infectivity, 29
Intralaboratory quality control, 205
Introns
    definition of, 315
    DNA and, 100, 318
Ionic interactions, antigen-antibody binding and, 220
Ionic strength, antigen-antibody reactions and, 221
IRMA; *see* Immunoradiometric assay
Isoelectric focusing, 243, 246-247
Isolation, DNA, 319-320
Isotopes, 115
Isotypes, 113
    definition of, 92
    immunoglobulin, 108
Isotypic variations, 115

J

J chain, 110, 111, 112
    definition of, 92
JCAHO; *see* Joint Commission on the Accreditation of
        Healthcare Organizations
Joint Commission on the Accreditation of Healthcare
        Organizations (JCAHO), 204
Junk DNA, 318

K

K; *see* Association constant
Karyotype, 318
Kidney transplants, 133
Kinetic method, radial immunodiffusion and, 235
Kits, commercial, laboratory testing and, 203

L

L chains; *see* LIght chains
Labeled antibodies, 223
Labeled antigens, 223
Labeled immunoassays, 270-289
    methods of, 279-286
    principles of, 272-279
    types of protocols in, 274-279
Labels
    antigen-antibody reactions and, 223-224
    chemiluminescence, 274
    definition of, 271, 316
    enzyme, 273, 274
    fluorochrome, 273-274
    radioisotopic, 273
    types of, 272-274
Laboratory immunology, diagnostic, 172-331

Laboratory personnel
  basic protective measures for, 195
  post-immunization testing of, 177
  vaccination against hepatitis B virus infection and, 28
Laboratory safety, 194-197
  regulatory government agencies for, 194
  and test quality assurance, 192-210
Laboratory testing; *see also* Tests
  allergic reactions and, 188
  autoantibodies and, 162
  bacterial infections and, 178
  hepatitis B virus infection and, 28
  histocompatibility in transplantation and, 184-185
  hypergammaglobulinemia and, 167, 168
  immunodeficiency and, 182, 183
  immunologic, indications for, 176-188
  inflammation and, 14
  multiple sclerosis and, 243-244
  plasma cell dyscrasias and, 187-188
  preparation for, 197-203
  pretransfusion, in renal transplants, 133
  pretransplantation, 140
  reagent antibodies and, 118-120
  scope of, 174-191
  viral infections and, 178
  Waldenstrom's macroglobulinemia and, 239-240, 241
Lattices, definition of, 255
Law of mass action, antigen-antibody reactions and, 221
LCR; *see* Ligase chain reaction
Legionella, antibody detection in, 177
Leukemia
  definition of, 175
  evaluation of, 183, 184
  lymphocytic, 184
Leukocyte circulation, alteration of, steroids and, 141
Leukocyte cross-matching, flow cytometry and, 298
Leukocytes
  passenger, 134
  polymorphonuclear, 73
Ligand, 272
  definition of, 271
Ligase chain reaction (LCR), 327
Light
  absorbed, immunoturbidimetry and, 248
  flash of, chemiluminescent labels and, 282
Light (L) chains, 105-106
Light scatter, 248
  definition of, 229
  flow cytometry and, 294
Light scattering immunoassays, 247-249
Linear regresson, statistical analysis and, 199
Lines, precipitin, 231, 232
  definition of, 229
Lipids, 42
List mode method, flow cytometry and, 295
Live viral vaccines, 30
Local alterations, autoimmunity and, 159
Localized reaction, immediate hypersensitivity and, 152-153
Lock and key fit, antigen-antibody reactions and, 217
Low stringency, hybridization and, 321
Luminols, 274, 282

Lyme disease, antibodies detection in, 177
Lymph nodes, 50, 66
Lymphocyte activation, 67, 304-306
Lymphocyte clones, 26
Lymphocyte diversity, specific immune response and, 25, 26
Lymphocyte matching technique using mixed lymphocyte reaction, 135-136
Lymphocytes, 58, 65, 66, 67, 68
  alterations in, autoimmunity and, 159
  B; *see* B lymphocytes
  CD8+, allograft recognition by, 135
  CD4+ T, recognition of allografts by, 134-135
  cytotoxic T, 306
  definition of, 4
  plasmacytoid, 187
  polyclonal stimulation of, 159
  pre-B, 70, 97
  T; *see* T lymphocytes
  types of, 67-71
Lymphocytic cells, 66-71
Lymphocytic leukemias, 184
Lymphocytotoxicity, 184-185, 309
Lymphoid tissue, 50, 57-66
  functional division of, 59
  generative, 60
  peripheral, 62-66
  primary, 60
    definition of, 5
  secondary, 62-66
    definition of, 5
Lymphokines, 80
  definition of, 5
Lymphoma, 184
  definition of, 175
  evaluation of, 183, 184
Lysis
  cell, 83, 86-87
    definition of, 125, 291
  osmotic cell, 86

M

M protein, 187
MAbs; *see* Monoclonal antibodies
MAC; *see* Membrane attack complex
Macroglobulin, 187
Macroglobulinemia, Waldenstrom's, 187, 239-241
Macromolecular proteins, 49
Macromolecules, 42, 49
Macrophage-activating factor (MAF), 139
Macrophages
  antigen processing by, 11
  impairment in, steroids and, 141
MAF; *see* Macrophage-activating factor
Magnetic separation, 303
Major cross-match, donor-specific alloantibodies and, 308
Major histocompatibility antigens
  donor, recognition of, 133-134
  in transplantation, 131-140
Major histocompatibility complex (MHC), 9, 42, 64, 67, 127-131
  definition of, 5, 39, 126, 292